D1483421

Monoclonal Hybridoma Antibodies: Techniques and Applications

Editor

John G. R. Hurrell, Ph.D.

Head, Immunochemistry R & D Group
Commonwealth Serum Laboratories
Parkville, Victoria
Australia

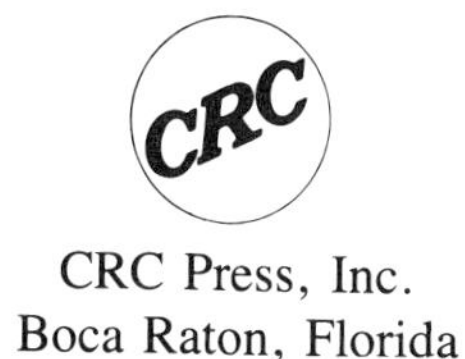

CRC Press, Inc.
Boca Raton, Florida

Library of Congress Cataloging in Publication Data
Main entry under title:

Monoclonal hybridoma antibodies.

Bibliography: p.
Includes index.
1. Antibodies, Monoclonal. I. Hurrell,
John G. R., 1949–
QR186.85.M663 616.07'93 81-18129
ISBN 0-8493-6511-2 AACR2

This book represents information obtained from authentic and highly regarded sources. Reprinted material is quoted with permission, and sources are indicated. A wide variety of references are listed. Every reasonable effort has been made to give reliable data and information, but the author and the publisher cannot assume responsibility for the validity of all materials or for the consequences of their use.

Direct all inquiries to CRC Press, Inc., 2000 Corporate Blvd., N.W., Boca Raton, Florida 33431.

International Standard Book Number 0-8493-6511-2

Library of Congress Card Number 81-18129
Printed in the United States

PREFACE

The landmark paper of Köhler and Milstein (*Nature (London)*, 256, 495, 1975) describing the production and characterization of the first somatic cell hybrids capable of indefinite production of antibody of predetermined specificity, heralded a new era in biology and initiated a virtual ''avalanche'' of scientific literature. The potential of the somatic cell hybridization (hybridoma) technique was quickly realized by investigators in many areas of biology and applied to a wide variety of antigens. The technique has been refined and many alternative protocols developed, but all with the same basic core element, the fusion of primed splenocytes with biosynthetically defective myeloma cells.

The first section of this volume was aimed to provide a comprehensive review of the many varied and often empirically derived techniques and procedures currently in use to produce monoclonal hybridoma cell lines and to characterize the antibodies secreted. This goal has been achieved with the chapter contributed by Zola and Brooks who, as each step in the process of hybridoma production and antibody characterization is reviewed, have provided an experimental procedure found to be satisfactory in their laboratory. Investigators about to begin a hybridoma program are thus presented with background information for the rapid assessment of alternative procedures. The advantages, faults, and known pitfalls of each method are discussed and, if confused by the numerous procedures in the literature, the investigator may choose the experimental procedure of the authors to serve as a starting point.

The second section of this volume was designed to provide a review of areas in which monoclonal hybridoma antibodies have been of particular advantage. This is a rapidly advancing field which could not be thoroughly reviewed in a single volume. The particular examples reviewed were selected from the broad areas of soluble antigens (somatotrophic hormones, cardiac myosin, alpha fetoprotein, and carcinoembryonic antigen), viral antigens (influenza virus and herpes simplex virus), parasite antigens, tumor associated human tissue antigens, and nontumor tissue antigens (macrophage membrane, lymphocyte membrane, and histocompatibility antigens). These specific applications of monoclonal hybridoma antibodies are intended as general reviews as well as illustrating and expanding on many of the points brought out by Zola and Brooks in the first chapter.

It is apparent that the surface has only just been broken regarding the information that monoclonal hybridoma antibodies will provide. The future will see the widespread development and use of monoclonal hybridoma antibodies for routine immunotherapy and diagnosis, and for furthering our understanding of the molecular biology of the cell and of disease processes. There is no doubt that this is an exciting time to be a biological scientist!

JOHN G. R. HURRELL
Parkville, Australia
December 1981

THE EDITOR

John G. R. Hurrell, Ph.D., is Head of Immunochemistry Research and Development at the Commonwealth Serum Laboratories in Parkville, Australia. He is also an Associate in the Department of Pathology and Immunology, Monash University, Melbourne.

Dr. Hurrell graduated from the University of Melbourne in 1971 with a B.Sc. in Chemistry and Biochemistry. In 1974, after 3 years as a Research and Development scientist at the Commonwealth Serum Laboratories, he returned to the University of Melbourne to study under Professor Sidney J. Leach in the Department of Biochemistry. Dr. Hurrell received a Ph.D. in 1977. After a postdoctoral year at the Commonwealth Serum Laboratories, Dr. Hurrell was awarded a Fulbright Fellowship in the Cellular and Molecular Research Laboratory, Massachusetts General Hospital, Boston. Following a short period as a Visiting Scientist at Centocor Inc., Philadelphia, Dr. Hurrell returned to Australia in July 1980 to take up his present position.

CONTRIBUTORS

Rosemary Betts, B.Sc.
Research Associate
Department of Pathology
University of Melbourne
Parkville, Victoria
Australia

D. A. Brooks, B.Sc.
Ph.D. Student
Department Clinical Immunology
Flinders Medical Centre
Bedford Park, South Australia

Paul Ehrlich, Ph.D.
Research Associate
Department of Medicine
College of Physicians & Surgeons
Columbia University
New York, New York

George M. Georgiou, B.Sc. Hons
Research Fellow
Royal Children's Hospital Research
Foundation
Royal Children's Hospital
Parkville, Victoria
Australia

Edgar Haber, M.D.
Professor of Medicine
Harvard Medical School
Chief, Cardiac Unit
Massachusetts General Hospital
Boston, Massachusetts

C. S. Hosking, M.D.
Director, Department of Immunology
Royal Children's Hospital
Parkville, Victoria
Australia

John G. R. Hurrell, Ph.D.
Head, Immunochemistry R & D
Group
Commonwealth Serum Laboratories
Parkville, Victoria
Australia

J. Ivanyi, Ph.D.
Head, Department of Experimental
Immunobiology
The Wellcome Research Laboratories
Beckenham, Kent
England

Hugo A. Katus, M.D.
Fellow in Internal Medicine
School of Medicine
University of Heidelberg
Heidelberg, West Germany

Ban-An Khaw, Ph.D.
Assistant Professor
Department of Pathology
Harvard Medical School
Associate Biochemist
Cellular and Molecular Research Lab
Massachusetts General Hospital
Boston, Massachusetts

Hilary Koprowski, M.D.
Director
The Wistar Institute
Philadelphia, Pennsylvania

Herbert Z. Kupchik, Ph.D.
Assistant Professor
Department of Microbiology
Boston University Medical Center
Member, Hubert H. Humphrey
Cancer Research Center
Boston University
Member, Special Scientific Staff
Mallory Institute of Pathology
Boston, Massachusetts

W. G. Laver, Ph.D.
Senior Fellow
Microbiology Department
John Curtin School of Medical
Research
Australian National University
Canberra City
Australia

Gary R. Matsueda, Ph.D.
Assistant Professor of Pathology
Harvard Medical School
Assistant in Biochemistry
Massachusetts General Hospital
Boston, Massachusetts

Ian F. C. McKenzie, M.D., Ph.D.
Department of Pathology
University of Melbourne
Parkville, Victoria
Australia

Graham F. Mitchell, Ph.D.
Laboratory Head
Laboratory of Immunoparasitology
The Walter and Eliza Hall Institute
of Medical Research
Melbourne, Victoria
Australia

Kenneth F. Mitchell, Ph.D., F.R.S.A.
Assistant Professor
The Wistar Institute
Philadelphia, Pennsylvania

Lenore Pereira, Ph.D.
Research Specialist
California State Department of Public
Health Services
Viral and Rickettsial Disease
Laboratory
Berkeley, California

Timothy A. Springer, Ph.D.
Chief, Membrane Immunochemistry
Sidney Farber Cancer Institute
Assistant Professor of Pathology
Harvard Medical School
Boston, Massachusetts

Zenon Steplewski, M.D., Ph.D., D.Sc.
The Wistar Institute
Philadelphia, Pennsylvania

H. Zola, Ph.D.
Chief Hospital Scientist
Flinders Medical Centre
Senior Lecturer, Immunology
Flinders University of South
Australia
Bedford Park, South Australia

Vincent R. Zurawski, Jr., Ph.D.
Vice President and Technical
Director
Centocor
Philadelphia, Pennsylvania

TABLE OF CONTENTS

Chapter 1

TECHNIQUES FOR THE PRODUCTION AND CHARACTERIZATION OF MONOCLONAL HYBRIDOMA ANTIBODIES

H. Zola and D. Brooks

TABLE OF CONTENTS

I. INTRODUCTION

When two cells are brought into close contact and their membranes caused to fuse together, the resulting fusion product contains both the nuclei. A cell with two or more dissimilar nuclei is called a heterokaryon and in due course the nuclei can fuse together producing a single nucleus with genetic information from both of the original cells. This fusion product is called a hybrid. The fusion of somatic cells has been carried out for many years with a variety of different aims. The hybrids usually lose some chromosomes but retain some of the properties of each of the parental cells. In 1975 Köhler and Milstein[1] fused antibody-producing mouse spleen cells with mouse myeloma cells. The hybrids they obtained secreted antibodies of the specificity dictated by the parent spleen cell, but in the quantity characteristic of a myeloma. This experiment has led to greatly increased use of somatic cell hybridization. Because many laboratories are now producing hybrids, there has been a rapid development and proliferation of techniques.

Several articles are available giving either detailed technical descriptions or overviews to enable the reader to make an informed choice of technique.[2–8]

In this chapter, we describe in detail the techniques used in our laboratory, while discussing some of the variations which can be used successfully. An attempt will be made to differentiate between procedures which are based on sound evidence and practices which appear to be beneficial but may turn out to have only ritual significance.

Successful fusion and selective growth of antibody-secreting hybrids depends on a complex interplay of experimental variables. The complexity of the interaction between variables can lead to contradictory results between laboratories. For example, it is conceivable that the beneficial effect of feeder cells (see Section VI) is much greater if the fetal calf serum and media are suboptimal. Thus, a laboratory using a good batch of serum may find feeder cells do not help very much, while another laboratory, using a batch of serum which is less able to support growth of hybridomas, will find feeder cells indispensable. Since there is no entirely satisfactory test to predict the suitability of the fetal calf serum, it is not easy to prove that the need for feeder cells is related to calf serum batch. Experiments to study all these variables are tedious and relatively uninteresting, at a time when most investigators are anxious to produce some useful antibodies, irrespective of the efficiency of the process. Thus, it is not surprising that successful procedures become entrenched, and that dogmatic statements about technical variables are accepted unchallenged. As the initial excitement wears off it is to be expected that much more work will be done on technical aspects and that the procedures will lose much of their empiricism and mysticism.

The newcomer to hybridization is well advised to learn the technique in a laboratory which is already practicing fusion. It has been a frequent observation that newcomers to the techniques are relatively unsuccessful initially and obtain many hybrids after some practice, although an experienced observer cannot see any difference between the technique used on the first day and in subsequent, successful experiments. The best approach therefore is to learn from an experienced laboratory and practice until hybrids are obtained. During this development stage all possible variables should be noted and controlled as far as possible, so that once a successful procedure has been established, it can be maintained.

The different stages in the production of monoclonal hybridoma antibody, starting from immunization and finishing with a characterized monoclonal antibody, are illustrated schematically in Figure 1. Each stage is dealt with in detail in subsequent sections of this chapter.

II. PREREQUISITES TO STARTING A HYBRIDOMA PROJECT

In this section, an attempt is made to list what is needed in order to successfully execute a hybridoma production exercise, in terms both of materials and expertise.

A. Major Equipment

Hybridoma work does not require any sophisticated equipment, but three major items of equipment are needed and they must be of good quality.

1. Cabinet for Sterile Work

The investment of time and effort into hybridoma production is such that the frequency of lapses in sterility must be kept low. An efficient cabinet in which sterile air is blown across the work area towards the operator is adequate, provided it is maintained well and disinfected after use. These cabinets incorporate ultraviolet lamps to sterilize the cabinet between use, but these lamps have a rapid fall-off in effectiveness and liberal use of alcohol to swab the surfaces is recommended.

If the project involves the use of pathogenic material, a laminar flow cabinet with a vertical curtain of sterile air separating the work from the operator is needed.[9] These cabinets are variable in performance, and are only effective if used properly.

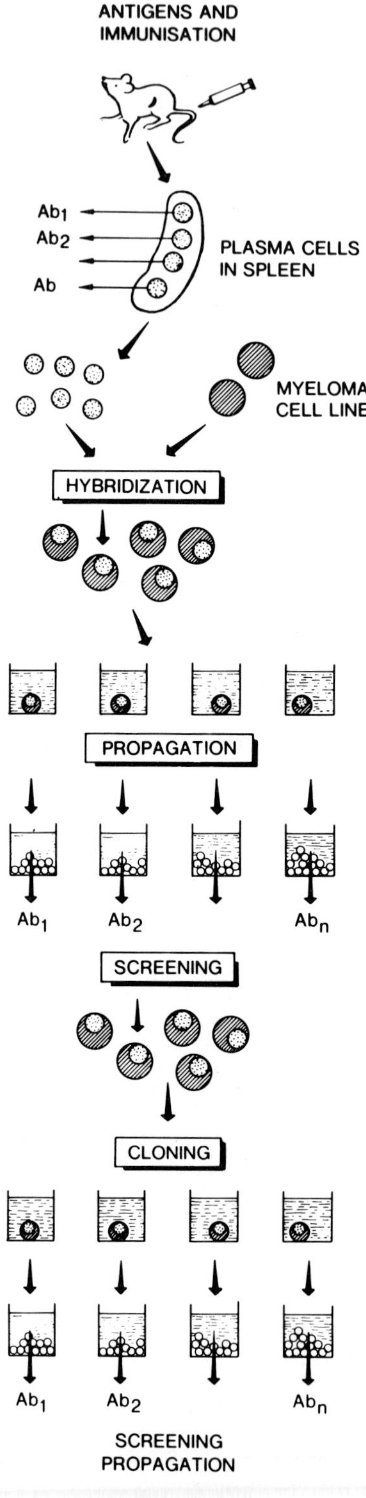

FIGURE 1. Schematic representation of the stages of a hybridization, from immunization to characterization of monoclonal antibody.

2. *Gassed Incubator*

Hybridoma cultures, in their early phase, are kept in unsealed culture vessels which depend on free and rapid exchange of CO_2 for pH control. Thus an incubator is needed with:

1. Temperature control
2. Arrangement for maintaining humidity
3. Arrangement for maintaining a stable CO_2 concentration

Many instruments are available commercially. The temperature control should be precise and large fluctuations (for instance, when the doors have been opened) are undesirable. Of particular importance is that the CO_2 concentration, which drops when the doors are opened, should be readjusted rapidly. This requires a method for rapid gassing. For the same reason, it is unsatisfactory to use an incubator which is shared for several different uses and is opened frequently.

3. *Liquid Nitrogen Storage Facility*

Once produced, hybridomas must be maintained and a low-temperature store for cryopreservation is essential (see Section IX). A simple but large cryogenic tank and a source of liquid nitrogen are needed. A programmed freezing instrument (see Section IX) is useful but not essential.

B. Minor Equipment

1. Animal holding facilities.
2. Sterile surgical equipment for mouse dissection.
3. Water baths, 37 and 56° C.
4. Centrifuges (bench top, preferably refrigerated).
5. Tissue culture ware (see Sections VI, VII, IX).
6. Inverted microscope (desirable but not essential).
7. Laboratory microscope, hemocytometers.

Further equipment needs will depend on the assay system to be used (see Sections VIII, XI) but typically a fluorescence microscope and a γ counter might be used.

C. Expertise

It is not necessary to have extensive cell culture experience or to be an immunologist to undertake hybridoma work, although it helps. On the basis that the hybridoma technique has many applications outside immunology, this chapter has been written in a style that does not assume an extensive familiarity with immunology. Hybridomas are rather fastidious cells and the chances of producing them and maintaining them are certainly higher if the worker has previous cell culture experience. This chapter is not intended to serve as a tissue culture primer and the reader who lacks experience is referred to available books.[10–13]

The most important prerequisite in terms of expertise relates to the antigen type to be used and the assay for antibody against the antigen. Hybridoma technology is secondary and can be learned, but it is essential to have experience working with the material which is the subject of the project, be it a virus or a peptide, a lymphocyte differentiation antigen or a pathogenic parasite. Specific examples of the production of hybridoma antibodies to each of these types of antigens are described in later chapters.

III. MATERIALS AND MEDIA

A. Materials/Chemicals to be Ordered

1. Cell Culture Medium: RPMI 1640, or Alternative (Dulbeccos; Iscoves)

2. Fetal Calf Serum: Selected Batch

Not all serum batches are suitable, and the critical stage is most probably the initial postfusion stage, when hybrids are present at low concentration in company with large numbers of dead or damaged cells. The only certain way of screening to select a batch is to do a fusion and plate out in the different serum batches (test 4 to 6 at a time), ensuring that the serum is the only variable. The plate that gives the most hybrids indicates the best serum batch.

This approach is not always used, for a variety of reasons. For the worker who is just starting fusion, it does not make sense to use a procedure with a variable chance of success to check his serum; failed hybridizations are as likely to result from other technical factors. The newcomer to fusion should try to get enough of a tested batch from an established fusion laboratory to get his technique working before he screens batches.

Even in the established fusion laboratory, serum selection by fusion essentially poses problems because it is difficult to ensure that the serum is the only variable (for instance, the different cell batches will inevitably be left to stand for different periods before plating out). Nevertheless this is the most relevant screen for selecting a batch of serum, and any simpler screen may, at least theoretically, not pick the right batch. The screening procedure that is used most often is simply to test the ability of serum batches to support cloning at limiting dilution (see Section IX) of either the parent myeloma or an established hybrid.

Some laboratories have used mixtures of fetal calf serum and horse serum for fusion, and established myeloma lines can be maintained in cheaper sera than fetal calf, including horse and calf sera (see Section VII).

3. HAT Selective Medium Components

1. Hypoxanthine
2. Aminopterin
3. Thymidine

4. Polyethylene Glycol (PEG)

This material varies according to manufacturer, batch, and molecular weight. For many fusions one 500 g bottle will suffice, so a batch number recommended by a colleague should be obtained. PEG is toxic to cells, and the toxicity probably depends on molecular weight. The molecular weight quoted on the label represents an average value, and the range of molecular weight will depend on the batch, even when the average molecular weight is the same. Successful fusions have been reported with batches ranging in nominal molecular weight from 500 to 6000. We have done all of our fusions with a single batch of PEG 4000 mol wt from British Drug Houses (BDH), Poole, U.K.

5. Dimethyl Sulfoxide

B. Working Solutions

1. Medium

RPMI 1640 is supplemented with: FCS 10%, Glutamine 2 mM, Penicillin 100 IU/mℓ, and Streptomycin 100 μg/mℓ.

Glutamine and penicillin/streptomycin mixture can be obtained as frozen stock solution, and should be kept frozen. Glutamine has a half-life of about 2 weeks in liquid media; thus, even though media can be obtained with glutamine already added, the level should be supplemented if the medium is stored for 2 weeks or more. Other media (e.g., Dulbecco's MEM, Iscoves) may be used. While these media are essentially equivalent and most cells can be grown in any of these media, changing from one to another can set the cell growth back or even cause cell death. Thus when receiving a new line from another laboratory, it is advisable to get it established in its original medium and change over to your own medium gradually. Other additives are used by some workers, for instance, pyruvate and 2-mercaptoethanol.

2. HAT Medium

Medium as above with added hypoxanthine (136 μg/mℓ), aminopterin (0.19 μg/mℓ), and thymidine (3.88 μg/mℓ). We make up 100x HAT stock with hypoxanthine (13.6 mg/mℓ), aminopterin (0.019 mg/mℓ), and thymidine (0.388 mg/mℓ), which we store aliquotted, frozen, and in the dark (aminopterin is light-sensitive). For use, add 1 mℓ stock to 100 mℓ medium.

3. HT Medium

This is prepared similar to the HAT medium but without the aminopterin. Again, we use a 100x stock HT, and dilute for use.

4. Phosphate-Buffered Saline (PBS)

The Ca^{++}/Mg^{++}-free Dulbecco's PBS is used because it generally does not cause cell clumping. It can be bought, or made up according to the following formula:

- Sodium chloride 8.0 g
- Potassium chloride 0.2 g
- Disodium hydrogen orthophosphate (anhydrous) 1.15 g
- Potassium dihydrogen orthophosphate (anhydrous) 0.2 g

Dissolve in sequence in 0.8 ℓ distilled water. Adjust pH to 7.3, make volume to 1 ℓ with distilled water. Sterilize by autoclaving at 15 lb/in.^{2} for 15 min.

5. Gey's Hemolytic Medium

This is not generally available commercially (another medium known as Gey's is a growth medium and cannot be used for hemolysis). Stock solutions made up as follows:

Gey's solution A

Ammonium chloride	35.0 g
Potassium chloride	1.85 g
Dipotassium hydrogen	

orthophosphate (KH_2 PO4)	0.119 g
Glucose	5.0 g
Phenol red	0.05 g
Gelatine (Difco®)	25.0 g
Distilled water	1000 mℓ

Gelatine is the variable component of this mixture, and not all gelatines will be effective. We have used Difco® gelatine successfully.

The mixture is dispensed into 20 mℓ aliquots in screwcap glass vials and autoclaved (15 lb/in.^{2}, 15 min). It can then be stored indefinitely at room temperature.

Gey's solution B

Magnesium chloride	($MgCl_2$ $6H_2O$)	4.20 g
Magnesium sulfate	($MgSO_4.7H_2O$)	1.40 g
Calcium chloride	($CaCl_2$)	3.40 g
Water		1000 mℓ

Dissolve salts with stirring, dispense in 10 mℓ aliquots in screwcap glass vials, and then autoclave (10 lb/in.^{2}, 10 min).

Gey's solution C

Sodium bicarbonate available commercially from media manufacturers, or make up:	
Sodium bicarbonate	5.6 g
Water	100 mℓ
Sterilize by membrane filtration.	

Working solution: Gey's hemolytic medium is made up from the stock solutions no more than 30 min before use.

Mix: 14.5 mℓ distilled water
4 mℓ Gey's solution A
1 mℓ Gey's solution B
add Gey's solution C (bicarbonate) to give pH 7.2 to 7.4 as judged by the indicator color.

Note: Bicarbonate solutions lose CO_2 and the amount to be added depends on the age of the solution. The volume required should be 0.1 to 0.5 mℓ.

6. PEG/DMSO Fusing Agent Contains 42% PEG W/V and 15% DMSO (V/V)

PEG will not dissolve unless heated, and the fusing mixture is made up as follows: weigh out 10 g PEG into a screwcap glass bottle; autoclave (15 lb/in.^{2}, 15 min) to sterilize and liquefy; while the PEG is still hot, add 14 mℓ of 15% DMSO in PBS; then store at +4° C.

7. Alternative Antibiotics or Antifungal Agents

Gentamycin may be used routinely in culture media at 0.2 mg/mℓ instead of penicillin and streptomycin. Fungal contamination will be experienced occasionally, and if this happens with a particularly important culture it is worth trying to recover the culture by the addition of fungizone (amphotericin B) at 5 to 10 μg/mℓ, or mycostatin at 100 μg/mℓ.

Occasionally other contaminants which are resistant to penicillin, streptomycin, and gentamycin are found. It is worth keeping a battery of alternative antibiotics in reserve for such occasions. The following antibiotics (with concentrations which cell cultures will survive) may prove useful: tylosin tartrate (25 μg/mℓ), neomycin (100 μg/mℓ), kanamycin (500 mg/mℓ), novobiocin (200 μg/mℓ), and mycostatin (100 μg/mℓ). Novobiocin and tylosin are particularly useful for Gram-positive organisms, while kanamycin and neomycin are active against Gram-negative organisms and staphylococci. Kanamycin is also useful in attempts to remove mycoplasma contamination.

IV. ANTIGENS AND IMMUNIZATION SCHEDULES

A. Introduction

The hybridoma technique has potential value in almost any situation where antibodies are used at present. Thus the range of antigens which will be used is wide and the best immunization procedure will clearly depend on the antigen in question. A protocol which works well with a membrane antigen will not necessarily be satisfactory with a soluble protein of low molecular weight or a lipid or polysaccharide antigen; thus immunization schedules cannot be considered separately from the antigens. A second general consideration is that in many instances the antigens of interest are not available pure. Indeed, one of the major advantages of the hybridoma technique is that it is possible to obtain highly specific antibodies against antigens which are not pure, and to use these antibodies subsequently to purify the antigens. If the antigen of interest is part of a mixture, then the strategy of immunization should recognize the relative immunogenicity of the antigen of interest and contaminating antigens. If the antigen of interest is highly immunogenic, it is sufficient to give a mild immunization protocol and hope thereby to stimulate a minimal response against contaminating antigens. On the other hand, where a mild immunization protocol will not stimulate sufficient antibody-producing cells against the antigen of interest, it is necessary to use a more vigorous protocol and to take steps to reduce the immunogenicity of the contaminating antigens.

B. Effectiveness of Immunization

It is not known with any certainty which cells from the spleen are involved in the formation of antibody-producing hybrids, but it seems very likely that the important cells are plasma cells or B cells in blast transformation. Empirically, the proportion of antibody producing hybrids depends on how well the mouse is immunized, although there is also a suggestion that overimmunization is unhelpful.[14] Some laboratories test the titer of antibody in the immunized mice and use only those mice producing high titers of antibody.

C. Enrichment of Antibody-Producing Cells

Measures which increase the number of cells in blast transformation, or at least enrich for these cells by depleting irrelevant cells, should in principle be helpful. Up to now, few laboratories have investigated such procedures, but it is likely that they will be used with increasing frequency.

Simple removal of T cells has been rather unhelpful,[7] perhaps because the process causes some trauma to the desired cells. An injection of LPS can be used to stimulate B cells to go into cycle, but this procedure may merely increase hybrid numbers in a nonselective way. More specific stimulation of B cells has been achieved by an immunization protocol involving repeated injections of soluble antigen (5 doses in the week before fusion).[15] This process leads to an increase in the proportion of cells with the size of blasts, and a concomitant increase in the number of specific hybrids.[15]

In another interesting approach to the problem of increasing the proportion of specific B cells taking part in the fusion, the cells from an immunized mouse are adoptively transferred to an irradiated second mouse to expand the B cell clones. If this procedure is combined with a specific enrichment step for the antibody-secreting cells, considerable improvement in the proportion of specific hybrids may be expected.[68]

D. Cell Membrane Antigens

When using particulate antigens such as cells with membrane antigens, the normal procedure is to give two injections separated by an interval of 4 weeks and to hybridize 4 or 5 days after the second injection. In xenogeneic systems, this works well although the number of antibody-producing hybrids might be increased by immunizing more vigorously. Trucco et al.[16] have shown that it is possible to obtain hybrids by fusing after a single injection of cellular material but in a subsequent paper,[17] the same group shows that the number of hybrids is greater after multiple injections. In order to stimulate the spleen, injections should be given either intravenously or intraperitoneally. Most laboratories prefer intravenous injections, although the i.v. route is technically more difficult and it is important to ensure that the total dose is in fact injected into the vein. In our laboratory, we inject 10^7 cells at each injection. There is a lack of information on the best immunization procedures in terms of yield of hybrids, but if we assume that the numbers of hybrids will correlate reasonably well with the antibody titer, it is possible to make use of the wealth of information on the best immunization protocols for making antilymphocyte sera. These earlier studies would suggest that two injections of 10^7 cells separated by 2 to 4 weeks would give good immunization, that more cells would not be necessary and that fewer cells, for instance 10^6, would give a slightly suboptimal response but would be worth trying if the cell in question is difficult to obtain. Adjuvants are generally not required when immunizing with whole cells and indeed the emphasis is normally on suppressing the immune response to unwanted dominant antigens. The need to do this is illustrated by attempts to make monoclonal antibodies against histocompatibility antigens. The reviews by Trucco et al.[17] and Brodsky et al.[18] indicate that the majority of monoclonal antibodies produced reaction either with antigens which are not HLA antigens or with determinants on HLA molecules which are common to all donors (nonpolymorphic or monomorphic determinants). There are a number of possible approaches to reducing the immunogenicity of unwanted antigens but again we have to rely largely on evidence obtained by comparing antibody titers before the start of hybridization. Although there are some data on the effect of various maneuvers on the relative proportions of hybridomas making antibody against different antigens, the results are not conclusive.[6]

E. Improving the Proportion of Hybrids Specific for the "Desired" Antigen

Conceptually, the simplest approach to improving the specificity is to use purified antigens. However, purifying glycoprotein membrane antigen requires specialized and complex techniques and only a small number of antigens of this type have been purified by classical means. The availability of monoclonal antibodies will help, but it is a difficult cycle to break into. Since solubilization of the antigens will immediately reduce their immunogenicity, there is a price to be paid for purification and the cost/benefit analysis will only be favorable if the purification can be carried through to a level giving pure or almost pure antigen. In most cases this is not possible and it is therefore more sensible to work with the whole cell. A few exceptions to this generalization must be allowed, in particular when there is a single dominant antigen which is not of interest in the particular experiment, any simple purification which can remove this antigen will be worthwhile. The second exception that can at present be readily recognized is that now that monoclonal antibodies against monomorphic parts of the HLA and Ia molecules are available, it is reasonably straightforward to use the antibodies to purify antigens from HLA-typed cells.[19] The antigen thus purified can be used as immunogen in experiments designed to prepare monoclonal antibodies against the polymorphic HLA and DRw antigens.

If we accept that purification is only likely to be worthwhile in exceptional circumstances, we must look for ways of reducing the immunogenicity of contaminating antigens. There are basically two immunological approaches available; one is to induce a state of partial tolerance to the antigens which are not required and the other is to suppress the antibody response to these antigens by the administration of specific antibody. The former approach has not been used very much in the hybridoma field or indeed in classical antibody preparation. Levy et al.[20] demonstrated a ''moderate advantage'' when they adoptively transferred cells from mice immunized with leukemic cells to animals which had previously been hyperimmunized with normal cells and then irradiated, in an attempt to induce a state of tolerance to the antigens of normal cells. This kind of maneuver is attractive in principle, but there is a scarcity of information on induction of tolerance to particulate antigens in adult mice. Rather more is known about the use of specific antibody against some antigenic components of the membrane to ''coat'' these antigens and specifically suppress the response against them, while allowing a full response against other ''uncoated'' antigens. Although the mechanism of this phenomenon is complex, and certainly involves more than the steric inhibition implied by the term ''coating,'' the procedure has been used successfully in preparing antisera of improved specificity in a number of laboratories.[21,22] In hybridoma preparation, coating antibody has been used by a number of groups[17,23] but the evidence that it helps is of an anecdotal nature. This method depends on the availability of antibody against the contaminating antigens free of antibody against the antigen of interest. For instance, when trying to make a T-cell specific antibody, the immune response to antigens which are common to T and B cells can be suppressed by using an antibody raised against B cells. Since there may be several common antigens to be suppressed, the polyspecific antiserum should be used in preference to monoclonal antibody as a source of coating antibody. Monoclonal antibodies could be used to block the response to certain specific antigens or a cocktail of monoclonal antibodies could be used.

These two approaches, tolerance induction or antibody-mediated suppression, are potentially useful in one particular situation where purification of the antigen will not help. The dominant ''contaminating'' antigenic determinant may be part of the same molecule as the antigenic determinant of interest. This is true, for instance, in the HLA system, where the monomorphic determinants seem to be dominant. No amount of purification will help in this case unless the molecule is broken up and only the polymorphic segment used for immunization. However, the use of coating antibody against the monomorphic determinants or the induction of tolerance to monomorphic determinants may reduce their relative immunogenicity. There is a further potential problem in that the monomorphic determinants may be required as carriers to stimulate a good immune response against the polymorphic determinants.

F. Soluble Antigens

Immunization with soluble antigens presents a totally different problem. In this case it is much more sensible to attempt at least partial purification since the antigen is already in solution and it is relatively easy to remove at least some of the undesirable material. In order to stimulate a good response to the antigen, adjuvant is usually necessary. All the adjuvant procedures that have been used in the preparation of classical antisera are potentially useful in the hybridoma area, but is should be pointed out that very few of the classical adjuvants even approach the efficacy of Complete Freund's adjuvant. *Bordetella pertussis* is often used as adjuvant,[2,4,8] and attention is drawn again to the studies of Stahli et al.[15] on the stimulation of a blast cell response before fusion.

G. Mouse Strain

One final consideration in the immunization is the choice of mouse. Basically any mouse strain will do, but if the hybrids are subsequently to be grown to produce ascites fluid it is helpful to use BALB/c mice because the myeloma cells used for fusion are of BALB/c origin. If a mouse other than BALB/c is used, the hybrids will carry some of the H2 antigens of the other strain and either an F1 hybrid mouse or an immunosuppressed mouse should be used to produce ascites fluid. With some antigens it is advantageous to use a strain of mice which is a good responder to the antigen of interest. The Biozzi strain of high-responder mice have been used in hybridoma production, but these mice give a high response to all antigens. In general, specificity is more difficult to achieve than sensitization, so that the use of these nonselectively high-responder mice is not likely to be helpful.

H. Examples of Immunization Protocols

In this section a number of successful protocols which relate to different types of antigen are described.

1. Production of Antibodies Against Human B Lymphocytes[23]

Animals	BALB/c male mice 6 to 8 weeks old
Antigen	BALM/1 (B cell line) 2×10^7 cell/mouse
Antibody coating	Mixture of monoclonal antibodies which reacted against T and B cells with a titer of 1/128 by immunofluorescence. Cells suspended at 2×10^7 in undiluted antibody preparation. Leave for 30 min at room temperature, inject mixture 1 mℓ per mouse.
Protocol	1. 2×10^7 coated cells i.p. day 0. 2. 2×10^7 coated cells i.p. day 28. 3. Hybridize 4 days after boost.
Notes	Dose: 10^7 has been used successfully, doses down to 10^6 or even lower will probably be effective. Route: i.v. route is as effective as i.p. and may be more effective. Coating antibody: may be omitted, see general discussion for merits of coating (Section III.E). Protocol: interval between injections is probably not critical, but 2 weeks is probably minimal. If mice are left more than 6 weeks it is desirable to give 2 boosters, 1 week apart. Mice which have received three or more injections give

more antibody-producing hybrids, but probably of a broader range of specificities.

2. *Production of Antibodies Against HLA Antigen*[24]

Animals	Female BALB/c mice.
Antigen	Papain-solubilized HLA antigen.
Protocol	1. 20 μg purified HLA antigen s.c. in Freund's Complete Adjuvant. 2. Boosted with similar dose after 1 month. 3. Mice tested for antibody production 2 weeks later; highest titer mice given 10 μg antigen without adjuvant i.v., fusion 5 days later.
Notes	Antigen: whole cells, membranes or soluble antigen have been used successfully for the preparation of anti-HLA antibodies. The proportion of colonies producing antibody which reacts with the HLA antigen is greater with soluble antigen. For reviews on the preparation of monoclonal antibodies against HLA antigens (including DRw antigens) see Brodsky et al,[18] Trucco et al,[17] and Zola.[6]

3. *Production of Antibody Against H2 Antigens*[25]

Animals	BALB/c mice
Antigen	CBA H2 antigens, in the form either of a skin graft or of lymphoid cells (see protocol).
Protocol	1. Skin graft or 1 to 2 $\times$ 10^7 lymphocytes i.p. and s.c. 2. After 15/25 days: boost with lymphocytes.
Notes	Immunized animal: several groups making antibody against H2 (or the rat equivalent, Ag B) antigens have used a cross-species immunization; i.e., mouse antigen into rat or rat antigen into mouse (see review by Howard et al.[26]). Protocol: the published protocol states an optional third injection of lymphocytes 10 to 15 days after the second.[25]

4. *Immunization with Substance P, a Peptide Neurotransmitter*[27]

Animals	Wistar Rats.
Antigen	Substance P coupled to bovine serum albumin.
Protocol	6 i.p. injections spread over 3 months; 3 mg immunogen per injection; in Freund's adjuvant. Final injection without adjuvant, i.v. 3 days before fusion. Rat selected for final boost/fusion on the basis of titer.
Notes	This is an example of immunization with a relatively nonimmunogenic soluble protein. Because of animal variation it is important in this situation to select animals on the basis of tests of sample bleeds. Further examples of protocols for low-immunogenicity combinations are the immunization of rat with mouse Ig[28] and the production of antibody against osteoclast activating factor.[29]

5. *Immunization with Rabies Virus Vaccine*[30]

Animals	BALB/c mice, female 10 to 12 weeks old.
Antigen	Concentrated, purified, inactivated virus, antigenicity determined.
Protocol	1. 0.1 mℓ vaccine i.p.

	2. After 3 to 4 months, boost i.v. with 1:5 dilution of vaccine.
Notes	Use of adjuvants: McFarlin et al.[31] immunized against measles virus using 15 μg virus in Freund's complete adjuvant, i.p. They boosted with 10 μg virus i.v. (no adjuvant) 4 weeks later, and hybridized after a further 2 days.

6. Immunization with Surface Antigen from Trypanosomes[4]

Animals	BALB/c mice, 10 to 12 weeks old.
Antigen	Purified soluble antigen.
Protocol	1. 20 mg antigen/CFA i.p.
	2. After 2 weeks, antigen in IFA i.p.; 5×10^8 *Bordetella pertussis* injected separately, but also i.p.
	3. 3 to 4 days before fusion, inject 20 mg antigen i.v. in PBS.

7. Immunization to Produce IgE Antibody[32]

Animals	BALB/c female mice.
Antigen	Ovalbumin: 1 to 2 mg with $Al(OH)_3$.
Protocol	3 to 4 injections i.p. at monthly intervals.
	Hybridize 3 to 17 days after last injection.

The following chapters in this volume describe immunization protocols found to be successful with other soluble, tissue, viral, and parasite antigens.

V. PARENT MYELOMA LINES

A. Properties Required

In order to be suitable for hybridoma work, a myeloma line must fulfill certain criteria. It must grow well, hybrids derived from it must grow well, and they must secrete high concentrations of immunoglobulin. The myeloma must express a feature which makes it possible to grow hybrids selectively in the presence of parent myeloma. In principle it should be possible to separate hybrids from parent cells, using physical methods such as differential sedimentation[33] or fluorescence-activated cell sorting (see Section IX.E.3). In practice it is very much easier to use a selective medium, particularly since the physical methods will give enrichment rather than pure fractions, and repeated fractionation will thus be necessary.

B. The HAT Selection System

The bulk of the hybridoma work done to date has been with HGPRT-deficient lines (the HAT medium system devised by Littlefield,[34]), and this works so well that it is likely to continue as the method of choice. The principle is illustrated in Figure 2. Aminopterin blocks the main biosynthetic pathway for nucleic acid synthesis. Cells can continue to multiply, utilizing the salvage pathway, if they are provided with hypoxanthine and thymidine. However, a mutant cell lacking an enzyme needed in this salvage pathway will not grow. In the most common version, myeloma cell mutants lacking hypoxanthine guanine phosphoribosyl transferase (HGPRT) are used. They cannot multiply in the presence of aminopterin, even when supplied with hypoxanthine and thymidine, because they cannot incorporate hypoxanthine. The fusion products, however, may have HGPRT from the spleen cell parent, and therefore can multiply in HAT medium. Strictly speaking this system is a half-selective medium, since the spleen cells are not selected against by the HAT medium, but die off naturally.

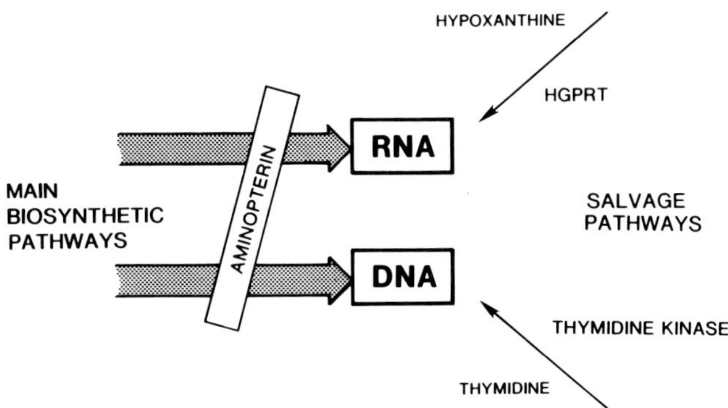

FIGURE 2. Principle of the HAT selection system. Main biosynthetic pathways are blocked by aminopterin (A). Cells can synthesize nucleic acids using the salvage pathways, if provided with hypoxanthine (H) and thymidine (T). Cells which lack the salvage pathway enzymes HGPRT or thymidine kinase cannot synthesize nucleic acids, and die out.

C. Alternative Selection Systems

Although all the myelomas which have been used so far are HGPRT-deficient, it is clear that a cell deficient in thymidine kinase could equally well be used in the HAT selection system. Other drug selections systems, so far not used in hybridoma work, involve the use of mutants lacking either adenine phosphoribosyl transferase or adenosine kinase,[35,36] or selective sensitivity to the antibiotic amphotericin B methyl ester[37] or to ouabain.[5] Other selection systems could be devised. In the production of mouse or rat hybridomas the existing HAT-sensitive cells work so well there is no incentive to try. It may however be that in other areas (e.g., T-T hybridization or human hybridoma production) a different selection system will be worth trying if suitable HAT-sensitive cells are not found.

D. Interspecies Hybridizations

Immunologists interested in mouse antigens have immunized rats with mouse antigen and fused spleen cells from these rats with mouse myelomas. The availability of a rat myeloma line may make this unnecessary, but it has been carried out successfully by several groups. Herzenberg and Ledbetter[38] obtained hybrid frequencies as good as those generally obtained in mouse/mouse fusions, though they did use a myeloma (spleen cell ratio of 1:1 instead of 10:1 used generally in mouse/mouse fusion).

There are several reasons why the preparation of human hybridoma immunoglobulin is highly desirable. While waiting for a suitable human myeloma line to become available (see Section V.E), several groups have fused human cells with mouse myelomas. The result obtained most frequently is a temporary growth of antibody-producing hybrids, followed by early loss of the ability to secrete antibody. It has long been known that mouse/human hybrids preferentially lose human chromosomes.

E. Human Myeloma Lines for Fusion

As indicated in the previous section, mouse/human hybrids are relatively unproductive, preferentially losing human chromosomes (including, frequently, the genes coding for the desired antibody). Furthermore the ability to produce human/human hybridomas offers greater potential in two areas in particular: (1) the production of antibody for in vivo therapeutic administration and (2) the immortalization of interesting antibody-producing clones obtainable from human donors, for instance clones producing autoantibody or alloantibody.

For these reasons there has been great interest in the derivation of suitable human myeloma line. To date one such line has been reported,[39] a HAT-sensitive mutant of the IgE myeloma line U266B1. Results with this line are preliminary but promising.[39]

F. Choice of Line

A number of HAT-sensitive lines are available (Table 1). The rationale for selecting lines is based on the following considerations.

1. Efficiency at Producing Hybrids

It is difficult to ascribe, as an intrinsic property of a line, good or bad efficiency at producing hybrids, since this property varies from culture to culture. A cell line obtained from a laboratory where it was productive may lose productivity through mutation, overgrowing, or contamination with mycoplasma. If fusions fail repeatedly it is advisable to use either another line or some cells of the same line obtained from another laboratory.

2. Immunoglobulin Synthesis

The original P3-X63-Ag8 produces its own immunoglobulin, and fusion products can thus secrete mixed molecules consisting of heavy chains from one parent and light chains from the other. A little calculation will reveal that only one immunoglobulin molecule in 16 produced by the hybrid will be entirely coded for by the spleen parent; the other 15 will have low or no binding affinity for the antigen. The use of the term monoclonal is inappropriate in describing such an antibody mixture, even though the cells may be monoclonal.

The NS1 variant does not secrete any immunoglobulin, but it does synthesize light chains and hybrids secrete molecules incorporating this light chain. In this case one molecule in four will be entirely coded by the spleen cell genome.

It is possible, by successive recloning, to select variant hybrid cells which have lost the myeloma parent chromosomes coding for light or heavy chain, and thus produce true monoclonality from X-63 or NS1 fusions.

However, with the advent of myeloma lines which synthesize neither heavy nor light chains, and therefore produce hybrids which make only the spleen cell antibody, there is no good reason to use X-63 or NS1. Of the three nonproducer myelomas described, we have experience only with P3-X-63/Ag8/653. This line is at least as good as NS1 or X-63 at producing hybrids. In a comparison between the nonsecreting SP2 line and P3-X63-Ag8 the SP2 line was found to produce many fewer hybrids than P3-X63-Ag8.[7] The variation between sublines discussed in the previous section suggests caution in accepting this conclusion as universally correct, although in this case the work originates from the same Institute as the line. The newest mouse myeloma, FO, appears to have all the necessary desirable properties but as yet experience with it is limited to one Institute.[7]

3. Species

Although rat/mouse hybridizations are effective, hybridizations across wider species differences are relatively unproductive. In particular, as has been mentioned, fusion of

Table 1
HAT-SENSITIVE MYELOMA LINES WHICH HAVE BEEN SUCCESSFULLY USED IN HYBRIDOMA PRODUCTION

Line	Species	Ig production	Ref.
P3—x63—Ag8	Mouse	Whole $IgG_1(\gamma_1, \kappa)$	1
P3—NS1/1—Ag4—1	Mouse	κ	41
P3—x63—Ag8.653	Mouse	—	41
SP2/0—Ag 14	Mouse	—	43
FO	Mouse	—	7
210—RCY3—Ag1	Rat	κ	28

human cells with mouse myelomas tend to produce unstable hybrids which rapidly lose the ability to make human immunoglobulin. An exception to this common finding is that when human CLL cells are fused with mouse myeloma cells some stable lines secreting human immunoglobulin are obtained.[40] This is clearly not a method for producing hybrids of known specificity, since the CLL cells are of unknown reactivity. The recent development of HAT-sensitive human myeloma line[39] is thus an important development.

G. Maintainance of Myeloma Line

Myeloma lines maintained in culture frequently lose the capacity to form hybrids. The reasons for this are not established, but it appears that contamination with mycoplasma or overgrowth to a high concentration may be responsible. In addition the possibility of reversion to an aminopterin-resistant line or mutation to a line that does not hybridize well is always present. A number of precautions will reduce the risks of prolonged periods of unproductive hybridization.

Store ampules of cells in liquid nitrogen—When the line is first received it should be grown to concentrations of 3 to 5 $\times$ 10^5/mℓ and several ampules stored in liquid nitrogen (Section X). Once the line has been used successfully more ampules should be stored, and the number of ampules should be maintained at around ten, always freezing fresh stocks from a healthy culture which has recently produced a good yield of hybrids.

Mycoplasma contamination—It is advisable to check cultures occasionally for mycoplasma contamination, and to use mycoplasma-free serum for culture. The spread of mycoplasma through cultures is easier to prevent if no mycoplasma-contaminated cultures are allowed into the laboratory. However, this is not easy to achieve, and we have (up to now) not taken any special precautions with regard to mycoplasma.

Overgrowth—It has been the subjective impression of several workers that if the myeloma cultures are allowed to overgrow, although the culture can be rescued by splitting and viability will return to high levels, hybrid productivity may be lost. For this reason we allow our myeloma lines to reach 3 to 5 $\times$ 10^5 cells per milliliter before splitting. If cultures have inadvertantly been allowed to reach 8 to 10 $\times$ 10^5 cells per milliliter and the viability drops below 85%, we thaw out a fresh ampule.

Nonproductive mutants and other causes of loss of productivity—It is always possible that a mutant which is incapable of giving rise to productive hybrids will arise in the myeloma culture, and will overgrow the productive cells. There are also probably other reasons for the myeloma to lose the ability to produce hybridomas. Without exploring the reasons, if hybridoma production suddenly fails, it is advisable to thaw out a fresh ampule of the myeloma. If after a few passages from cryopreserved stocks productivity always falls off, it may be necessary to reclone the myeloma, but selection of clones will clearly be difficult, and a more practical solution is to get cells from another laboratory.

Revertants—Although we have never experienced this, it is possible for a proportion of the myeloma cells to revert to aminopterin-resistant cells. If the proportion remains small, it will not be apparent, since the only effect will be an increase in the proportion of colonies which do not secrete antibody. If the revertants reach a significant proportion of the myeloma culture, colonies will appear profusely and, soon after, fusion. If this happens, a return to an ampule of cells stored in liquid nitrogen should solve the problem. Alternatively, some workers regularly passage their myelomas through medium containing 6-thioguanine (40 μg/mℓ) or 8-azaguanine (20 μg/mℓ) to kill revertants.

Preparation of myeloma for fusion—It seems to be important to have the myeloma cell line in log phase, with as many cells as possible in G_2 + M phase of the cell cycle. This is the subjective impression of most workers in the field, although there is little hard evidence. We scale up our myeloma cultures before fusion and give them a 50% feed with fresh medium (taking them ideally from 5×10^5 to 2.5×10^5 cells/mℓ) 24 hr before fusion. The volume required may be calculated knowing the number of spleens to be used (approximately 100 mℓ per spleen, see Section VI). We are currently carrying out lifecycle analysis to determine the proportion of cells in G_2 + M phase before fusion, in order to see if this is variable and correlates with hybrid yield.

VI. FUSION PROCEDURES

A. Introduction and Rationale

Fusion of cell membranes occurs with a very low frequency when cells are brought together, and the frequency can be increased to useful levels by the addition of various substances, sometimes referred to as fusogens. Fusing agents have been used of two general types; viruses (Sendai virus in particular) and agents such as lysolecithin and polyethylene glycol which affect the membrane, in a poorly understood manner, to cause fusion. Polyethylene glycol is the agent most commonly used.

The Sendai virus method does not appear to offer any advantages over polyethylene glycol in hybridoma production, and requires the handling of a virus of doubtful safety. Variations of the polyethylene glycol method are now used almost universally and the virus method will not be described.

A successful fusion procedure should bring cells together, with an optimal frequency of interactions between the two "parent" cell types, allow fusion to occur at a sufficiently rapid rate, and cause minimal damage to the cells. The potential problems relate to the frequency of interactions between like cells (producing useless hybrids) and cell damage. Inevitably an agent which enables membranes to "flow" together is likely to affect membrane integrity adversely.

The variables, assuming a population of immune cells and healthy myelomas, are as follows: cell ratio, medium used (particularly presence or absence of serum and pH control), conditions for achieving contact, fusing agent and stablilizing additives, conditions for fusion (time, temperature, physical handling), and processing after fusion up to the plating out stage. An additional variable is the operator; it is a common observation that success with fusions increases with experience even though there is no change in technique detectable to the trained "hybridizer."

The conditions which favor successful fusions are not unique, and there are several variations which seem equally successful. The procedure used by the authors is set out below. Variations which may be important are discussed subsequently.

B. Materials and Preparation

1. Immunized mice which have been boosted with antigen 4 days prior to the day of hybridization (see Section IV).
2. Myeloma cells, subcultured (split) the day before the hybridization, to a concentration of 2 to 3 $\times$ 10^5/mℓ. These cells are routinely passaged in culture and are not allowed to grow above a concentration of 8 $\times$ 10^5/mℓ (see Section V).
3. Medium RPMI 1640 which is supplemented with penicillin, streptomycin, glutamine and 10% FCS (see Section III).
4. 24 well cluster plates (COSTAR) which are pregassed and warmed on the day of hybridization.
5. 70% alcohol.
6. Sterile surgical equipment.
7. Petri dishes (28 cm diameter) tissue culture grade, sterile.
8. 23-gauge needles and 10 mℓ syringes.
9. Sterile pasteur pipettes.
10. 1 mℓ and 10 mℓ sterile pipettes.
11. 20 to 30 mℓ "V" bottom centrifuge tubes.
12. Gey's hemolytic medium (Section III).
13. Polyethylene glycol solution (Section III). Prewarmed to 37° C before fusion.
14. HAT selective medium: (hypoxanthine, aminopterin, thymidine) consists of 100 mℓ of RPMI 1640 (supplemented) to which is added 1 mℓ of 100x HAT concentrate (Section III).

C. Method

1. Mice are killed by CO_2 asphyxiation (dry ice in closed container). The abdominal skin is liberally wetted with 70% alcohol, resected well out of the way, and the abdominal wall cut with sterile scissors to expose the spleen.
2. Spleens are removed and placed in a petri dish containing 20 mℓ of medium.
3. Using a 10 mℓ syringe and 23 gauge needle medium is injected into the spleens causing swelling and the release of cells. The spleens are then teased apart using sterile forceps and the tip of the needle, using a gentle scraping motion.
4. The spleen cells are pipetted into 20 mℓ conical tubes, leaving large clumps of tissue behind. The cells are allowed to stand for 5 min, during which time clumps settle out. The single cell suspension is transferred to a new tube, leaving behind clumps, and the cells are centrifuged at 200 g for 5 min.
5. Gey's medium: this is made up less than 30 min before use. To 14.5 mℓ of sterile distilled water is added 4 mℓ of solution A, 1 mℓ of solution B and 0.1 mℓ bicarbonate solution (5.6%). More bicarbonate is added if the pH of the Gey's solution is less than 7.2 (titrated by color of indicator).
6. The pelleted cells from 1 spleen are resuspended in 5 mℓ of Gey's medium to lyse the RBC. After 5 min the cells are centrifuged at 200 g for 5 min and then washed once in culture medium.
7. The spleen cells are then resuspended in 10 mℓ of culture medium and counted in

trypan blue solution to determine the viability. Cells are only used in hybridization if the viability is greater than 85%.

8. Myeloma cells are centrifuged at 200 g for 5 min and resuspended in culture medium. The viability of the cells is determined using trypan blue exclusion. Cells are only used if viability is greater than 90%. The myeloma cells are then diluted such that 10 mℓ of medium contain 1/10 of the number of spleen cells to be used in the fusion.
9. The spleen cell suspension is then mixed with the myeloma cell suspension in a 20 to 50 mℓ conical-bottom tube (i.e., 10 mℓ of spleen cell suspension +10 mℓ of myeloma cells to give a final cell ratio of 10 spleen cells: 1 myeloma cell). The mixture is centrifuged to a common pellet (200 g for 5 min) and the supernatant discarded. It is important at this stage to remove all supernatant.
10. Add 1 mℓ of warm (37° C) PEG solution to the cell pellet. Using a 1 mℓ pipette the mixture is then aspirated once to give a suspension which still retains clumps. The suspension is then gently mixed using the tip of the pipette, until 1 min has elapsed from the initial addition of the PEG.
11. At the end of the 1 min incubation, the fusion mixture is diluted by slowly adding medium at 37° C dropwise at a rate of 3 mℓ over 10 min. During this time the fusion mixture is gently agitated to ensure an even dilution.
12. Following this first dilution stage a further 10 mℓ of medium is added over a further 10 min with frequent gentle mixing.
13. The cells are then centrifuged at 200 g for 5 min and resuspended in 20 mℓ medium. The cell suspension is poured into a petri dish and placed in the gassed incubator.
14. After 1 to 3 hr in the incubator the cells are collected using a pasteur pipette and transferred to a 20 mℓ conical tube. Gentle repeated aspiration is required in order not to leave behind too many cells.
15. The cells are centrifuged at 200 g for 5 min, and resuspended in HAT medium. The volume is calculated to give a cell concentration of 2×10^5 myeloma cells/mℓ, based on the original cell counts.
16. The fusion mixture is plated out into 24 well cluster plates (flat bottom wells) by adding 1 mℓ of cell suspension per well. These wells may already contain feeder cells (see Notes).
17. The plates are then placed in the humidified 5% CO_2 incubator at 37° C.

D. Notes

The method that we have described is derived from the original PEG technique described by Galfre et al.[44] with minor modifications. The following notes emphasize the points of importance in the method and discuss the merits of various alternative procedures.

1. Spleen Cells

The procedure used to prepare the spleen cells from the mice must be a gentle method which preserves viability and function. Loss of viability as seen by uptake of trypan blue may only be a minimal indication of the damage caused to the cells.

2. Red Cell Lysis

Some workers do not remove red cells. We do so on the assumption that the resultant increased collision frequency between spleen leukocytes and myeloma will be beneficial, in other words red cells would get in the way of useful interactions. The lysis method gives somewhat variable results and we do not aim for absolute purity; the aim being to drastically reduce red cell contamination. As a rule of thumb red cell:white cell ratio should be <1. Geys hemolytic medium is recommended because it probably affords the white cells a greater degree of protection than do other lytic procedures.

3. Myeloma Cells

The myeloma cell line should clearly be viable and functional. The conditions considered optimal for the growth of myeloma cells for fusion have been considered in Section V.G.

We routinely use the X63 variant P3/653 as this neither secretes nor produces immunoglobulin molecules; thus the only immunoglobulin produced by hybrids comes directly from the spleen cell genome (see Section V for a detailed discussion of the myeloma lines available).

4. Presence of Serum

In the washing procedures before hybridization we maintain both the spleen cells and the myeloma cells in media supplemented with FCS. While it has been suggested that FCS may be undesirable in the fusion mixture, producing protein precipitation when PEG is added, FCS allows us to maintain the cells in optimal condition immediately prior to fusion. The medium containing FCS provides a well-buffered system during the critical fusion procedure and if FCS is omitted HEPES buffer is generally added. HEPES is, however toxic to some degree. Fusion products can be obtained in serum free conditions, but no evidence has been presented to indicate that FCS is harmful, and when we have compared the use of serum-free with serum-supplemented media we have obtained more hybrids in serum-supplemented fusions.

5. Temperature

The instinct of anyone trained in biochemistry is to maintain everything on ice until ready for use. However, it is general experience with other procedures which require preservation of cell function (for instance cell-mediated cytotoxicity) that function is best preserved by leaving the mouse cells at room temperature in a good medium. We have followed this procedure and data presented by Fazekas de St Groth and Scheidegger[7] indicates that cooling on ice is clearly detrimental. The fusion process itself is thought to be optimal at 37° C. We maintain our PEG/DMSO and medium for dilution at 37° C up until the time they are used. We have also attempted to keep the fusion tube in a 37° C water bath during dilution, but this has not brought about any noticeable improvement and does render sterile handling more difficult.

6. Fusing Agent

The introduction of PEG as a fusogen has been one of the major changes in method since Köhler and Milstein[1] first described the preparation of monoclonal antibody by cell fusion. The mechanism of action of fusing agents is not well understood but some explanations have been proposed.[45,46] Briefly it has been suggested that cell fusion occurs in three distinct phases. The plasma membranes of the fusing cells are first brought into close contact by centrifugation, and the fusing agent induces agglutination. In the second stage, the membranes of the two cells fuse over a larger area, to form the heterokaryon. Finally, the nuclei fuse to form the hybrid cell. In using PEG as a fusogen cells are thought to agglutinate in the first stage, giving rise to large areas of plasma membrane contact. Cell shrinkage in the presence of PEG is also thought to increase the exposure of glycoprotein. The second stage, the formation of the hetrokaryon, is thought to follow more slowly, so that agglutinated cells can still be disrupted during handling after fusion.

Some workers favor the use of DMSO in the fusion mixture. While it is not an essential component, experiments described by Fazekas de St Groth and Scheidegger[7] indicate that it does no harm and is beneficial if other conditions are not optimal.

7. Time of Fusion

The length of exposure of the cells to the fusing agent seems to be critical. The time of exposure is a compromise to achieve sufficient fusion while keeping cell damage to an acceptable level.

8. Dilution

The dilution procedure is critical and fast addition of fresh medium is detrimental. At this stage it is probable that the aggregated cells which will eventually fuse can still be dissociated by vigorous treatment. Centrifugation and resuspension should be kept to a minimum immediately after fusion. Our procedure, intended as a compromise solution to the conflicting needs, is to exchange the medium by a single gentle wash (to remove PEG and DMSO, thus minimizing toxicity) and then place the cells in a petri dish in the gassed incubator for 1 to 3 hr. This is intended to allow the fusion process to proceed while also allowing DMSO to leach out of the cells. The medium is then exchanged once more by a gentle wash, to finally remove DMSO and PEG and introduce HAT.

9. Feeder Cells

Feeder cells are added to the hybridized cells by some groups, and there is some disagreement about their usefulness. On the basis of experimental evidence, we can make two points. First, feeder cells are not essential, since fusions carried out without feeders frequently work very well. Second, feeder cells can greatly improve the yield of hybrids, in some but not all experiments. These two apparently contrasting statements can be reconciled by the suggestion that if conditions are ideal, feeder cells are not necessary, but if one of the many factors influencing the growth of hybrids after fusion is not optimal, feeder cells can help make up the deficiency.

Fazekas de St Groth and Scheidegger[7] favor using feeder cells on the basis of results which show a variable yield of hybrids if feeder layers are not used and a constant success rate if feeder layers are used. Their conclusion that feeder cells should be used if only as a harmless precaution is difficult to argue with, and probably agrees with the intuitive feeling of most groups. Our own experience has been that in most experiments done without feeder cells, we obtain enough hybrids to keep us gainfully employed, but we use feeder cells occasionally.

Our procedure is to make a spleen cell suspension from an unimmunized mouse exactly as for fusion, and add 1 mℓ of suspension at 10^5 cells per milliliter to each well. This is usually done the day before fusion, although the cells can be prepared on the same day as the fusion and the cells mixed before plating out.

Alternative sources of feeder cells are thymocytes,[2] peritoneal macrophages,[7] and irradiated human fibroblasts.[18] There is evidence suggesting macrophages are particularly important as feeder cells, and subjectively it seems that in experiments (whether given a feeder layer or not) where healthy, spread-out adherent cells are seen, more colonies form than in experiments where few adherent cells are seen.

Recently Astaldi et al.[47] have introduced the use of a supernatant material derived from human epithelial cell cultures. Admixture of this material improves the recovery of hybrids after fusion, when compared with cultures given no feeder supplement or cultures with feeder cells. The use of this type of material could be very helpful, particularly if it was produced on a commercial scale. The effectiveness of this cell-free

supplement indicates that the main function of feeder cells is to add unknown growth factor to the medium, rather than to remove waste products and dead cells, as has been suggested.

VII. PROPAGATION PROCEDURES

A. Introduction and Rationale

For the sake of convenience, we will discuss under "propagation" the procedures subsequent to fusion and washing, i.e., from plating out onwards, up to the point when screening is complete and the hybrids are ready for cloning and cryopreservation.

The objectives are self-evident—to place the hybrids into a medium which will allow hybrids to grow, prevent growth of unfused cells, and support the hybridoma colonies while their antibody products are tested.

This stage in the production of monoclonal antibody is perhaps the most difficult and complex. Fusion products have been formed, but at this stage the cultures are unstable, in several different ways. The fusion products themselves are genetically unstable. A mouse diploid cell has 40 chromosomes, so that a nucleus formed from the fusion of 2 such cells has 80 chromosomes. Such a nucleus is unstable, and over the first few days in culture chromosomes will be lost. In mouse/mouse hybrids there is no evidence that this chromosome loss is anything other than random, although in hybrids between human and mouse the loss is highly selective, human chromosomes being lost preferentially. It is too early to rule out the possiblity that the loss of chromosomes in mouse/mouse hybrids is also in some way selective. When a cell loses a chromosome which is involved in the production or secretion of immunoglobulin, but retains the ability to grow, it becomes a nonsecretor. Thus in a culture well which originally contained only one hybrid cell, an antibody secretor, after several divisions we may have several nonsecreting clones in addition to the secretor. Since the nonsecretors may outgrow the secretor, the result is a gradual loss of antibody production.

If a cell loses a chromosome involved in cell replication, it no longer contributes to the culture and such chromosome loss is thus not important unless it happens before the original hybrid has divided. This is possible, since extrapolation of the kinetics of colony growth back to the early stages of the culture indicates that hybrids may sit in culture for several days before cell division starts.

The chromosomal loss gradually stops, hybrids stabilizing at a chromosome number somewhere between the diploid and tetraploid number; the stable number being different for different hybrids. The stabilization is an asymptotic process, and can never be deemed to have reached completion. Thus hybrids which have been in culture for months can gradually lose antibody secretory activity, due probably to the development of a nonsecretor which outgrows the secretor. Cloning (see Section IX) is important early in the life of a hybridoma, and may be necessary at later stages.

Quite apart from this chromosomal instability, the cultures are unstable in other ways during the early postfusion days. Unfused myeloma cells are dying out as a result of the aminopterin block. Spleen cells are dying out, with the exception of macrophages and/or fibroblasts which may be establishing themselves and beginning to divide. As noted above, the fusion products may remain dormant for several days, before beginning to divide. It is easy to imagine that during this time they are on a knife-edge, and can be pushed into division, or die, depending on the state of the culture. Established, growing, hybridomas will tolerate culture conditions which an early culture will not.

Chromosome loss cannot be controlled by the experimenter, but the other factors leading to instability of the cultures can. Much more information is needed before this stage of hybridoma production can be approached more rationally. For the present, we

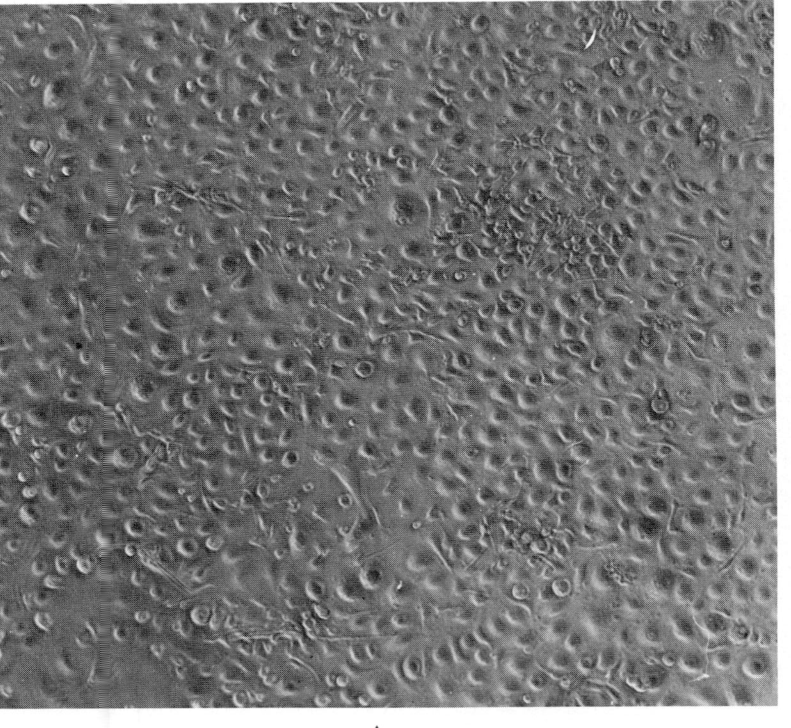

A

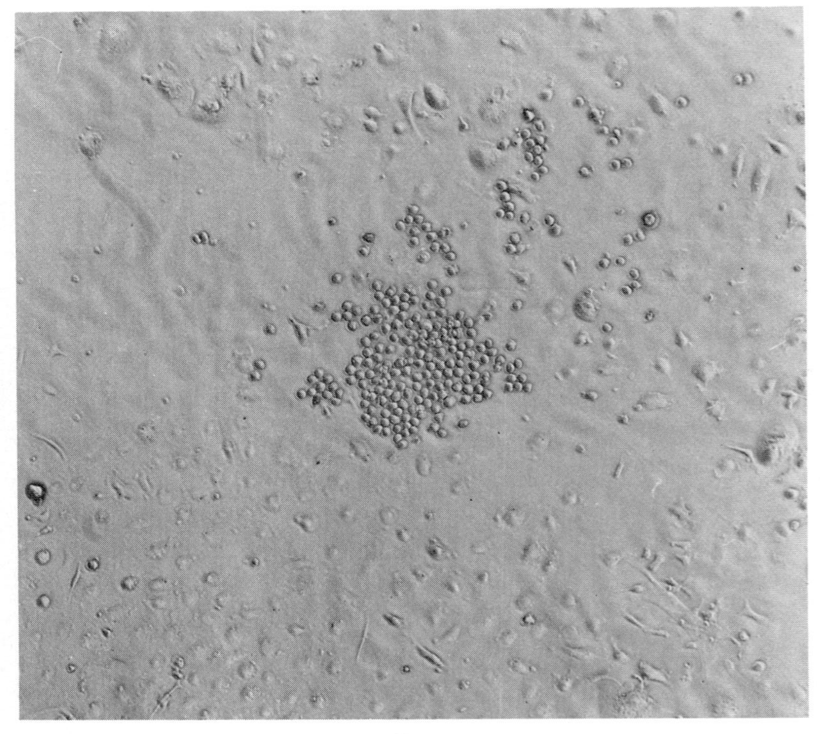

B

FIGURE 3. Appearance of cultures during propagation stage. (A) Spreading colony of macrophage or fibroblast-like cells. These are seen occasionally and appear macroscopically as rather thin colonies, which should not be confused with hybridoma colonies. The latter appear macroscopically as white, opaque colonies, and are quite different microscopically. Small numbers of spread-out adherent cells are often seen in the first week after fusion. These derive either from the spleen cells used in the fusion or the feeder cells, if used. There appears to be a correlation between the appearance of such cells and subsequent good yields of hybrids. If no adherent macrophage-like cells are seen this may be an indication that fusion conditions were toxic and the hybrids are also dead. (B,C) Hybridoma colonies at different stages of growth. The small colony might just be visible macroscopically, the large one would be readily visible. The cells are characteristically round with a membrane which shows up very clearly under phase contrast. The cells are larger than small lymphocytes.

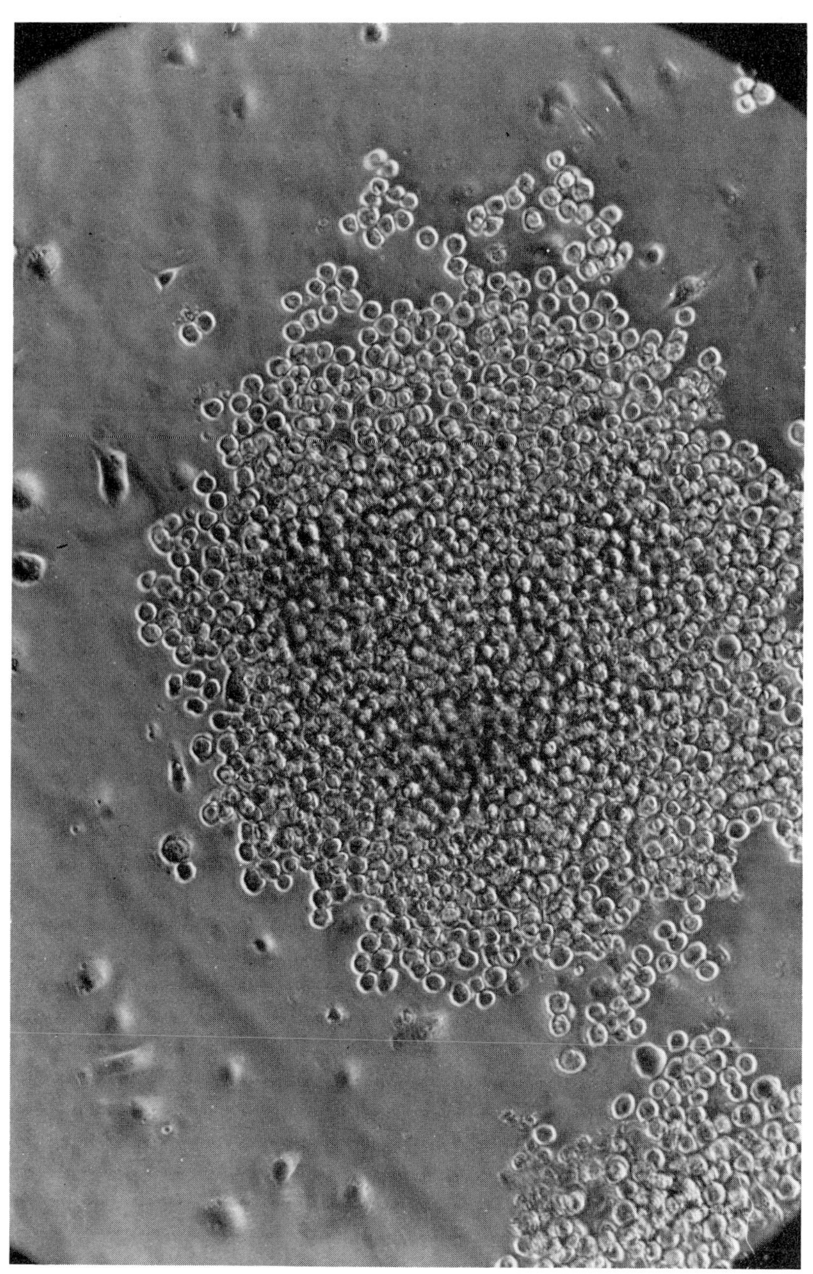

FIGURE 3C.

will discuss the methods which have been arrived at empirically for the handling of early cultures after fusion. As in the other aspects of hybridoma technology, there are many alternative solutions to the problems.

B. Handling of Hybrids After Hybridization

1. *After hybridization* the culture plates are usually examined daily to check for colony growth and condition of the culture medium. (color, pH).
2. *Hybrids are fed* 7 days after fusion. To each 2 mℓ culture well (which has 1 mℓ of hybrid mixture) is added 1 mℓ of HT medium. This addition of fresh medium is carried out as gently as possible so as to reduce the risk of generating multiple colonies which are derived from a single parent colony and to reduce the probability of mixing of cells from adjacent colonies. If the culture wells already contain 2 mℓ (as is the case if 1 mℓ of fusion mixture was added to 1 mℓ of feeder layer) gently aspirate off approximately 1 mℓ of culture supernate before feeding.
3. *Over the next 7 days* the color of the medium is examined. If undue yellowing occurs, then plates are fed with fresh HT medium. This yellowing may result from revertant HAT-resistant myeloma (see Section V.G.), spreading fibroblast-like cells (see Figure 3a), an excessive number of feeder cells, and growth of hybrids (see Figures 3b and c).
4. *Colony growth*. When colonies are macroscopic and the medium is yellowing, they are fed by removing 1 mℓ of spent medium (which can be used for screening, see next section) and replacing it slowly with 1 mℓ of HT medium. This further reduces the concentration of aminopterin and appears to enhance colony growth.
5. *Samples for screening*. If the sample is taken early there is a risk of missing positive hybrids because the antibody concentration in the supernatant is too low. Conversely, it is important not to allow the colony to overgrow (excess yellowing of the medium) as this may result in death of the hybrids; thus on balance it is best to test samples before the cultures are very crowded, but to retest wells giving negative results at a later stage, when the medium is yellow. A further problem results from the presence of small amounts of antibody produced not by hybrids but by surviving spleen cells. This is occasionally manifested as a weak positive result which disappears when the cultures are fed and retested after a further period of growth.
6. *Picking of positive colonies*. Supernatants taken from appropriately growing cultures are tested for antibody activity (see Section VIII). The colonies producing positive antibody are selected for further expansion. Colonies are removed by carefully placing a sterile pasteur pipette on/in the colony and withdrawing the cells plus medium in to the pipette. These cells are transferred to a 2 mℓ well of a 24 well cluster plate containing 1 to 2 mℓ of fresh HT medium already equilibrated to temperature and pH in the incubator. In cases where wells have more than one colony growing, each individual colony is picked for further expansion and testing.

   Some of the cells should be used to clone the hybrid at this stage (Section IX). If on transfer to new wells the cells do not continue to grow well growth can be stimulated by the addition of feeder cells,[48] which can be prepared and used exactly as at the outset of the fusion (see Section V.D.).

   While waiting for the clones to grow the uncloned hybrid should be grown up by expansion of the culture into bottles and cells should then be stored in liquid nitrogen (Section X). Difficulty will be experienced with scaling up if the hybrids are diluted excessively (to below 10^4/mℓ). Hybrids do not always transfer well to growth in bottles. The reason for this is not clear but it may help to wash the bottles out with medium (incubate them full of medium overnight) in order to remove any toxic plasticizers, etc. and to add feeder cells for the initial growth in bottles. When growth is established, care must be taken not to allow the cultures to die off by overcrowding. Hybrids seem to be variable in respect of the maximum cell concentration they will tolerate; some grow well up to 10^6/mℓ while others lose viability if they exceed 5×10^5/mℓ. Furthermore, the same hybrid seems to tolerate higher concentrations when it has been in culture for a few months than it does earlier; thus early in the life of a culture it should be split frequently and the concentration maintained between 10^5 and 4×10^5/mℓ.

Cryopreservation of the uncloned hybrid is not essential since all subsequent work will be done on the cloned cells, but we have found it to be a useful insurance against failure of the cloning experiment.

7. *Use of HT*. The cells grow initially in HAT medium. If, after selection against the unhybridized myeloma is completed, the HAT constituents are all omitted from the medium, the hybrids will die out. This is because the hypoxanthine and thymidine are used up faster than the aminopterin, and the cells then have neither main nor salvage pathways for DNA synthesis. The cells are thus maintained in HT, allowing the salvage pathways to operate. After splitting a few times the aminopterin concentration will have fallen sufficiently for the main pathway to operate, and H and T could be omitted from the media. This has to be done gradually, and after experiencing difficulty with some hybridomas, we have stopped trying to wean cells off HT. All subsequent operations are thus carried out in HT medium.

VIII. SCREENING METHODS

A. Rationale

Having successfully immunized, hybridized, and propagated the fusion products, the experimenter is faced with a large number of rapidly growing colonies. The medium in the culture is beginning to turn yellow, and it is time to screen the cultures in order to determine which ones are producing interesting antibody.

The aims of screening are twofold: to identify positive cultures as early as possible in order to clone early and to identify uninteresting cultures early in order not to waste time and materials propagating them.

For example, let us suppose we are looking for antibodies specific for human T cells. Clearly we must first screen with T cells and only those cultures reacting with T cells are examined further. However, many of the antigens of the T cell membrane are also found on B cells and other cells. If we are interested in T cell-specific antibodies to the exclusion of others, and if we are reasonably certain that each well contains only one colony, we should follow the primary T-cell screen with a secondary screen using B cells, and discard any colonies positive in the second assay.

Clearly interesting clones may be lost in this way and the experimenter must make a conscious decision whether he is looking very specifically for certain products, or is going to investigate any positive hybrids. The second approach has been very productive. However, as more and more monoclonal antibodies become available, the potential of this approach to finding useful new specificities dwindles and a more directed approach becomes necessary.

B. Choice of Screening Test

In principle any test for antibody can be used to screen hybrid supernatants. However, the very properties that make monoclonal antibodies useful render them unsuitable for some assay systems which depend on secondary interactions (for instance, immunoprecipitation). The suitability of different test systems will be discussed in greater detail later in this section.

Clearly the most important factor in selecting an assay is the nature of the antigen. Since the hybridoma techniques can be applied in so many areas and in most cases antigen-antibody assays were already well established before the use of hybridization, we will not attempt to describe assays. Rather the principles will be set out in detail, with particular emphasis on the peculiarities of monoclonal antibodies, in order to help the potential user to make a rational choice of test. Tests which have been used successfully in screening hybridomas against various types of antigen will then be tabulated, with references.

1. Speed and Convenience

Hybrid colonies mature and grow at different rates and, typically, there will be a few new samples to test almost every day in the 3rd and 4th weeks after fusion. Samples can be accumulated for batch testing to a limited degree, but any delay entails the risk of loss of clones, either due to overcrowding or selective growth of nonsecreting cells; thus the assay used should be quick and capable of being set up on a daily basis.

2. Primary Interaction vs. Secondary Interaction

There is an important distinction between assays which detect binding of antigen to antibody (primary interaction) and assays which depend on a secondary reaction following after the binding of antigen to antibody. The second reaction may be the binding of complement in cytotoxicity or complement fixation tests, the formation of large lattices in precipitation reactions, or the use of a second antibody in immunofluorescence or radio-labeled antiglobulin tests.

Tests measuring the primary interaction should always work provided the affinity of binding is adequate. In tests involving a secondary interaction it is important to consider the requirements for this second step. Provided the second step is automatically successful, the distinction is unimportant; thus Farr assays, in which soluble complexes are precipitated by ammonium sulfate, are considered as measurements of primary interaction. Indirect immunofluorescence or radio-labeled anti-immunoglobulin tests may be considered in the same way, provided the second antibody (fluorescence- or isotope-labeled antimouse immunoglobulin) reacts with all subclasses of mouse immunoglobulin. However, the corresponding assay using labeled protein A will, under normal conditions, only detect IgG 2a, 2b, and 3 and some IgG 1 antibodies, and is thus not suitable for screening.

Similarly, only IgM and IgG 2a and 2b fix complement and assays based on complement are thus not suitable for screening, unless the purpose of the experiment is to find only cytotoxic antibodies.

More examples of the distinction between screens based on primary interactions and secondary interactions will become clear during the subsequent discussion. The point being made is not necessarily that secondary interactions should not be used; it is difficult to avoid using them. However, it is important to think through the various stages of a potential screening assay in evaluating its suitability.

3. Single and Multiple Determinants

Antibodies against macromolecular or cellular antigens do not react with the entire antigen, but with relatively small molecular conformations, referred to as antigenic determinants or epitopes. A particular epitope may occur only once in each antigen molecule (common in polypeptide or glycolipid antigens) or, alternatively may occur several times in the same antigen (in proteins composed of several identical chains, in polysaccharides, and on cell membranes).

An antibody against a single, nonrepeating determinant can at most bind two antigenic molecules. The resulting complex is not very large, and will generally stay in solution. If the antigen contains two determinants, a long chain antigen-antibody complex can form and if more than two determinants are present a lattice can form. These large structures are much more likely to precipitate.

This reasoning leads us to one of the major differences between a normal antiserum and a monoclonal antibody, a difference which must be borne in mind when selecting an assay. An antiserum is a mixture of antibodies, and can be expected to contain antibodies against several antigenic determinants on each antigen. Even if each determinant occurs once on each antigen molecule, the mixture of antibodies renders the system multideterminant and precipitation should occur, at appropriate concentrations. A monoclonal antibody, in contrast, contains antibody against only one determinant and will therefore not precipitate an antigen consisting of nonrepeating determinants.

This means that immunoprecipitation in its various forms is not a suitable screening test for monoclonal antibodies, except where the antigen consists of multiple copies of determinants.

Cytotoxicity assays suffer from a similar problem. Although the reason is not as clear as in the case of immunoprecipitation, the failure of some complement—binding monoclonal antibodies to produce lysis on their own has been clearly demonstrated.[49] Mixtures of antibodies which react noncompetitively with different determinants on the same molecule synergise to produce lysis, and the reason is probably that each antibody by itself does not provide a sufficient density of complement fixing sites to cause lysis.

4. The Prozone Phenomenon

Consideration of the process of cell agglutination shows that at high antibody concentrations, agglutination will not occur, because there will be enough antibody to saturate all of the antigenic determinants without linking cells to each other. As the antibody is diluted, agglutination is observed, while at high dilutions of antibody there is insufficient antibody to crosslink cells—the agglutination ''titrates out.'' The zone in which agglutination is not found because there is too much antibody is called the prozone; when the test is used to detect antibody it will give a false-negative result in the prozone region.

Clearly assays which exhibit prozones have disadvantages for use in hybridoma screening, because samples cannot be tested at a single concentration but must be titrated. Prozones occur somewhat unpredictably, suggesting that simple explanations such as that given above do not tell the whole story.

Agglutination, precipitation, and cytotoxicity reactions all show prozones. Assays based on binding of a fluorochrome- or isotope-labeled second antibody should not show a prozone. We have observed a prozone in indirect immunofluorescence using very concentrated ascites—derived monoclonal antibody. This probably results from the presence of excess mouse immunoglobulin after the first stage of the test, reacting with the conjugated antimouse antibody. An extra wash between antibody treatments should prevent this prozone, but it is in any case not seen with culture supernatants or diluted ascites fluid.

5. The Screen Should be Appropriate to the Intended Use of the Antibody

This statement may seem self-evident, but deserves emphasis. If, for instance, the purpose is to make antibody for use in cell subpopulation identification in a routine clinical immunology laboratory, indirect immunofluorescence or rosetting assays will be used in routine practice and are suitable for use in screening hybridoma cultures. A radio-labeled anti-immunoglobulin method may be more sensitive and may detect some clones not seen by immunofluorescence or rosetting. Such clones may be producing antibody which reacts either with low affinity or with an antigen which is scarce on the cell membrane. It may indeed be a very interesting antigen, but if the antibody is not detected by the assays which are available in the routine diagnostic laboratory, it will not be of use in the context for which it was intended.

6. Background Staining and Affinity of Binding

A further point to be considered in selecting an assay is that conventional sera usually include some high-affinity antibody and also usually give some nonspecific (background) binding. Assays are often tailored for these conditions, by favoring only high-affinity binding (low concentration, high temperature, presence of mild detergent). These conditions reduce nonspecific binding, which is usually of a low affinity. Monoclonal antibodies usually suffer much less from nonspecific binding so that these precautions are not necessary. Furthermore, since the use of such conditions will preclude the detection of all but the most avid monoclonal antibodies, they should be avoided.

7. Screening for Antibody-Producing Cells Rather than Secreted Antibody

If the antibody-secreting cells in a fusion mixture can be identified and selected this will be more direct than screening for antibody in the supernatant. This approach was used in the original hybridoma paper[1] and is particularly suited to agar cloning. The agar procedure has been described in detail;[3] however, in its original form (as an erythrocyte plaque assay) it is only suitable for erythrocyte antigens or antigens which can readily be coupled to erythrocytes. Even with erythrocyte antigens, plaques will not always be found; thus Howard and Corvalan[49] have demonstrated that cells secreting antibody against rat MHC antigens do not lyse rat erythrocytes, even though the cells express MHC antigens. The reason is probably an insufficient density of complement-fixing sites.

Selection of antibody-secreting cells reaches its greatest level of sophistication in the use of fluorescent beads coated with antigen to pick out and clone antibody secreting cells on the cell sorter[50] (see also Section IX.C.3). It is interesting that the method works, since it has generally been held that antibody-producing cells, unlike their B cell precursors, do not have significant amounts of immunoglobulin actually resident in the membrane at any time. Indeed it appears that surface membrane Ig (SMIg) and secreted Ig differ structurally, the former having a hydrophobic region which interacts with the lipid bilayer. Clearly, since the method does work, there is enough Ig sufficiently tightly bound to the membrane to take up the antigen-coated beads. It is however, possible that the method detects only a proportion of clones, and that others secrete antibody but do not have enough bound to the membrane to show up in the assay.

8. Screening for Immunoglobulin Production

Clearly only colonies which are secreting immunoglobulin are of potential use. When the screen for the specific antibody activity being sought is difficult, time consuming, or expensive it may be worthwhile to screen first for immunoglobulin in the supernatant, thus eliminating from further testing those clones which are not secreting antibody. Suitable methods for detecting mouse immunoglobulin in the culture supernatant would include radioimmunoassay and enzyme-linked immunoassay. It is of course important to ensure that the assays do not miss any subclasses, as would happen either if the antiglobulin used in the assay did not react with a minor subclass, or if the labeled mouse immunoglobulin used in a competitive-binding assay was deficient in a minor subclass.

Table 2
SPECIFIC ANTIBODY ASSAYS USED FOR SCREENING HYBRIDOMAS

Test	Antigen type	Ref.
Indirect immunofluorescence	Cell membrane	23
Fluorescent microspheres bearing antigen, analyzed by flow microfluorometry	Immunoglobulin allotypes (soluble antigens available pure)	50
^{125}I-labeled anti-immunoglobulin or protein A	Cell membrane	51
^{125}I-labeled anti-immunoglobulin-replica method	Virus, polysaccharide, DNA	35, 36, 52, 53
Passive cutaneous anaphylaxis for	Ovalbumin	32
IgE antibodies	DNP	54
Bioassay	Osteoclast-activating factor (biologically active substances for which radioimmunoassay is not available)	29

No estimate is available on the proportion of colonies which do not secrete immunoglobulin, and, unless this proportion is high and the specific antibody assay very difficult, it is unlikely that such a preliminary screen would be worthwhile.

C. Compilation of Screening Tests in Use

As has already been emphasized, the number of available tests is large and the primary consideration is the nature of the antigen. Furthermore the screens are mostly derived from well-established assays. We have therefore not attempted to describe each assay in detail. Table 2 contains a list of assays successfully used in screening hybridomas, with appropriate references. It will be noted that in several cases the general groundrules for selection of a test, as outlined above, have been successfully disregarded.

D. Control of Assay Conditions

Mosmann et al.[55] have recently pointed out that, since binding affinity depends on the physical conditions (especially pH and temperature) the apparent specificity of an antibody can vary as these conditions are altered. In particular, a high-affinity interaction would give a positive result over a wide range of temperature and pH, whereas a low-affinity binding would only be detectable at low temperature and optimal pH. Thus a single antibody might bind two determinants at optimal conditions but only one at suboptimal conditions. The data of Mosmann et al.,[55] showing that such specificity changes with pH do happen, suggest that it is important to control the physicochemical conditions under which screening is carried out, in order to obtain reproducible results.

IX. CLONING

A. Introduction and Rationale

Approximately 10 to 20 days after a successful fusion, hybrids are growing as colonies in a proportion of culture wells. At this stage, the cultures are screened for antibody production and positive colonies are selected for expansion and cloning. It is essential to clone as early as practicable, to ensure that a given culture contains only one cell type and that it is producing only one immunoglobulin specificity.

Immediately after hybridization, the fusion products will have approximately 80 chromosomes, and as these cells proceed to divide they will randomly lose some of these chromosomes. By cloning early, it is possible to select those cells which still have the chromosomes coding for antibody production. If cloning is not carried out at this stage there is a risk that variants not producing immunoglobulin will appear and overgrow the culture. In addition hybridization culture wells often have multiple colonies, which may become disturbed and mixed during the course of feeding. The process of cloning allows the selection of a positive hybrid which is derived from a single cell; thus any colonies which are composed of a mixture of cell types can be separated into pure populations. Wells containing two or more colonies may still produce only one antibody, if the other hybrids in the well are nonsecretors. It is nevertheless necessary to clone and isolate the secretor hybrid, as the nonsecretors may overgrow the culture.

Essentially, cloning is achieved by seeding single cells into culture wells and allowing them to proliferate into colonies. However, hybridoma cells placed in culture at very high dilution have a tendency to die out. In order to stimulate colony growth it is necessary either to co-culture other (nonhybridoma) cells as a ''feeder cell layer,'' or to culture the hybrid in semisolid agar. Even in the case of agar cloning, feeder layers improve the cloning efficiency considerably. The precise function of feeder cells is not fully understood and is probably complex. Feeder cells probably secrete ''growth factors'' which stimulate the growth of the hybridoma, and may also remove toxic byproducts from the medium. The simple increase in overall cell concentration is also important.

B. When to Clone and How Often

As has already been emphasized, the first cloning should be performed as soon as possible in order to reduce the chance of overgrowth by negative hybrids. If there is any doubt about the monoclonality after cloning (for instance if the antibody reacts with two apparently unrelated antigens) the cloned culture should be recloned. The probability of obtaining the same mixture from a mixed colony on two successive clonings is low.

Once a satisfactory clone has been obtained, it may still produce mutants in culture; thus if the hybridoma is kept in continuous culture the antibody activity should be monitored. If there is an indication of a fall in activity the hybrid should be recloned. The frequency of chromosome loss decreases with time in culture, but the possibility never disappears completely.

C. Methods

Three essentially different techniques are used.

1. Cloning by the Technique of Limiting Dilutions

This method relies on diluting cells out to a stage where there is, statistically, only one viable cell per well in a culture plate. Unstimulated spleen cells are added to the culture system to act as feeder cells. Dispensing single cells into wells is clearly a random process, and in order to obtain wells with colonies derived from single cells it is necessary to put up several wells, and advisable to use several different cell concentrations. Consideration of the statistics of the procedure (see notes) has led to the use of concentrations which place a nominal 0.5, 1, and 5 cells per well.

a. Materials

1. Sterile HT medium and RPMI medium (see Section III.B).
2. Sterile 24 well cluster tissue culture plates.
3. Gey's hemolytic medium.

4. Spleen from normal, unimmunized mice (1 spleen per 2 cloning plates).
5. Cell suspension of hybrids, preferably with viability >80%.

b. Procedure

1. After isolation of the spleen cells in RPMI medium clumps are removed by settling out and RBC are lysed using Gey's hemolytic medium (see Section VI.C for detailed description of method used for preparation of spleen cells).
2. The spleen cells are then washed twice in RPMI medium, and resuspended in HT medium. The cell viability is determined by dye exclusion.
3. The hybrid cells are washed once in HT medium and the cell viability determined by dye exclusion.
4. The cell suspensions are then mixed to give the following final concentrations in HT medium:
   a. Spleen cells at 1×10^6 viable cells/mℓ
   b. Hybrid cells at 0.5, 1 and 5 cells/mℓ
5. The resulting cell mixtures are then plated out in 24 well cluster plates (pre-equilibrated in 5% CO_2 at 37° C), seeding 1 mℓ per culture well. Generally, 12 or 24 wells are set up for each hybridoma and placed in the gassed (5% CO_2 in air) 37° C humidified incubator.
6. After 7 days from the initial seeding, microscopic colonies should be visible. At this stage examine colonies microscopically and reject any wells containing more than one colony, or a colony that appears asymetric, suggesting it may consist of two adjacent colonies. Monoclonal colonies are usually circular.
7. Cloning wells are fed with HT medium as necessary (judging from the color of the medium). When macroscopic colonies are present, supernatants can be tested and positive clones harvested and set up in expanded culture.

c. *Notes*

Cloning plates and cell concentrations—We have used mainly the 2 mℓ wells for cloning, and a hybrid cell concentration of 1 cell per well usually gives some wells with single, positive colonies. Occasionally the cell concentration is too low, resulting in a lack of positive colonies, or is too high, leading to multiple colonies. The cloning then has to be repeated. A method widely used to get around this (in our experience infrequent) problem, is to set up larger numbers of wells and cover a range of cell concentrations. The concentrations used are 0.5, 1 and 5 cells per well and in order to obtain sufficient wells with monoclonal growth a 96-well flatbottom tissue culture microtiter plate is used; 24 wells are seeded at the lowest dilution and 36 wells at each of the higher dilutions. The disadvantage of the smaller wells is that once colony growth starts, testing and transfer must be done rapidly, before the small volume of culture medium and small growth area are used up.

Handling of cloning plates—Colonies arising in cloning wells remain circular and the cells are slightly adherent and so remain in position if handled carefully. However, rough handling of the plates or rapid feeding causes cells to detach and establish subsidiary colonies. It then becomes impossible to determine whether the well has multiple different colonies, or one colony which has given rise to subcolonies. For this reason plates should be handled gently, feeding should be kept to a minimum and carried out very slowly, with every effort made to minimize disturbance of the colony.

2. *Cloning Using Semisolid Agar*

The method of cloning cells in semisolid agar also relies on diluting the hybrid cells to a level where colonies grow at distinct sites; however, in this case the cells are suspended in agar and are not free to move in the culture vessel. Proponents of the agar method have argued that monoclonality is more assured in this system, because the cells are not free to move. Cloning efficiencies, however, are much lower in agar than in liquid media requiring the use of much higher cell concentrations (typically 10^3 to 10^4 cells per milliliter instead of 0.5 to 5 in the limiting dilutions method). This higher concentration clearly increases the chances of having two adjacent cells initiating a colony.

In practice most users find the limit-dilution method satisfactory, and we will not describe the agar method. The technique is described in several reviews.[4,8]

3. Cloning and Selection Using the Fluorescence-Activated Cell Sorter

Herzenberg and co-workers[38,50] have used the FACS instrument to select positive hybrids and clone. This has been discussed under screening (Section VIII.B.7). In order to clone using the FACS a single-cell deposition accessory is available from the two principal manufacturers of flow cytometers. The single-cell deposition accessory allows the FACS to place a single cell in a well of a microtiter tray, containing medium and feeder cells. The cell stream automatically stops while the tray is repositioned and the sorter is reactivated to sort a drop in the next well. Cloning is either done using fluoresceinated antigen (Section VIII.B.7) so as to select positive cells and clone in one operation, or alternatively cells are deposited individually in cloning wells without selection for antigen binding. The first method offers the clear advantage of selecting positive hybrids only, whereas cloning on an unselective basis using the FACS offers no significant advantage over cloning by manual dilution and dispensing.

X. CRYOPRESERVATION

A. Introduction

The maintenance of hybridoma cells lines in culture is subject to many pitfalls including:

1. Contamination of cultures
2. Loss of chromosomes coding for growth or antibody production
3. Overgrowth by nonsecreting mutants
4. Cell death due to overgrowth

Cryopreservation of cells is an essential safeguard against loss of valuable lines. It is important to freeze down a hybridoma line as soon as possible, even before it has been cloned. This then gives a source of the original line if the cloning fails. After cloning the clones selected for antibody production are also frozen down. Thus both the original line and a line which has stabilized with respect to chromosome loss are maintained in frozen storage.

While there are many variations on the basic method for cryopreservation and thawing of cells, we described the methods used in our laboratory. These methods are adapted from well-established procedures for cryopreservation of human cells.

B. Freezing Cells Down

1. Hybrid cells are washed once in culture medium and resuspended at 6 × 10^6/mℓ in HT medium containing 50% fetal calf serum.
2. To this cell suspension an equal volume of unsupplemented RPMI medium con-

taining 30% DMSO is added dropwise with continuous gentle mixing. The medium is added at a rate of approximately 1 mℓ/min.

3. After thorough but gentle mixing, 2 mℓ of cell suspension is transferred to a 2 mℓ freezing ampule (NUNC).
4. The ampules are sealed tightly and frozen using a programmed freezing device. This is a machine in which the ampules are cooled from room temperature to −100°C by admitting vapor from a liquid nitrogen reservior at a rate which is controlled by a cam. Different cams are available, designed to cool the cells according to programs regarded as optimal for particular cell types. Most programs take the cells from ambient to −10°C at a rate of 1 to 2°/min; the rate increases briefly at −10°C to take up the latent heat of fusion which is emitted by the mixture freezing at that temperature; and cooling continues at 1 to 2°C/min to −25°C. From here to −100°C the cooling rate increases gradually to 5 to 10°/min.

   This type of program was not initially designed for hybridomas but works well enough with them. It is not essential to use a programmed cooler, but it is important to cool the cells relatively slowly to −25°C. This can be achieved using special polystyrene chambers which fit into the neck of the liquid nitrogen container, where the temperature does not reach liquid nitrogen levels.
5. When the cells are at a temperature of −100°C the vials are removed from the freezing chamber and stored in a liquid nitrogen container. Ampules do not have to be immersed in liquid nitrogen, but can be in the vapor phase above liquid nitrogen. The temperature will be between −190 and −150°C.

C. Thawing Cells Out

1. The ampule to be thawed is removed from N_2 storage and placed in a 37°C water bath.
2. Care must be taken to completely thaw the frozen sample but the ampule should not be left in the water bath for longer than necessary.
3. The contents of the ampule are diluted by slow dropwise addition of an equal volume of HT medium. Approximately 2 mℓ of medium is added over 10 min, and the suspension is mixed gently during dilution.
4. The cell suspension is left undisturbed at room temperature for 15 min.
5. The suspension is further diluted by adding another 6 mℓ of medium over 10 min.
6. The cell suspension is again left for 15 min at room temperature without being disturbed.
7. The cells are washed twice in HT medium.

The importance of gradual dilution is not clear. Some laboratories thaw rapidly and transfer the contents of the ampule immediately into 5 volumes of medium. We have compared the two procedures and obtained better viability by the slow dilution process.

D. Notes

1. The importance of obtaining cryopreserved ampules of hybrids and clones early cannot be emphasized too often. A hybridization experiment yields a new and useful combination of genes, and this new combination cannot readily be reproduced to order. In view of the multiplicity of potential pitfalls in tissue culture, this new set of genes should be cryopreserved so that it can be readily recovered.
2. Storage in mechanical refrigerators at −80°C is not effective, except for very short times.

Table 3
CHARACTERIZATION OF MONOCLONAL ANTIBODIES

Characteristic	Useful techniques
Specificity	Screening test applied to different antigens
Titer	Screening test applied quantitatively coupled with immunoglobulin concentration determination
Affinity of binding	Kinetic studies of binding
Stability on storage	Storage and testing of titer
Immunoglobulin class/subclass	Immune precipitation, radio-immunoassay or enzyme—linked immunoassay, using subclass-specific antisera.
Monoclonality	Isoelectric focusing, cross-absorption studies, subcloning and analysis of products, flow cytofluorometry with DNA-binding dyes
Immunochemical identification of antigen detected	Coprecipitation of antibody with radiolabeled antigen followed by one- or two-dimensional electrophoresis in gel.

3. It is clearly important to introduce a proper system of responsibilities and contingency plans to ensure that the liquid nitrogen store does not run dry. Holidays, sickness of the person primarily responsible, and even nondelivery of liquid nitrogen should be planned for. In the event of a failure of liquid nitrogen supplies, due for instance to strike action, the safest solution would be to transfer ampules to a −80°C mechanical freeze and put one ampule of each important hybrid into culture.
4. There are many technical variations of the procedures described in this section; some of them have already been discussed. When considering a variation of procedure it is relatively easy to assess the relative merits of two methods, simply by measuring the viability after the procedures. Not all cellular damage is immediately apparent in terms of dye exclusion, however; thus, the growth of ice crystals within internal organelles could produce damage not apparent until the cells are allowed to go through the cell cycle.
5. In the media formula given above we have included HT, because we maintain our hybrids in HT (see section VII.B.7). This practice is not universal, and if the hybrids are not grown in HT these constituents should be omitted from the freezing and thawing media.

XI. CHARACTERIZATION OF MONOCLONAL ANTIBODIES

A. Introduction

The most interesting characteristic of a monoclonal antibody is its specificity. This will be determined to some degree during screening or by using the same antibody assay on different target antigens. This section is concerned more with additional information which may be of interest concerning a monoclonal antibody (Table 3).

B. How Much Information Do We Need?

A few moments of thought into the reasons for obtaining such information are worthwhile. Clearly the *specificity* needs to be established in order to evaluate the usefulness of the antibody. Specificity can never be established absolutely since it is not possible to test every alternative source of tissue. Rather, specificity should be established in the context of the potential use of the antibody. For example, a monoclonal antibody against a parasite antigen should be tested against other parasites with which the target antigen might be confused, and with tissue antigens which may be found together with the parasite. There is, however, little point in screening against exhaustive panels of other, unrelated parasites with which it cannot be confused.

The *titer* is useful in telling us how much material we have available, and allowing us to work with saturating concentrations of antibody or lower concentrations, depending on the experiment in hand. For example, studies aimed at determining the number of copies of a particular antigenic determinant must be carried out using saturating amounts of antibody.

The *affinity* of binding is of less obvious importance, and a monoclonal antibody may be used successfully without knowing anything about the binding kinetics. However, the studies of Williams and co-workers[56] have shown that kinetic studies with monoclonal antibodies can provide an insight into the processes of binding of antigen and antibody.

Stability on storage is of purely practical significance. One of the (justifiably) most eulogized virtues of monoclonal antibodies is that they will provide standardized reagents which can be used internationally to allow different laboratories to compare results. This has been rendered (in our experience) a little difficult by problems in international exchange of antibodies, and these problems must be solved if the full potential of monoclonal antibodies is to be realized. Antibodies can be shipped frozen, but the cost is prohibitive for individual samples. Commercial undertaking can make savings by shipping large quantities frozen. We have generally freeze-dried our materials for international exchange, but some antibodies are damaged by freeze-drying.

For storage in the laboratory, frozen storage is recommended. We have not experienced any significant loss of activity at −20°C, but in principle −80°C or liquid nitrogen storage are preferable. Repeated freezing and thawing can damage most proteins, and samples should be aliquotted before freezing to avoid this. An aliquot in use may be kept refrigerated (+4°C) for weeks, especially if azide (0.02 M) is added to inhibit bacterial growth.

Determination of the *class* and *subclass* of antibody is useful in predicting the properties of the antibody (for instance, complement fixation and protein-A binding). It is also a first indication of monoclonality.

Monoclonality clearly should be established if the theoretical advantages of using monoclonal antibodies are to be claimed for a particular preparation. Unfortunately, it is not possible to prove monoclonality, only to demonstrate it beyond reasonable doubt. The amount of effort required to do this depends on the specificity of the antibody. Thus an antibody with specificity for a defined subpopulation of lymphocytes (e.g., FMC1[23] reacting only with B cells in peripheral blood) will readily be accepted as monoclonal on the basis that it has been cloned and shows a specificity which relates to a known classification of cells. On the other hand, an antibody which reacts with blood cells in a way which does not fit existing classification (e.g., FMC3,[57] which reacts with some B and some T cells) requires more intensive study to allay doubts that it may contain two antibodies, one against a subpopulation of B cells and one against a subpopulation of T cells.

This situation is not desirable, since it means that preconceptions of expected specificity determine the amount of evidence required to establish monoclonality beyond reasonable doubt.

In practice, it is not unreasonable to accept that an antibody is monoclonal if: (1) it is produced by a hybridoma which has been put through a technically satisfactory cloning procedure; or (2) it shows exquisite specificity, which correlates with a preconceived classification. There may still be "silent" immunoglobulin present, but this will not affect the specificity.

In the long term, the hybridoma community should move towards generally acceptable minimal requirements for demonstration of monoclonality. It is unfortunate that the technique which might be expected to be most useful in this regard, isoelectric focusing, is of limited value because multiple bands can be obtained with antibodies that are generally regarded as monoclonal. It is even more unfortunate that this limitation is not widely realized.

The *immunochemistry* of the antigen will be of interest to a degree which depends on the purpose of the study. However, even when the main purpose is to find markers for identifying different cell populations, characterization of the antigen will help different laboratories to determine whether their antibodies detect the same or different markers. An antibody distinguishing, for instance, between two related viruses, or between T and B cells, can be very useful without knowing the molecular identity of the antigen, but in the long term identification of the antigen is desirable.

C. Techniques

1. Specificity

The tests selected for screening (see Section VIII) can be applied to the determination of specificity. The choice of antigens to be used has been discussed (Section XI.B).

2. Titer

The antibody titer can be determined by using the assay selected for screening and determining the highest dilution at which a positive result is obtained. Serial doubling dilutions, are generally used, giving a titer in the form $1/2^n$, e.g., 1/128.

Such a value is useful internally, for instance in following loss of activity on storage, and also to outside users of the antibody, giving them an idea of the dilution at which they can use it. The titer however, tells us nothing about the specific activity of the antibody, which should be expressed in units of activity per milligram antibody. The amount of antibody in milligrams can be determined in a number of ways and, since the titer is determined by doubling dilutions, there is little point in determining the concentration of immunoglobulin protein to a very high degree of precision. Thus determination of the percent immunoglobulin by scanning of zone electrophoresis and total protein by a Lowry or Biuret method would be adequate. If a more accurate and precise assay system, such as radio-immunoassay or enzyme-linked immunoassay is available, it can of course be used.

A convenient way of expressing the specific activity of the antibody is to express the reciprocal of the titer as units of activity; thus if our antibody preparation has a titer of 1/128 and immunoglobulin content of 0.01 mg/mℓ we can say it has 128 units in 0.01 mg, i.e., 12,800 units per milligram.

a. Example A: Determination of Specific Activity of FMC12, a Monoclonal Antibody Reacting with Human Granulocytes[58]

Antibody titer is determined by indirect immunofluorescence: 1/1600. Antibody concentration requires two items of information:

1. Total protein: Biuret method[59]: 1.98 mg/mℓ.
2. Fraction of protein which is immunoglobulin: separate ascites by electrophoresis on agarose gel (or similar material, e.g., cellulose acetate). Stain, and scan in a scanning densitometer (Figure 1). Ensure that staining intensity is not too high, otherwise the stain will not be proportional to the amount of protein.
   % of protein which is Ig: 18.2%
   Total Ig: 18.2% of 1.98 mg/mℓ = 0.36 mg/mℓ

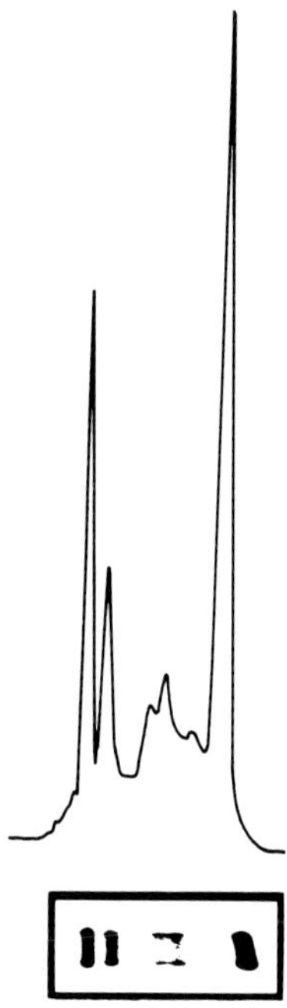

FIGURE 4. Zone electrophoresis of ascites fluid from hybridoma-bearing mouse. Monoclonal antibody band is at left (nearest cathode).

Specific activity = reciprocal of titer ÷ Ig concentration = 1600/0.36 = 4444 units per milligram

This method does not depend on the use of an antiserum against mouse γ-globulin to quantitate the antibody; however the method of estimating the proportion of total protein in the form of immunoglobulin lacks precision.

An alternative procedure, based on quantitation of precipitate produced by adding antimouse γ-globulin, is given below.

b. Example B: Estimation of Immunoglobulin Concentration in Hybrid Culture Supernatants Using the Laser Nephelometer

Materials

(1) Phosphate-buffered saline (PBS) filtered through 0.45 μ membrane filter;
(2) Mouse Ig (γ-globulin) standard at a concentration of ~100 μg/mℓ in PBS (filtered through 0.45 μ membrane filter);
(3) Culture supernatant to be tested (filtered);
(4) Rabbit antimouse-Ig precipitating antibody; and
(5) Laser Nephelometer (Behring).

Procedure

(1) Set up dilutions of Ig standard and culture supernatant in PBS to give final volume of 0.5 mℓ. The following standard concentrations should be set up: 30, 25, 20, 15, 10, 5, 2, 1, and 0.5 μg/mℓ. (NB All adjusted to a final volume of 0.5 mℓ in

filtered PBS). Set up doubling dilutions of the culture supernatants to be tested, i.e., NEAT, 1/2, 1/4, 1/8, 1/16, 1/32, 1/64. (NB All adjusted to a final volume of 0.5 mℓ in filtered PBS).

(2) To each tube add 20 μℓ of rabbit antimouse-Ig, mixing each tube individually on a vortex mixer.
(NB Care must be taken not to froth the sample).

(3) After 30 min incubation at room temperature the tubes are remixed. The laser nephelometer is turned on at this point to allow it to warm up.

(4) After a further 30 min incubation the samples can be read.

(5) Using a 1 mℓ pipette the sample is mixed and placed in the cuvette for reading. The cuvette should be prerinsed with filtered PBS multiple times. A PBS blank should be read before and after each set of samples. Care must be taken not to get bubbles in the samples.

(6) Plot the values obtained for the standards, on graph paper, i.e., Ig concentration in μg/mℓ vs. nephelometer reading. Estimations of Ig concentrations of supernatants are obtained from this standard curve.

This method is more precise than the electrophoretic method. However, the results depend on the use of a standard mouse immunoglobulin and an antiserum. Since the monoclonal antibody contains only one subclass, the apparent concentration will depend on the amount of antibody in the antiserum which reacts with the particular subclass, and on the proportion of the subclass in the standard. There are two general points which should be emphasized: (1) the ''unit of activity'' is arbitrary and a different assay could produce a different result and (2) the way the results are expressed does not assume that the immunoglobulin is all specific antibody. If the monoclonal antibody is separated from other immunoglobulin present is ascites fluid the specific activity should rise in consequence.

3. *Affinity of Binding*

Few people preparing monoclonal antibodies will be sufficiently concerned with affinity to wish to measure it. The reader is referred to the excellent studies of Mason and Williams[56]

4. *Storage and Stability*

Sequential determination of titer or specific activity is all that is required to assess stability on storage, or effect of such manipulations as lyophilization.

5. *Immunoglobulin Class/Subclass*

The class or subclass can be identified by any of the various immunological tests for identifying an antigen, provided specific antisera are available. Sets of antisera available commercially for identification of IgG1, IgG2a, IgG2b, IgG3, and IgM have in our experience not been adequately specific, allowing the unequivocal identification of some, but not all subclasses. However, specific antisera are available and it is a matter of shopping around the commercial antisera and obtaining others either from colleagues or by preparing them in the laboratory.

Having obtained the sera, the simplest method of using them to identify class/subclass is double diffusion in gel. This is wasteful in terms of antisera, and alternative techniques, requiring less material but more expertise are radio-immunoassay and enzyme-linked immunoassay.

Class and subclass should be determined on monoclonal antibody prepared in culture rather than in mice, since the latter will contain the other classes and subclasses, originating from the mouse rather than the hybridoma.

6. Monoclonality

As has been discussed earlier, monoclonality is impossible to prove, but a number of techniques can be used to establish a reasonable degree of confidence in the monoclonality of an antibody preparation.

Only one subclass of antibody should be present—It is theoretically possible for one cell clone at a particular time to switch class or subclass in which case, at least for a time, there will be two subclasses with the same idiotype. This is a special case, and it is doubtful that such a preparation could be called monoclonal even though the antibody is monospecific.

Only one cell type should be present in the hybridoma—Analysis of chromosomes or DNA content by flow cytometry[69] may reveal mixed populations with different chromosomal content. Such a mixture may consist of one secreting hybrid and one "silent" one, which does not secrete immunoglobulin. In this case the antibody produced is monoclonal; however, such a hybridoma mixture could prove troublesome, since the amount of antibody secreted would vary as the relative numbers of secretor and nonsecretor cells change. A cell mixture of this type should be recloned, so that the hybridoma, as well as the antibody, is monoclonal.

A method for analyzing the DNA profile on hybridomas is set out below:

Staining solution:[60]

Stock solutions:

1. Mithramycin (Mithracin®, Chas. Pfizer & Co); 100 μg/mℓ in 150 mM $MgCl_2$.
2. Ethidium bromide (Sigma®) 200 μg/mℓ aqueous.
3. Triton®-X-100: 1% aqueous.

Working solution (make up within 30 min of use): 1 volume ethidium bromide +2 volumes Mithramycin; make up to 20 volumes with Triton®-X-100 solution.

Staining of cells—Cells harvested from culture are adjusted to a concentration of 1 to 2×10^6/mℓ. Add 1 volume of stain solution to 4 volumes of cell suspension, on ice. Stained cells are kept on ice and in dark until analyzed. Analysis should be carried out within 30 min of staining.

Flow cytometry—DNA stained by mithramycin and ethidium bromide emits fluorescence at wavelengths above 550 nm when excited with light at 410 to 460 nm. The fluorescence intensity is proportional to the amount of DNA. Samples are run in a flow cytometer, using 457 nm laser excitation or a mercury vapor lamp filtered to transmit at 410 nm and a detector filtered to collect emission at wavelengths longer than 550 nm. Figure 5 shows the trace obtained on a FACS IV (Becton Dickinson) flow cytometer for two cloned hybridomas and a mixture of the two hybrids. It can be seen that if a hybridoma culture contains two clones of different DNA content this may be detected as complexity or broadening of the G_1 peak. However the sensitivity of this method, in terms of the number of chromosone differences required to show up as a change in the DNA profile, has not been determined.

Physiochemical analysis—Isoelectric focusing of radiolabeled antibody may be carried out in cases where there is any doubt about monoclonality. Unfortunately, the technique is unlikely to give a definite answer.

Method

1. Intrinsic labeling of antibody. Hybridoma cells are cultured at 5×10^5 cells per milliliter for 16 hr in leucine-free RPMI medium, supplemented with FCS, anti-

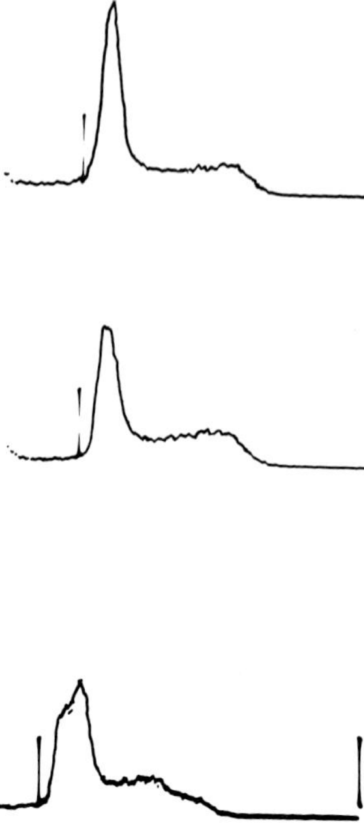

FIGURE 5. Fluorescence Activated Cell Sorter (FACS IV) tracings obtained with hybridoma cell lines after staining of DNA (refer to text). Life cycle patterns of FMC1 hybridoma (top), FMC4 hybridoma (centre) and mixture of FMC1 and FMC4 (bottom trace), illustrate the potential of this method for detecting mixed clones.

biotics, and (if the cell line is usually grown in HT) HT (see Section III.B.3). The medium contains 5 μCi ^{14}C-leucine per milliliter.

2. Isoelectric focusing: ^{14}C-labeled culture supernatant is dialyzed against 1% glycine or ampholine mixture and concentrated to 50 to 100 μℓ (from 1 to 5 mℓ culture supernatant). The sample is applied to the anodal end of a polyacrylamide electrofocusing gel with a pH gradient from 5 to 9.

When an analysis of separated light and heavy chains is required (see notes on interpretation below) the immunoglobulin is first gently reduced and alkylated. This may be done as described by Hoffman et al.[61] by dialyzing and concentrating the supernatant to 0.6 mℓ in 0.66 *M* Tris®-HCl pH 7.7, and adding 0.1 mℓ of 0.15 *M* dithiothreitol in the same buffer, in a nitrogen atmosphere. The solution is maintained at room temperature under nitrogen for 1 hr and 0.1 mℓ of 0.3 *M* iodoacetamide in Tris® buffer is added to alkylate the reduced chains. The pH is maintained between 7.0 and 8.0 for a further 1 hr; 56 μℓ of propionic acid added to prevent association of the chains, and the mixture dialyzed against two changes of 10 *M* urea. The material is applied to a pH 5 to 9 focusing gel containing 8 *M* urea.

Details of the preparation and running of focusing gels may be found in specialized texts[62] or general immunology methods manuals.[63–65]

Interpretation

If the hybrid is derived from a myeloma line which secretes immunoglobulin at least two heavy and two light chains can be obtained (one of each from the myeloma and the spleen cell partner of the fusion). If the myeloma line manufactures light chain only (as is the case for the NS1 myeloma) the hybrid may produce two light chains and one

Table 4
CROSS-ABSORPTION EXPERIMENT TO DETERMINE IF ACTIVITY AGAINST TWO DIFFERENT ANTIGENS IS DUE TO A COMMON DETERMINANT OR THE PRESENCE OF TWO ANTIBODIES

	Reactivity with target cell	
Absorption	**A2**	**A10**
Unabsorbed	+	+
Absorbed with A2 cells	—	—
Absorbed with A10 cells	—	—

heavy chain. Hybrids derived from myeloma parents which do not make light or heavy chains should produce only one immunoglobulin species, and one heavy and one light chain.

There are two problems which may complicate interpretation. First, the cells are likely to be incorporating ^{14}C-leucine into other proteins which may be released into the medium. Thus, although immunoglobulin is the major secreted product of hybridomas, a minor second component may either by evidence of contamination by a second hybridoma or may not be immunoglobulin at all.

Secondly, monoclonal antibody may produce a series of closely-related polypeptides, due probably to modification (deamidation) during isolation.

Cross-absorption studies—When an antibody reacts with two apparently unrelated antigens, cross-absorption studies may be used to answer the question: is the reaction due to one antibody (reacting with a shared antigenic determinant) or two antibodies (produced by a hybrid which has not been properly cloned)? An example is FMC5[70] which in general shows specificity for the HLA antigen HLA-A2. Some donors with the HLA-A10 antigen react. The appropriate cross-absorption experiment is set out in Table 4.

Clearly if two antibodies were responsible, absorption with A2 (A10-negative) cells could not have removed A10 reactivity and absorption with A10 (A2-negative) cells would not have removed A2 reactivity.

Absorption was done with platelets, and using an antibody dilution determined by prior titration such that absorption with an equal volume of platelets would remove reactivity against the absorbing cells. The antibody tests were performed by cytotoxicity in a standard tissue typing system.

Subcloning—If the hybridoma is monoclonal then all subclones should have identical specificity. If the hybridoma is not monoclonal, the probability of obtaining subclone cultures which contain the same mixture of cells, and thus produce an antibody mixture with the same specificity, must be low; thus subcloning can be used to provide evidence of monoclonality.

7. *Immunochemical Characterization of the Antigen*

a. Principle

Detailed studies of the antigen detected by a monoclonal antibody are outside the scope of this chapter. However, it is frequently desirable to obtain some preliminary characteristics of the antigen, in order to compare different monoclonal antibodies.

Methods for the characterization of protein and glycoprotein antigens are relatively well developed, whereas if the antigen is glycolipid or polysaccharide in nature more complex procedures will be needed.

We describe here methods for the characterization of protein or glycoprotein antigens found on the membrane of mammalian cells. Similar methods would be used for protein antigens which are either nonmembranous or of different origin, and the modifications to the method which would be required would need to be determined by experiment.

The principle of the method to be described is as follows: the antigen (along with many other components of the cell) is labeled with a radioactive isotope, to facilitate detection in small quantities. ^{125}I is commonly used, but in some situations it is preferable to use intrinsic labeling, by growing the cells in the presence of amino-acid or sugar precursors, labeled with ^{3}H, ^{14}C, or ^{35}S. The antigen mixture is solubilized (if possible using a selective procedures which solubilizes only the plasma membrane and leaves nuclei intact).

The soluble extract is now mixed with the monoclonal antibody, and the complex between the antibody and its homologous antigen is isolated, usually by precipitation. Careful washing is needed to ensure that the antigen is the only labeled component of the precipitate.

The precipitate is now redissolved and examined, usually by polyacrylamide gel electrophoresis in the presence of the detergent sodium dodecyl sulfate (SDS). In this detergent proteins and glycoproteins are all highly negatively charged, and migration in acrylamide gel is a function of molecular size, and not charge, of the protein.

b. Methods

1. *Cell membrane iodination material and preparation:*

Polythene bottle for hot waste
Plastic disposable waste bag
Disposable rubber gloves
Bench top centrifuge
10 mℓ centrifuge tubes
Timer
1 to 5 μℓ Micropipette and plastic disposable tips
5 to 25 μℓ Micropipette and plastic disposable tips
50 to 100 μℓ Micropipette and plastic disposable tips
Cold PBS (4°C)
Ice
PBS containing glucose (20 mM) and KI ($6 \times 10^{-6} M$)
Lactoperoxidase
  stock solution (5 mg/mℓ; SIGMA®; 70 units per milligram protein)
  dilute stock 1/10 in PBS for working strength
Glucose Oxidase
  stock solution (1400 u/mℓ; SIGMA®, type V)
  dilute stock 1/1000 (1.4 u/mℓ) in PBS to give working solution
Na ^{125}I:
0.5 to 1 mCi (as fresh as possible; 100 mCi/mℓ)
Portable radiation monitor

Procedure

1. Lymphocytes/lymphoblastoid cell lines to be labeled are washed 3 times in PBS (200 g for 10 min).

2. 4 to 6 × 10^6 cells are resuspended in 10 mℓ of PBS in a 10 mℓ centrifuge tube.
3. The cells are then recentrifuged at 200 g for 10 min. The supernatant is removed and the cells resuspended in 1 mℓ of PBS containing 20 mM glucose and 6 × 10^{-6} *M* KI.
4. The following reagents are added in sequence:
   a. 10 μℓ of lactoperoxidase enzyme (1/10 dilution of stock solution).
   b. 4 μℓ of glucose oxidase (1/1000 dilution of stock solution).
   c. 100 μCi of carrier free ^{125}I (~ 1 μℓ of carrier free Na ^{125}I).
5. The cells are then incubated at room temperature for 30 min (~ 20°C).
6. The reaction is stopped by placing the reaction mixture on ice and by the addition of 9 mℓ of cold PBS. The cells are washed 3 times in cold PBS (200 g for 10 min) and finally resuspended in 50 μℓ of PBS.

2. *Preparation of membrane extracts, immune precipitation, and washing*

Materials

Lysis buffer:

1% Nonidet P40 detergent, 10 mM Tris® pH 7.4, 1 mM EDTA, 0.15 *M* NaCl, 1 mM phenyl methyl sulfonyl fluoride (made up as 0.2 *M* stock in propanol), 1 mg/mℓ bovine serum albumin.

Hypotonic buffer

0.01 *M* NaCl, 0.01 *M* Tris® pH 7.4, 1.5 m*M* $MgC1_2$,

Sample Buffer

6 mℓ of 10% SDS, 3 mℓ glycerol (A.R.), 2.4 mℓ Tris® 0.1 *M* pH 6.8, 15.6 mℓ water

2 *M* Dithiothreitol (stock solution, stored frozen) Bromophenol blue.

Procedure

1. To 100 μℓ of labeled cell suspension (~10^8 cells per milliliter) is added 900 μℓ of lysis buffer.
2. After 1hr at 4°C the extract is centrifuged at 200 g for 10 min to remove cell debris and nuclei.
3. The extract is then ultracentrifuged at 100,000 g for 1 hr at 4°C to remove residual subcellular particles.
4. To 100 μℓ of the centrifuged extract is added 100 μℓ of 10 times concentrated hybridoma supernatant (or 10 μℓ of ascites).
5. After 2hr at 4°C, 0.5 mℓ of a precipitating goat antimouse serum is added and the mixture incubated at 4°C overnight.
6. The precipitate is pelleted by centrifugation at 500 g for 20 min at 4°C, then washed 3 times in cold hypotonic buffer. The effectiveness of the washing may be determined by monitoring radioactivity after each wash. The radioactivity of the precipitate should plateau after 2 to 3 washes.
7. The precipitate is then resuspended in 45 μℓ of sample buffer and dithiothreitol (0.2 *M*, containing 0.2% bromophenol blue) added.
8. The sample is then boiled and reduced for 4 min by incubation in a sealed glass tube, suspended in a boiling water bath.
9. Samples are then run on a 10% SDS polyacrylamide SDS slab gel in conjunction with molecular weight standards.

3. *Polyacrylamide electrophoresis in SDS (SDS/PAGE)*

SDS/PAGE is generally carried out using the two-gel system and buffers of

Laemli.[66]
Stock solutions
Acrylamide: Acrylamide 30 g, bis-acrylamide 0.8 g, water to make 100 mℓ. Store in dark bottle in refrigerator.
Tris®/HCl buffers:
1 *M* Tris®/HCl pH 8.8
1 *M* Tris ®/HCl pH 6.8
(make up 1 *M* Tris® and adjust pH using strong HCl solution)
Sodium dodecyl sulfate (SDS)
10% in water
(Precipitates on cooling—redissolve by warming)

Running buffer

Tris® (base)	3.03 g
Glycine	14.42 g
SDS	1 g

Water to make 1 liter. Adjust pH to 8.3 if necessary.

Gel mixtures

Running gel	5%	7.5%	10%
Acrylamide stock (mℓ)	5	7.5	10
1 *M* Tris® pH 8.8 (mℓ)	11.2	11.2	11.2
10% SDS (mℓ)	0.3	0.3	0.3

Stacking gel	5%	3%
Acrylamide stock (mℓ)	1.67	1.0
1 *M* Tris® pH 6.8 (mℓ)	1.25	1.25
10% SDS (mℓ)	0.1	0.1
Water (mℓ)	7.03	7.7

Make up mixture, degas, add freshly dissolved aqueous ammonium persulfate solution (100 mg/mℓ) (100 μℓ for running gel; 50 μℓ for stacking gel); mix, add TEMED (20 μℓ for running gel, 10 μℓ for stacking gel); mix, pour immediately.

The above quantities are suitable for the slab apparatus in common use; quantities may need to be altered for different apparatus.

The sample is loaded on top of the stacking gel (most systems cast sample troughs in the stacking gel). Electrophoresis (toward the anode) is carried out at constant current. The current used will depend on the dimensions of the apparatus and the efficiency of the cooling system. The aim should be to achieve separation in the shortest time without distortion of bands due to overheating. Electrophoresis is stopped when the marker dye reaches the bottom of the gel, or shortly before.

4. *Fixing, staining, drying, and autoradiography*

After electrophoresis the gel is detached from the glass plates under a solution of stain and fixative. The gel is stained and destained. The dye most commonly used for staining proteins is Coomassie® Brilliant Blue, and the following series of steps gives good staining and clear background:
Solution 1:
0.05% Coomassie® blue
25% Propan-2-ol (isopropyl alcohol)
10% Acetic acid in water
Stain overnight

Solution 2:
0.005% Coomassie® blue
10% Propan-2-ol
10% Acetic acid in water
Stain for 2hr
Solution 3:
0.0025% Coomassie® blue
10% Acetic acid in water
Stain for 2hr
Solution 4:
10% Acetic acid in water
Destain until background level adequately reduced (overnight should be adequate)
Drying: in order to obtain autoradiographs it is necessary to dry the gel onto a rigid support. This is usually done with heat at low pressure, and apparatus is available commercially. If the drying process is not adequately controlled distortion or splitting of the gels occurs.

Procedure:

a. Soak gel in 10% acetic acid per 1% glycerol, in water, for 30 min (at least).
b. Float gel onto a sheet of presoaked filter paper (Whatman® 3m*M* or similar). Place the sheet of paper, with the gel uppermost, onto the metal grid of the drying apparatus, cover either with Mylar® sheet or with thin cellophane "sandwich wrapping"; avoid trapping air bubbles.
c. Establish vacuum, covering the gel with the rubber sheet of the drying apparatus. A good Venturi® pump is adequate, and if a motorized vacuum pump is used it is necessary to take precautions to avoid corrosion of the motor or damage to the oil by the acetic acid vapor given off.
d. Switch on heater. Drying time will vary but will be around 2 hr with heat, followed by 1 hr without heat.

Autoradiography: autoradiographic exposures can be considerably shortened by using scintillation screens. If these are used exposure must be carried out at −70°C, to obtain good scintillation. Suitable screens are available from most manufacturers of X-ray film, but it is important to match the screen to the spectral response of the film.

We use Ilford® Fast Tungstate intensifying screens, and Kodak® XPR-5 X-ray film. The dried gel is laid on the darkroom bench face up, followed by a sheet of thin paper (to prevent contamination of the screen), one screen (scintillant uppermost); the film (emulsion both sides); the second screen (scintillant down). The entire sandwich is firmly pressed between two steel plates (to maintain close contact and cut down external radiation), the plates clipped together using strong "bulldog" clips, and the whole assembly placed in a light-tight bag and transferred to a −70°C freezer. The film may be developed manually or using automatic X-ray film processing equipment. Using this system, a sample with activity producing 10,000 cpm will produce a clear band after autoradiography for 1 week.

XII. PRODUCTION, PURIFICATION, AND LABELING OF MONOCLONAL ANTIBODIES

This section is concerned with the preparation of monoclonal antibody in useful quantities, its purification, and labeling.

A. Production

Monoclonal antibody may be prepared either in culture or by growing the hybridoma as a tumor in mice. Production in cell culture is easier, since the hybrids are always available in culture, and the antibody produced is strictly monoclonal. Production in animals may be advantageous for the preparation of large amounts of antibody. However antibody made in this way will be contaminated by other mouse immunoglobulin, including possibly antibodies against viruses or other antigens, which may lead to artifactual reactions of the "monoclonal" antibody. These factors must be considered when selecting the method of preparation for a particular purpose.

1. Tissue Culture

Cultures may be maintained for long periods, removing 80 to 90% of the culture when it becomes yellow. The cells are removed from the harvested culture by centrifugation and the supernatant stored frozen. In this way it is easy to accumulate large volumes without using large-scale culture apparatus. Alternatively, roller cultures or stirred/gassed culture apparatus may be used to produce larger volumes.

The immunoglobulin concentration of monoclonal antibody produced in this way is in the region of 1 to 10 μg/mℓ, sometimes higher. When higher concentrations are required it may be concentrated by membrane ultrafiltration. Use of an appropriate membrane porosity (e.g., 50,000 mol wt nominal cut-off Diaflo® Membranes, Amicon Corp. Lexington, Mass.,) will avoid concentrating some of the tissue culture media constituents. Ideally, a 100,000 mol wt cut-off membrane would allow the removal of the bulk of the fetal calf serum protein, but in our experience some immunoglobulin also passes through these membranes, at least in stirred-cell apparatus. For small volumes the "Minicon® B-125" (Amicon Corp.) serum concentrator retains most of the immunoglobulin, while removing some (approximately 20%) of the albumin.

2. Hybridoma Growth in Mice

Hybridomas may be injected into mice subcutaneously, in which case a tumor forms locally and antibody is released into the serum, or intraperitoneally, in which case an antibody-rich ascites fluid develops. Antibody concentrations range from under 1 mg to 10 mg/mℓ. Hybridomas do not always grow easily in vivo, and a number of precautions are necessary

a. The Tumor and Mouse Should be Syngeneic

The myelomas in current use for fusion are BALB/c so that, provided the mouse which supplied the spleen cells for the fusion was also a BALB/c, hybridomas can be grown in BALB/c mice. Even in this syngeneic combination, large doses of cells (10^6 to 10^7) are required to initiate a tumor. This may be due to minor histocompatibility differences between the mice known as BALB/c in different laboratories around the world. There are however marked differences between different hybrids in terms of their ability to grow in mice, indicating that other factors are involved. When producing large amounts of antibody it may be helpful to passage mouse-produced tumor to fresh mice, rather than going back to cultured cells, since most tumors show adaptation to animal or culture conditions. If the hybrid is not syngeneic to the mouse being used for tumor growth, a larger inoculum should be used and it may be necessary to immunosuppress the mouse using irradiation (350 rad), antilymphocyte globulin, or drugs such as methotrexate or cyclophosphamide.

b. Pretreatment of the Peritoneal Cavity.

The production of ascites fluid is facilitated by pretreatment of the mouse with an intraperitoneal injection of an irritant substance. The material most widely used for this purpose in hybridoma production is pristane (2, 6, 10, 14—tetramethylpentadecane). Mice are injected with 0.5 mℓ pristane i.p. and cells are injected at least 7 days subsequently. The tumor may take 7 to 14 days to grow, and ascites fluid is removed when the mice show sufficient abdominal swelling. Serum and ascites fluid may be obtained from the same mouse.

Serum or ascites fluid should be allowed to clot (a fibrin clot occasionally forms in withdrawn ascites fluid) and clarified by centrifugation. Inactivation of complement and proteolytic enzymes is carried out by heating at 56°C for 30 min, in glass tubes.

Electrophoresis of ascites fluid (see Figure 4, Section XI.C.2) shows a characteristic myeloma band, but also indicates that many other proteins are present.

B. Purification

For many purposes culture or ascites fluid may be used without purification; however it may be necessary to purify the monoclonal antibody, for example for labeling with radioactive or fluorescent tags. Depending on the purity required, the antibody may be precipitated with ammonium sulfate or a higher degree of purity may be obtained by ion-exchange chromatography or affinity separation using protein A.

1. Ammonium Sulfate Precipitation

1. Prepare saturated ammonium sulfate solution: dissolve 100 g ammonium sulfate in 1ℓ distilled water at 50°C. Allow to cool overnight at room temperature and adjust pH to 7.2 using 2N H_2SO_4.
2. Add ammonium sulfate to the antibody containing culture supernate (undiluted) or ascites/serum (diluted 1 + 2 with saline). Add sufficient ammonium sulfate to give a final concentration of 45% saturated (i.e., 45 volumes saturated ammonium sulfate + 55 volumes antibody).
3. Stir at room temperature for 30 min; collect precipitate by centrifugation (1000 g for 15 min) and wash precipitate once in 45% saturated ammonium sulfate.
4. Redissolve precipitate in PBS to the original volume, and reprecipitate at 40% saturated ammonium sulfate.
5. Wash precipitate once in 40% ammonium sulfate, and redissolve in a minimal volume of PBS or other buffer as required. Dialyse at 4°C against two changes of buffer. Clarify by centrifugation.

Note: Sodium sulfate (16%) may be used as an alternative to ammonium sulfate.

2. Ion Exchange Chromatography

The fact that the γ-globulins are the least-negatively charged of the serum proteins makes them relatively easy to purify using positively charged ion exchange matrices (diethylaminoethyl cellulose or Sephadex®). The optimal buffers may depend on the immunoglobulin subclass, but the method has been used to purify monoclonal antibody from ascites fluid.[56] In this particular instance the normal immunoglobulin separated from the monoclonal antibody on the column.

Details are not given here since the experimenter may need to vary buffers. Experimental details may be obtained from the paper of Masters and Williams already referred to[56] or from general compendia of methods.[63] It is important to note, however, that the best buffer system will depend on the species producing the immunoglobulin, and methods published for rabbit or human immunoglobulin may not be suitable for mouse monoclonal antibody.

3. Affinity Separation on Protein-A-Sepharose

Materials

Protein-A-Sepharose CL 4B (Pharmacia, Uppsala).

Buffers: a. 0.05 M Tris®/0.15 M NaCl, pH 8.6, containing 0.02% sodium azide. 6.06 g Tris® (base) + 8.76 g NaCl dissolved in 800 mℓ water. Adjust pH to 8.6 using strong HCl and make volume to 1 ℓ including stock sodium azide solution to give final 0.02% azide.

b. 0.05 M phosphate/0.15 M NaCl, pH 7.0. 2.17 g $Na_2H\ PO_4$ + 1.35 g $Na_2H\ PO_4$ + 8.76 g NaCl dissolved in turn in 1ℓ water. Check pH (7.0).

c. 0.05 M citrate/0.15 M NaCl, pH 5.5. 2.68 g citric acid monohydrate + 10.96 g tri-sodium citrate dihydrate + 8.76 g NaCl + 1ℓ water. Check pH (5.5).

d. 0.05 M acetate/0.15 M NaCl pH 4.3. 6.8 g CH_3COO Na + 8.76 g NaCl + 800 mℓ water. Add CH_3COOH to bring pH to 4.3 and make up to 1ℓ with water.

e. 0.05 M glycine/0.15 M NaCl, pH 2.3. 5.6 g glycine-HCl + 8.76 g NaCl + 800 mℓ water. Adjust pH to 2.3 with strong HCl and make up to 1ℓ with water.

Method

1. Swell 1.5 g protein-A-sepharose in buffer (a.) and pack a small column (a 10 mℓ syringe is suitable, with glass wool at the bottom end; alternatively a more sophisticated column of capacity 5 to 6 mℓ may be used).
2. Adjust pH of antibody to 8.6 with dilute NaOH (note: add NaOH with mixing to avoid local high pH).
3. Apply to column (capacity is about 50 mg of antibody). Wash off unbound protein with buffer (a.) (Use a UV monitor to follow elution).
4. Elute successive fractions with buffers (b), (c), (d), (e). The monoclonal antibody should be located in only one of the fractions, depending on its subclass. Collect the appropriate fraction, neutralize immediately if in acid buffer, dialyze and concentrate as necessary.
5. Regenerate column by washing with buffer (d) and then reequilibrating in buffer (a.)

C. Labeling

Depending on the use to be made of the monoclonal antibodies he has prepared, the experimenter may wish to label his antibodies with a radioactive tag or a fluorescent chromophore. The need to label may be avoided by using indirect immunofluorescence or radio-labeled second antibody; but this is not always desirable. Generally second antibody procedures give higher sensitivity and higher backgrounds than direct-labeling techniques.

The methods for labeling monoclonal antibodies do not differ in essence from those used widely for labeling immunoglobulin, with one significant exception—that monoclonal antibody can readily be intrinsically labeled by growing the hybridoma in the presence of radioactively labeled amino acids.

1. Radioisotopic Labeling

a. Iodination

^{125}I is the isotope most commonly used in radioisotope labeling in immunology. It is a γ-ray emitter, which makes for easy detection and quantitation, and methods for coupling ^{125}I or ^{131}I to proteins have been worked out in detail. It is, however, important to be aware of the risk of conformational damage to the protein resulting from iodination. This may be assessed by competitive binding experiments between the labeled and unlabeled antibody-competition should be stoichiometric.

There are many iodination procedures in use, and these will not be described here. The "Iodogen" method[67] and a variant of the chloramine T method[56] are two that have been used for monoclonal antibodies.

b. Intrinsic Labeling

The fact that monoclonal antibodies are produced in tissue culture provides an opportunity to label them intrinsically. This has the advantage over extrinsic labeling (such as iodination) that the product is native unmodified (apart from isotopic substitution of a few atoms) antibody and should behave in precisely the same way as unlabeled antibody in its reaction with antigen.

The disadvantage, compared with iodination, is that most of the labels which can be used are β-particle emitters and the detection methods are more complex. However, since many laboratories are already equipped with liquid scintillation counting equipment the use of intrinsically labeled monoclonal antibodies is attractive and will probably increase in popularity.

^{14}C or ^{3}H labeled amino acids may be used, either singly or in mixtures to label monoclonal antibody. ^{35}S-methionine can be used if a relatively high specific activity is required, but the half-life is correspondingly short. ^{75}Se-methionine can also be used, and this has the advantage of being a γ emitter. However in this case the substitution (^{75}Se for ^{32}S) is much greater than simple isotope substitution and it is possible that the properties of the protein will be affected.

Techniques for intrinsic labeling are varied, depending on the specific activity required. Labeling using ^{14}C-leucine and leucine-free medium has already been described (Section XI.C.6).

2. Labeling for Fluorescence

Fluorescein and rhodamine are the two dyes most often used in immunofluorescence, and microscope filter systems have been developed to analyze these two dyes effectively. In flow cytometry quantitation of fluorescein and rhodamine together poses some problems, unless a dual-laser system is used. Instruments which use only one laser for immunofluroescence are equipped with an electronic "compensation" system to subtract the overlapping emission spectra of the two dyes. This reduces the signal strength very considerably. A partial solution is to use a modified rhodamine chromophore (XRITC, available from Research Organics, Cleveland, Ohio). The emission spectrum of this dye overlaps less with that of fluorescein.

Various methods for conjugating fluorescein and rhodamine to antibodies have been described. For monoclonal antibodies, the antibody should first be purified (see Section XII.B) and then labeled according to published methods.[8]

A method which has recently become popular is to label the antibody with biotin and use fluorescein, or rhodamine-conjugated avidin as the labeled ligand. This is analogous to an indirect immunofluorescence method, except that avidin, which has a high affinity for biotin, is used instead of the second antibody. There are two principal reasons for using this procedure. First, the degree of amplification of fluorescence tends to be higher than in second-antibody methods. Since many monoclonal antibodies are directed against antigens which are present at low densities on the cell, this is a distinct advantage. Second, the use of biotin-avidin makes possible double-marker assays with two monoclonal antibodies, which would otherwise be difficult. Thus if we wish to label two antigens, A and B, we treat the cells first with monoclonal anti-A, followed by fluoresceinated antimouse immunoglobulin. Biotin-labeled monoclonal anti-B is now added, followed by rhodamine-labeled avidin.

Biotin conjugation is relatively straightforward,[8] provided the biotin-succinimide ester is available. The preparation of this ester requires some organic chemistry not generally used by immunologists, but is is now available commercially (Calbiochem®).

XIII. SUMMARY

The preparation of a monoclonal antibody requires the successful achievement of a series of procedures (illustrated schematically in Figure 1). Mice must be immunized, and a myeloma cell line suitable for fusion must be obtained and maintained in culture. Immune cells from the mouse (or other species) are fused with myeloma cells, and the fusion products, which form a very small proportion of the cells, are induced to grow in culture in the absence of other dividing cells. If this is achieved, a number of growing hybridoma colonies arise and must be screened to pick out the ones which are making the desired antibody. The interesting hybrids must be cloned (perhaps several times) to ensure monoclonality. Cloned hybrids producing interesting antibodies are scaled up to provide useful quantities of antibody, and the cells are cryopreserved so that their unique assortment of immunoglobulin genes are preserved in perpetuity. The monoclonal antibody produced is examined to establish its essential characteristics, and, in order to use the monoclonal antibody, it may be necessary to purify it and label it.

In this chapter methods have been presented for the achievement of all these steps. The chapter was not intended as an all-embracing compendium of methods; rather, it was designed to present adequate methodology with which the authors have actual experience, and to provide the reader with sufficient background information to enable him to make a rational choice between alternative techniques.

REFERENCES

1. **Köhler, G. and Milstein, C.,** Continuous cultures of fused cells secreting antibody of predefined specificity, *Nature (London)*, 256, 495, 1975.
2. **Oi, V. T. and Herzenberg, L. A.,** Immunoglobulin-producing hybrid cell lines, in *Selected Methods in Cellular Immunology,* Mishell, B. B. and Shiigi, S. M., Eds., W. H. Freeman, San Francisco, 1980, 351.
3. **Herzenberg, L. A., Herzenberg, L. A., and Milstein, C.,** Cell hybrids of myelomas with antibody forming cells and T-lymphomas with T cells: a new means of making large amounts of monoclonal antibodies and a potential means of making large numbers of cells carrying out specific T cell functions, in *Handbook of Experimental Immunology*, Vol. 2, 3rd ed., Weir, D. M., Ed., Blackwell Scientific, Oxford, 1978, 25.1.
4. **Pearson, T. W., Pinder, M., Roelants, G. E., Kar, S. K., Lundin, L. B., Mayor-Withey, K. S., and Hewett, R. S.,** Methods for derivation and detection of anti-parasite monoclonal antibodies, *J. Immunol. Methods,* 34, 141, 1980.
5. **Kennett, R. H.,** Cell Fusion, in *Methods in Enzymology,* Vol. 58, Colowick, S. P. and Kaplan, N.O., Eds., Academic Press, New York, 1979, 345.
6. **Zola, H.,** Monoclonal antibodies against human cell membrane antigens: a review, *Pathology,* 12, 539, 1980.
7. **Fazekas de St Groth, S. and Scheidegger, D.,** Production of monoclonal antibodies: strategy and tactics, *J. Immunol. Methods,* 35, 1, 1980.
8. **Goding, J. W.,** Antibody production by hybridomas, *J. Immunol. Methods,* 39, 285, 1980.
9. **Barkley, W. E.,** Safety considerations in the cell culture laboratory, in *Methods in Enzymology,* Vol. 58, Colowick, S.P. and Kaplan, N. O., Eds., Academic Press, New York, 1979, 36.
10. **Whitaker, A. M.,** *Tissue and Cell Culture,* Williams & Wilkins, Baltimore, 1972.

11. **Hall, D. O. and Hawkins, S. E.,** *Laboratory Manual of Cell Biology,* English Universities Press, London, 1975.
12. **Colowick, S. P. and Kaplan, N. O., Eds.,** *Methods in Enzymology,* Vol. 58, Academic Press, New York, 1979.
13. **Paul, J.,** *Cell and Tissue Culture,* Churchill Livingstone, Edinburgh, 1975.
14. **Oi, V. T., Jones, P. P., Goding, J. W., Herzenberg, L. A., and Herzenberg, L. A.,** Properties of monoclonal antibodies to mouse Ig allotypes, H-2, and Ia antigens, in *Current Topics in Microbiology and Immunology,* Vol. 81, Melchers, F., Potter, M., and Warner, N. L., Eds., Springer-Verlag, New York, 1978, 115.
15. **Stahli, C., Staehelin, T., Miggiano, V., Schmidt, J., and Haring, P.,** High frequencies of antigen-specific hybridomas: dependence on immunization parameters and prediction by spleen cell analysis, *J. Immunol. Methods,* 32, 297, 1980.
16. **Trucco, M. M., Stocker, J. W., and Ceppellini, R.,** Monoclonal antibodies against human lymphocyte antigens, *Nature (London),* 273, 666, 1978.
17. **Trucco, M. M., Garotta, G., Stocker, J. W., and Ceppellini, R.,** Murine monoclonal antibodies against HLA structures, *Immunol. Rev.,* 47, 219, 1979.
18. **Brodsky, F. M., Parham, P., Barnstable, C. J., Crumpton, M. J., and Bodmer, W. F.,** Monoclonal antibodies for analysis of the HLA system, *Immunol. Rev.,* 47, 3, 1979.
19. **Parham, P., Barnstable, C. J., and Bodmer, W. F.,** Use of a monoclonal antibody (W6/32) in structural studies of HLA-A,B,C antigens, *J. Immunol.,* 123, 342, 1979.
20. **Levy, R., Dilley, J., Fox, R. I., and Warnke, R.,** A human thymusleukaemia antigen defined by hybridoma monoclonal antibodies, *Proc. Natl. Acad. Sci. U.S.A.,* 76, 6552, 1979.
21. **Reif, A. E. and Robinson, C. M.,** A method for determination of the relative specificity of antisera prepared against cells, *Immunology,* 28, 199, 1975.
22. **Zola, H.,** Antisera with specificity for human T lymphocytes. Preparation by selective suppression of the antibody response against shared antigens, *Transplantation,* 24, 83, 1977.
23. **Brooks, D. A., Beckman, I., Bradley, J., McNamara, P. J., Thomas, M. E., and Zola, H.,** Human lymphocyte markers defined by antibodies derived from somatic cell hybrids. I. A hybridoma secreting antibody against a marker specific for human B lymphocytes, *Clin. Exp. Immunol.,* 39, 477, 1980.
24. **Parham, P. and Bodmer, W. F.,** Monoclonal antibody to a human histocompatibility alloantigen, HLA-A2, *Nature (London),* 276, 397, 1978.
25. **Gotze, D. and Vollmers, H. P.,** Reactivity of monoclonal antibodies specific for H-2 antigenic determinants with cells of wild mice, *Immunol. Rev.,* 47, 207, 1979.
26. **Howard, J. C., Butcher, G. W., Galfre, G., Milstein, C., and Milstein, C. P.,** Monoclonal antibodies as tools to analyze the serological and genetic complexities of major transplantation antigens, *Immunol. Rev.,* 47, 139, 1979.
27. **Cuello, A. C., Galfre, G., and Milstein, C.,** Detection of substance P in the central nervous system by a monoclonal antibody, *Proc. Natl, Acad. Sci. U.S.A.,* 76, 3532, 1979.
28. **Galfre, G., Milstein, C., and Wright, B.,** Rat × rat hybrid myelomas and a monoclonal anti-Fd portion of mouse IgG, *Nature (London),* 277, 131, 1979.
29. **Luben, R. A., Mohler, M., A., and Nedwin, G. E.,** Production of hybridomas secreting monoclonal antibodies against the lymphokine osteoclast activating factor, *J. Clin, Invest.,* 64, 337, 1979.
30. **Wiktor, T. J. and Kiprowski, H.,** Monoclonal antibodies against rabies virus produced by somatic cell hybridization: detection of antigenic variants, *Proc. Natl. Acad. Sci. U.S.A.,* 75, 3938, 1978.
31. **McFarlin, D. E., Bellini, W. J., Mingioli, E. S., Behar, T. N., and Trudgett, A.,** Monospecific antibody to the haemagglutinin of measles virus, *J. Gen. Virol.,* 48, 425, 1980.
32. **Bottcher, I. and Hammerling, G.,** Continuous production of monoclonal mouse IgE antibodies with known allergenic specificity by a hybrid cell line, *Nature (London),* 275, 761, 1978.
33. **Lewis, D. and Williams, H.,** Nonselective isolation of human somatic cell hybrids by unit-gravity sedimentation, *Nature (London),* 278, 168, 1979.
34. **Littlefield, J. W.,** Selection of hybrids from matings of fibroblasts in vitro and their presumed recombinants, *Science,* 145, 709, 1964.
35. **Kusano, T., Long, C., and Green, M.,** A new reduced human-mouse somatic cell hybrid containing the human gene for adenine phosphoribosyltransferase, *Proc. Natl. Acad. Sci. U.S.A.,*68, 82, 1971.
36. **Chan, R. S., Creagen, R. P., and Reardon, M. P.,** Adenosine kinase as a new selective marker in somatic cell genetics: isolation of adenosine kinase-deficient mouse cell lines and human-mouse hybrid cell lines containing adenosine kinase, *Somatic Cell Genet.,* 4, 1, 1978.
37. **Goldstein, N. I. and Fisher, P. B.,** Selection of mouse x hamster hybrids using HAT medium and a polyene antibiotic, *In Vitro,* 14, 200, 1978.

38. **Herzenberg, L. A. and Ledbetter, J. A.,** Monoclonal antibodies and the fluorescence-activated cell sorter: complementary tools in lymphoid cell biology, in *Proc. of 13th Leucocyte Culture Conf.* Kaplen, J. G., Ed., Elsevier/North-Holland, Amersterdam, 1979.
39. **Olsson, L. and Kaplan, H. S.,** Human-human hybridomas producing monoclonal antibodies of predefined antigenic specificity, *Proc. Natl. Acad. Sci. U.S.A.,* 77, 5429, 1980.
40. **Levy, R. and Dilley, J.,** Rescue of immunoglobulin secretion from human neoplastic lymphoid cells by somatic cell hybridization, *Proc. Natl. Acad. Sci. U.S.A.,* 75, 2411, 1978.
41. **Kohler, G., Howe, C. S., and Milstein, C.,** Fusion between immunoglobulin secreting and nonsecreting lines, *Eur. J. Immunol.,* 6, 292, 1976.
42. **Kearney, J. F., Radbruch, A., Liesengang, B., and Rajewsky, K.,** A new mouse myeloma cell line that has lost immunoglobulin expression but permits the construction of antibody-secreting hybrid cell lines, *J. Immunol.,* 123, 1548, 1979.
43. **Shulman, M., Wilde, C. D., and Kohler, G.,** A better cell line for making hybridomas secreting specific antibodies, *Nature (London),* 276, 269, 1978.
44. **Galfre, G., Howe, S. C., Milstein, C., Butcher, G. W., and Howard, J. C.,** Antibodies to major histocompatibility antigens produced by hybrid cell lines, *Nature (London),* 266, 550, 1977.
45. **Knutton, S. and Pasternak, C. A.,** The mechanism of cell-cell fusion, *Trends Biochem. Sci.,* 4, 220, 1979.
46. **Pontecorvo, G., Riddle, P. N., and Hales, A.,** Time and mode of fusion of human fibroblasts treated with polyethylene glycol (PEG), *Nature (London),* 265, 257, 1977.
47. **Astaldi, G. C. B., Janssen, M. C., Lansdorp, P., Willems, C., Zeijlemaker, W. P., and Oosterhof, F.,** Human endothelial culture supernatant (HECS): a growth factor for hybridomas, *J. Immunol.,* 125, 1411, 1980.
48. **Levy, R., Dilley, J., and Lampson, L. A.,** Human normal and leukemia cell surface antigens. Mouse monoclonal antibodies as probes, in *Current Topics in Microbiology and Immunology,* Vol. 81, Melchers, F., Potter, M., and Warner, N. L., Eds., Springer-Verlag, New York, 1978, 164.
49. **Howard, J. C. and Corvalan, J. R. F.,** Demonstration of MHC-specific haemolytic plaque-forming cells, *Nature (London),* 278, 449, 1979.
50. **Parks, D. R., Bryan, V. M., Oi, V. T., and Herzenberg, L. A.,** Antigen-specific identification and cloning of hybridomas with a fluorescence-activated cell sorter, *Proc. Natl. Acad. Sci. U.S.A.,* 76, 1962, 1979.
51. **Eisenbarth, G. S., Haynes, B. F., Schroer, J. A., and Fauci, A. S.,** Production of monoclonal antibodies reacting with peripheral blood mononuclear cell surface differentiation antigens, *J. Immunol.,* 124, 1237, 1980.
52. **Sharon, J., Morrison, S. L., and Kabat, E. A.,** Detection of specific hybridoma clones by replica immunoadsorption of their secreted antibodies, *Proc. Natl. Acad. Sci. U.S.A.,* 76, 1420, 1979.
53. **Andrzejewski, C., Jr., Stollar, B. D., Lalor, T. M., and Schwartz, R. S.,** Hybridoma autoantibodies to DNA, *J. Immunol.* 124, 1499, 1980.
54. **Eshhar, Z., Ofarim, M., and Waks, T.,** Generation of hybridomas secreting murine reaginic antibodies of anti-DNP specificity, *J. Immunol.,* 124, 775, 1980.
55. **Mosmann, T. R., Gallatin, M., and Longenecker, B. M.,** Alteration of apparent specificity of monoclonal (hybridoma) antibodies recognising polymorphic histocompatibility and blood group determinants, *J. Immunol.,* 125, 1152, 1980.
56. **Mason, D. W. and Williams, A. F.,** The kinetics of antibody binding to membrane antigens in solution and at the cell surface, *Biochem., J.,* 187, 1, 1980.
57. **Zola, H., Beckman, I. G. R., Bradley, J., Brooks, D. A., Kupa, A., McNamara, P. J., Smart, I. J., and Thomas, M. E.,** Human lymphocyte markers defined by antibodies derived from somatic cell hybrids. III. A marker defining a subpopulation of lymphocytes which cuts across the normal T-B-null classification, *Immunology,* 40, 143, 1980.
58. **Zola, H., McNamara, P., Thomas, M. E., Smart, I. J., and Bradley, J.,** The preparation and properties of monoclonal antibodies against human granulocyte membrane antigens, *Br. J. Haematol.,* 48, 481, 1981.
59. **Pesce, M. A. and Strande, C. S.,** A new micromethod for determination of protein in cerebrospinal fluid and urine, *Clin. Chem., Winston-Salem, NC,* 19, 1265, 1973.
60. **Taylor, I. W. and Milthorpe, B. K.,** An evaluation of DNA fluorochromes, staining techniques and analysis for flow cytometry; 1. Unperturbed cell populations, *J. Histochem. Cytochem.,* 28, 1224, 1980.
61. **Hoffman, D. R., Grossberg, A. L., and Pressman, D.,** Anti-hapten antibodies of restricted heterogeneity: studies on binding properties and component chains, *J. Immunol.,* 108, 18, 1972.

62. **Righetti, P. G. and Drysdale, J. W.,** Isoelectric focusing in *Laboratory Techniques in Biochemistry and Molecular Biology,* Vol. 5, Work, T. S. and Work, E., Eds., Elsevier/North-Holland, Amsterdam, 1976, 335.
63. **Hudson, L. and Hay, F. C., Eds.,** *Practical Immunology,* Blackwell Scientific, Oxford, 1976.
64. **Weir, D. M., Ed.,** *Handbook of Experimental Immunology,* Vol. 1, 3rd Ed., Blackwell Scientific, Oxford, 1978.
65. **Lefkovits, I. and Pernis, B., Eds.,** *Immunological Methods,* Academic Press, New York, 1979.
66. **Laemli, U. K.,** Cleavage of structural proteins during assembly of the head of bacteriophage T4, *Nature (London),* 227, 680, 1970.
67. **Ballou, B., Levine, G., Hakala, T. R., and Solter, D.,** Tumor location detected with radioactively labeled monoclonal antibody and external scintigraphy, *Science,* 206, 844, 1979.
68. **Kenny, P. A., McCaskill, A. C., and Boyle, W.,** Enrichment and expansion of specific antibody-forming cells by adoptive transfer and clustering, and their use in hybridoma production, *Aust. J. Exp. Biol. Med.,* 59, 427, 1981.
69. **Gardner, I. and Zola, H.,** unpublished.
70. **Beckman, I. G. R., Bradley, J., Macardle, P. J., Wolnizer, C. M., and Zola, H.,** A hybridoma monoclonal antibody which reacts with cells carrying the HLA-A2 antigen: evidence for heterogeneity in the expression of HLA-A2, *Tissue Antigens,* in press.

Chapter 2

ANALYSIS OF MONOCLONAL ANTIBODIES TO HUMAN GROWTH HORMONE AND RELATED PROTEINS

J. Ivanyi

TABLE OF CONTENTS

I. INTRODUCTION

Human pituitary hormones have been classified into three structural categories, namely proteins, glycoproteins, and peptides. The protein hormones represent a family with structural and functional homologies, comprising growth hormone (hGH), chorionic somatomammotropin (hCS), and prolactin (hPRL). These molecules built of a single polypeptide chain with a molecular weight of 22,000 (hGH) or 21,000 (hCS, hPRL) daltons are globular in shape but there is only scant information about their three-dimensional structure (see reviews).[1–3] The nucleotide sequence of the DNA complementary to hGH messenger RNA was determined recently.[4] Homologies in the amino acid sequences of growth hormones, chorionic somatomammotropins, and prolactins of various mammalian species indicate their origin from a common ancestral molecule.[5] A primordial peptide probably of smaller size diverged structurally at an early stage of evolution into two major lines which functionally overlap and manifest both somatotropic and lactogenic activities. In the phylogenic tree, hCS is placed very close to hGH but distant from hPRL, since 86% of amino acid sequences of hGH are shared with hCS but only 16% are homologous with hPRL. Accordingly, studies with polyclonal antisera demonstrated strong cross-reactivity between hGH and hCS[6] but no evidence of shared antigenicity with hPRL.

Multiple biological activities are manifested by this group of hormones (see reviews).[1–3, 7–9] The main function of hGH is somatotropic and its action is demonstrable in various species including rats which are commonly used to monitor the growth-promoting potency of hGH preparations. On the other hand, it is of interest to note that nonprimate growth hormones are ineffective in man. The mechanism of action of hGH is a subject of intensive experimental studies which are centered on the mediatory role of somatomedins represented by a group of small molecular weight peptides, (see reviews).[3,10] The liver has been considered as the main site of somatomedin production and important advances have been achieved on the purification of the growth hormone receptor from liver membranes.[11] The main biological function of prolactin is lactogenic, i.e., control of milk secretion and growth of the mammary gland, but there is a range of several other regulatory endocrine functions.[9] hCS is produced in large quantities by the placenta and the hormone's lactogenic effects are stronger than its growth-promoting activity (1 to 10% of hGH). However, the hormone disappears rapidly after parturition and its true physiological function is not yet clear.[8]

The introduction of radioimmunoassay (RIA) of hGH as one of the first sensitive hormone immunoassays[12,13] greatly contributed towards the rapid expansion in experimental and clinical research. The clinical significance of blood hGH levels is relevant not only for the diagnosis of growth disorders but also as a general index of pituitary function.[7,14] The levels of hCS rise during pregnancy, reaching peak levels at 38 weeks of gestation. Subnormal concentrations are generally considered to be a sign for "at risk" subjects, but its relative value has not been clearly established.[8] Hyperprolactemia is of diagnostic interest in patients with amenorhea, pituitary adenomas, in a broad spectrum of hypothalamic-pituitary-gonadal dysfunctions and also following the usage of a variety of neuroleptic drugs.[9]

The radioimmunoassay of hGH is one of the most reliable and most frequently used hormone assays. Various procedures using radioiodinated hGH[11] or antibodies, i.e., immunoradiometric assays[13] were employed. Rabbits respond readily to immunization with hGH or hCS and antisera of satisfactory titer and avidity are readily available. Only very little variation was observed when blood hGH levels were determined using different antisera;[7] however, cross-reactivity of rabbit antisera with hCS has been commonly observed and this invalidates their usage for RIA in pregnant women unless cross-absorbed. RIA tests have become indispensable not only for quantitative determinations of serum hormone levels but also for monitoring hormone concentrations during the various stages of hormone purification and in numerous experimental studies. The use of antibodies as immunoadsorbents represents another important contribution of immunological techniques. Prolactin was separated from growth hormone by affinity chromatography of monkey pituitary extracts using an anti-hCS antibody cross-reactive with monkey growth hormone.[16] Finally, immunofluorescent techniques have been used to demonstrate hormone secreting cells in sections of pituitary glands, tumors or placental tissues.[17,18]

The antigenic relatedness of human somatotropic/lactogenic hormones to homologous proteins from other species has been studied by various investigators. Rabbit, guinea pig, and rat anti-hGH sera showed strong cross-reactivity with growth hormones from primates but only weak reactions with porcine and to an even lesser extent with bovine and ovine growth hormone.[19–21] Similarly, rabbit anti-hCS sera cross-react strongly with primate hCS but only marginally with various nonprimate species.[22] The lack or short supply of purified hPRL led several investigators to raise antisera against prolactins from mammalian species and utilize them for RIA testing of hPRL levels. The most effective antibodies were obtained from guinea pigs or rabbits immunized against ovine PRL,[23,24] thus indicating a possibly closer antigenic relationship between man and nonprimate mammalian species for PRL than for GH and CS hormones. Comparison of hPRL levels estimated by RIA using antisera to human or ovine PRL were in good agreement and sometimes the assay based on the heterologous antibody seemed to be even more sensitive.[24,25]

Preparations of "clinical grade" hGH reveal various degrees of size heterogeneity, but it is not clear how much of it is physiological or the result of aggregation which had occurred during the extraction procedure. The conditions of hormone purification and the degree of protein aggregation has been implicated in the aggravation of immunogenicity of hGH when used therapeutically in children with hereditary hormone deficiency.[26] Sera of individual hGH-deficient patients were reported to have antibodies with different specificities towards the antigenic determinants of hGH.[27] This was indicated by the fact that antibodies from some patients reacted poorly with carbamido- or carboxy-methylated hGH whereas antibodies from other patients reacted equally with reduced/alkylated or native hGH. Another study of "autoantibodies" following hGH therapy suggested the presence of at least two different antibody populations directed to distinct antigenic sites.[28] The authors detected low titers of antibodies binding to ^{125}I-hGH only in few patients following long-term therapy (2 years); however, higher titers of antibodies binding to ^{125}I-pig GH were detected in more patients and also following short-term therapy. The binding of ^{125}I-pig GH could not be reduced by unlabeled hGH, thus indicating that the immunogenic structure of hGH which triggered the synthesis of antipig GH antibodies is normally "cryptic" and becomes expressed as a result of some form of hGH aggregation or in vivo degradation.

Although antibodies served as invaluable tools for sensitive immunoassays, their use for immunochemical analysis of the antigenic structure of hormones was limited by the heterogeneity of antibody specificities in conventional antisera. Thus, monoclonal antibodies secreted by hybridoma cell lines indicated an opportunity of a novel and more advanced approach towards the various yet unresolved questions.

II. GENERATION OF HYBRIDOMA CELL LINES

BALB/c mice respond with high antibody titers to immunization with either hGH or hCS. Priming with 10 to 100 μg antigen in complete Freund's adjuvant (intraperi-

Table 1
SUMMARY OF FUSION RESULTS

			No. of primary wells			Stable clones	
Strain	**Antigen**	**Immunization**[a]	**Total**	**Growing**	**Active**	**No.**	**Code**
BALB/c	hGH	3 × 100 μg	48	46	12	3	NA39, NA71, NA27
BALB/c	hGH	3 × 100 μg	96	84	36	1	QA68
BALB/c	hCS	4 × 10 μg	96	32	3	2	EB1, EB4
BALB/c	hCS	4 × 10 μg	96	34	9	2	EB2, EB3
Ab/H	hPRL	5 × 1 μg	96	57	1	1	QB1

Note: All antibodies are of IgG1 isotype. Preliminary results were reported.[32,33]

[a]Priming with emulsion in complete Freund's adjuvant followed by challenge with soluble antigen over a period of 5 months.

toneal or subcutaneous) was followed by 2 to 3 challenge injections (intraperitoneal or intravenous) of the same dose of soluble antigen given at 3 to 6 weekly intervals. Serum samples taken from mice 7 days after challenge were titrated for antibody levels by RIA and high responder individuals with ABT_{50} values above 1000 (for techniques see legend to Table 2) were challenged 3 to 4 days prior to fusion.

The efforts to immunize mice to hPRL have been hampered by the notorious short supply of adequate antigen. The antigenicity of hPRL is apparently unstable upon storage since various preparations lost their activity when tested by displacement RIA. Consequently, mice were immunized with a low dose, i.e., 1 μg hPRL per injection. BALB/c mice failed to respond but satisfactory antibody responses were obtained in mice of the AB/H strain which has been bred for multiple generations by selecting from each progeny individuals with a sheep erythrocyte high-responder phenotype.[29]

Spleen cell suspensions from individual high-responder mice harvested 3 to 4 days after challenge were fused with 1×10^7 P3NS1/1-Ag4-1 nonsecretor myeloma cells (obtained from Dr C. Milstein) in the presence of 42% polyethylene glycol 1500.[30–31] The cell suspension was distributed into 96 wells containing 2 mℓ of selective HAT RPM1-1640/10% fetal calf serum medium and incubated in 5% CO_2 at 37°C. Media from wells which contained macroscopically discernible colonies were assayed by radioimmunoassay (see legend, Table 2).

Colonies from positive wells were transferred into microtiter plates containing 0.2 mℓ of HT-medium and gradually expanded into 2 to 4 mℓ wells. Subsequently, cells were cloned and when necessary recloned by the limiting dilution technique in microtiter plates. As a rule, cells were grown prior to cloning until good viability and growth activity was reached. It is apparent from the summary of the results (Table 1) that the rate of success was variable. Several hybrids which were initially active ceased either growth or antibody secretion upon subsequent culture or cloning. Nevertheless, the QBI anti-hPRL hybridoma was successfully established from a single positive primary well.

Established hybridoma cells at a dose of 2×10^6 per mouse were injected i.p. into BALB/c or (BALB/c × AB/H)F1 hybrid mice which had been given 0.5 mℓ Pristane (−10 days) and 25 mg/kg cyclophosphamide (−1 day). Ascitic fluid and serum were harvested 10 to 20 days later. Monoclonal antibody (MAb) titers in tissue culture media varied between 10^2 to $10^3 \times ABT_{50}$ whereas ascites/serum (A/S) batches varied between 10^4 to $10^5 \times ABT_{50}$. In contrast with polyclonal murine anti-hGH sera which gave precipitin lines with hGH (0.5 mg/mℓ) by double diffusion in agar gel, none of

Table 2
TITRATION OF MONOCLONAL ANTIBODIES TO hGH AND hCS BY RIA

Monoclonal antibodies	$Log_{10} \times ABT_{50}$[a]		Cross-reaction (%)
	^{125}I-hGH	^{125}I-hCS	
NA39	4.9	4.3	87.7
NA71	4.7	<0.0	<1.0
NA27	4.4	<0.0	<1.0
QA68	5.2	<0.0	<1.0
EB 1	3.8	4.6	82.6
EB 2	3.4	3.0	88.2
EB 3	3.2	3.7	86.5
EB 4	<0.0	2.8	<1.0

[a]100 $\mu\ell$ samples of ascites/serum serially diluted in 1% normal mouse serum (NMS)/PBS plus equal volumes of ^{125}I-hormone (0.1 mC/μg) were incubated 20 hr at 4°C. Complexes were precipitated with 100 $\mu\ell$ sheep antimouse Ig serum and radioactivities counted in centrifuged and drained precipitates. Specific binding was related to the "high control" value obtained in the presence of a saturating amount of antibody and corrected for binding in the presence of normal mouse serum ("low control"). Antibody concentrations are expressed as reciprocal values of the dilution giving 50% specific binding (ABT_{50}).

the monoclonal antibodies showed a precipitin reaction when tested alone or in mixtures of as many as four MAbs.[32]

III. SPECIFICITY OF ANTIBODIES TO hGH, hCS, AND hPRL

Considering the extensive homology in the primary structure of hGH and hCS[1] and the previously reported cross-reactivity of rabbit antisera,[6] it was conceivable to expect that certain MAbs should be directed against the shared determinants. Indeed hybridoma antibodies NA39 (hGH immune spleen) and EB1, EB2, and EB3 (hCS immune spleen) reacted equally with both hormones (Table 2). A weak or marginal degree of cross-reactivity with hCS was previously reported for antibodies NA71 and NA27.[32] At the extreme ends, QA68 antibody showed specific binding to hGH and EB4 antibody to hCS since incubation with as much as 5 to 50 μg of the heterologous antigen failed to compete with binding with the respective homologous ^{125}I-labeled hormone (Table 3). None of the anti-hGH or anti-hCS antibodies showed any binding with hPRL.[33] Furthermore the binding of the four tested antibodies with ^{125}I-HGH could not be displaced by an excess of either bovine or sheep growth hormone (Table 3). The species specificity of these antibodies was confirmed in immunohistological assays by their failure to stain porcine, dog, or rat pituitary sections.[34] Growth hormone producing cells in pars anterior of several human pituitary glands were readily stained by monoclonal antibodies[34] although NA71 antibody in some experiments was at least ten times less effective than NA39, NA27, or QA68.[35]

The anti-hPRL antibody QB1 failed to react with ^{125}I-hCS or ^{125}I-hGH and the binding to ^{125}I-PRL could not be displaced with 10 μg of the respective unlabeled heterologous hormones. This is not surprising, considering the great distance between hPRL and hGH/hCS in the evolutionary tree of this family of hormones and the small number (15%) of homologous amino acid residues. It was unexpected to find that QB1 did not

Table 3
SPECIFICITY ANALYSIS OF MONOCLONAL ANTIBODIES BY DISPLACEMENT RIA

Monoclonal antibody	RIA assay	Inhibitor	ID_{50} (μg)
QA68	^{125}I-hGH	hGH	0.02
		hCS	>10.00
		bGH,oGH	>10.00
EB 4	^{125}I-hCS	hCS	0.15
		hGH	>10.00
QB 1	^{125}I-PRL	hPRL	0.05
		hGH,hCS	>10.00
		bPRL,oPRL	>50.00
		pPRL	>5.00

Note: h = human, b = bovine, o = ovine, p = porcine.

International reference preparations of hGH (66/217) and hPRL (75/504) were obtained from Dr. D. R. Bangham, National Institute for Biological Standards; bGH, oGH, bPRL, and oPRL from Dr. M. Wallis, University of Sussex, and pPRL from Dr. C. R. Hopkins, University of Liverpool.

react with bovine, ovine, or porcine prolactins (Table 3) which apparently have a closer relationship to hPRL in evolution and structure.[5] The strict specificity of QB1 allowed us to determine the presence of 0.1 to 1% hPRL as a contaminant in clinical grade and other imcompletely purified hGH preparations.

IV. AFFINITY OF ANTI-hGH ANTIBODIES

The affinity of anti-hGH antibodies under equilibrium conditions was determined by displacement RIA analysis. Significant displacement of ^{125}I-hGH binding at the 1 ng cold hGH level was demonstrable only with NA71 antibody whereas binding of NA39, NA27, and QA68 was displaced only at higher hormone concentrations (Figure 1). These results indicated a low affinity of binding which would not satisfy the requirements of clinical RIA for testing hormone levels. Using these criteria, the specific anti-hCS (EB4) and anti-hPRL (QB1) antibodies are also of low affinity (Table 3). The equilibrium affinity constants were calculated by Scatchard plot analysis and the results confirmed the highest affinity constant for NA71 followed by NA39 > QA68 > NA27 (Figure 2).

Dissociation rates were determined by RIA whereby the sequence of reaction was modified in the following way: various concentrations of cold hGH were added either 1 hr prior to or 1 hr after mixing of MAb plus ^{125}I-hGH (Figure 1). Similar results were obtained when cold hGH was added to MAb 1 hr in advance or simultaneously with ^{125}I-hGH. When preformed ^{125}I-hGH-MAb were dissociated by adding the increasing amounts of unlabeled hGH, the differences between the four MAbs appeared in a different light as compared with equilibrium constants. Only poor dissociation (20 to 30%) was achieved by 1000- or 20-fold excess of NA71 and NA39, respectively; somewhat higher (50%) dissociation was observed for QA68 complexes. However, extreme dissociative properties were observed for the NA27 bound ^{125}I-hGH: the labeled hormone was displaced from preformed complexes as readily as in the reaction without a priority in the incubation sequence.

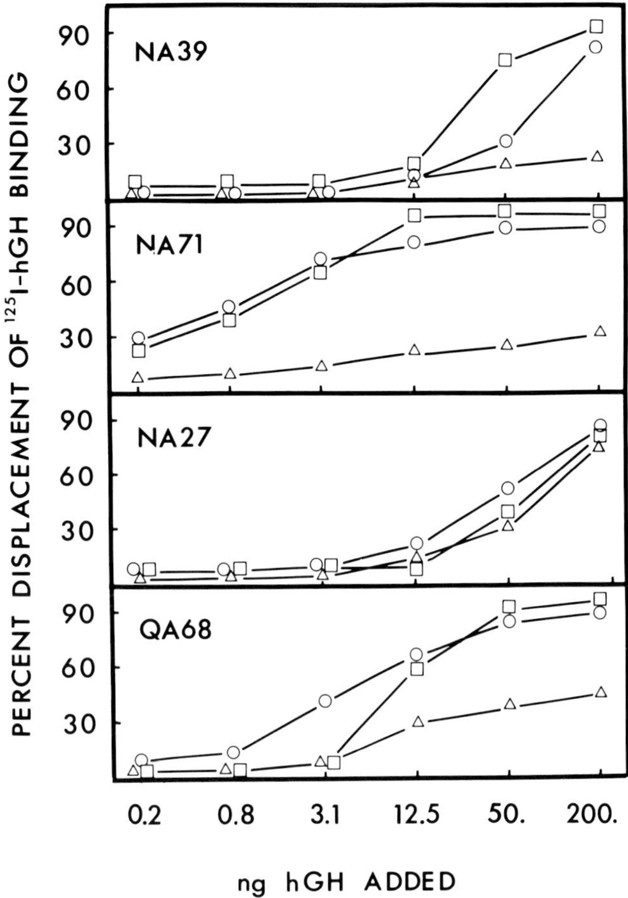

FIGURE 1. Displacement—dissociation RIA of anti-hGH antibodies. □-Preincubation of MAb plus various doses of hGH for 1 hr followed by 1 hr incubation with ^{125}I-HGH; ○-Simultaneous incubation of MAb plus unlabeled hGH and ^{125}I-hGH for 2 hr; △-Preincubation of MAb plus ^{125}I-hGH for 1 hr followed by 1 hr incubation with various doses of hGH. All samples were coprecipitated for 20 hr at 4°C as described in legend to Table 2.

Similar ranking of MAbs was determined by assessment of the dissociation rates in a solid-phase RIA. ^{125}I-hGH bound to MAB-coated microtiter plates was displaced by incubation at 37°C in the presence of increasing concentrations of unlabeled HGH (Figure 3). The most effective dissociation of ^{125}I-hGH resulted from NA27 coated plates, followed by lower values for QA68; however, dissociation of NA71 and NA39 complexes did not occur under these conditions.

V. ISOELECTRIC FOCUSING OF ANTIBODIES AND IMMUNE COMPLEXES

It was considered that isoelectric focusing spectra[36] may qualify as characteristic "markers" for individual hybridoma MAbs, all being of the IgG1 isotype. Analysis of anti-hGH antibodies showed that NA71 and NA27 had identical spectrotypes composed of five bands with fast mobilities, NA39 bands were of somewhat slower mobility

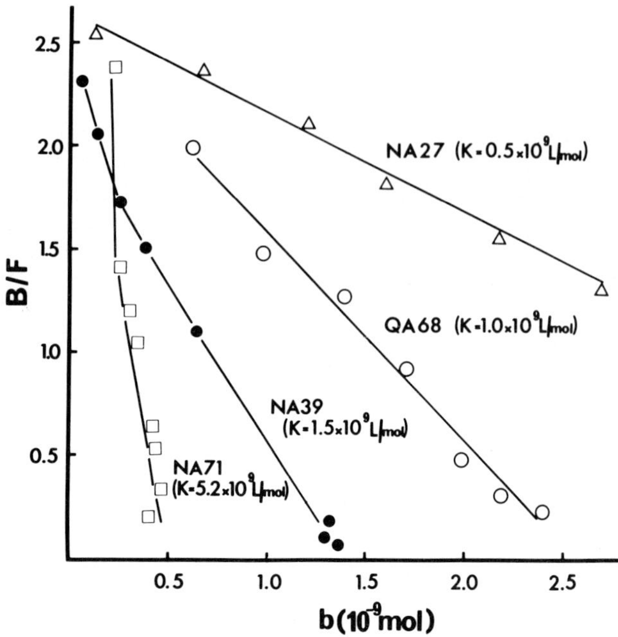

FIGURE 2. Scatchard plot analysis of anti-hGH antibody affinities. B/F—bound/free ^{125}I-hGH; b—amount of bound hGH; RIA technique: see legend to Table 2.

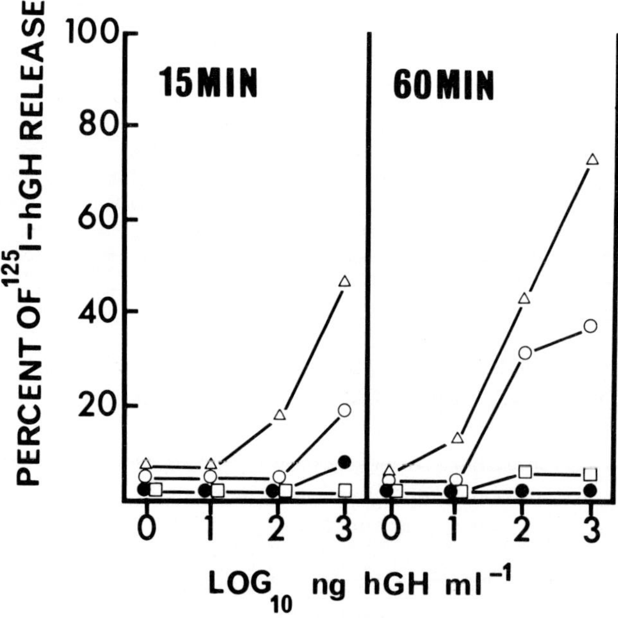

FIGURE 3. Dissociation rate of ^{125}I-hGH from immune complexes NA39 (●), NA71 (□), NA27 (△), or QA68 (○) antibody-coated microtiter plates were complexes with ^{125}I-hGH and washed (see legend to Figure 7.2). The radioactivity released upon incubation for 15 or 60 min with 100 μℓ of unlabeled hGH at 37°C was counted.

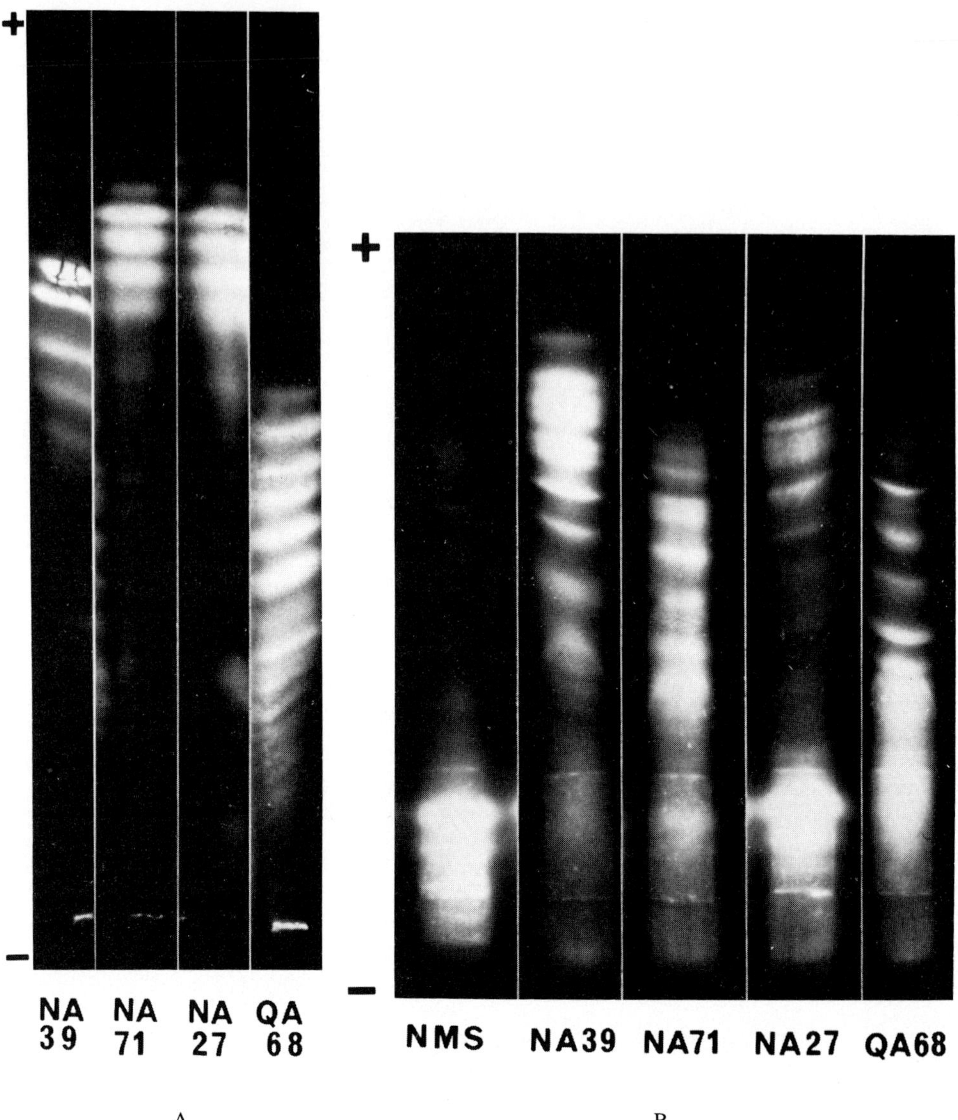

FIGURE 4. Isoelectric focusing of anti-hGH antibodies and immune complexes Separation in slabs of 5% polyacrylamide gels containing Ampholine® (LKB) pH 3.5–10 and 3*M* urea. Plates were run for 2 hr at 150V, 16 hr at 300V, and 2 hr at 500V per plate at 4°C and then immersed in 18% NA_2SO_4 for 1 hr. (A) Samples (15 μℓ) of MAb ascites/serum ($10^4 \times ABT_{50}$) were applied: bands were developed by incubation of plates with ^{125}I-hGH (2×10^5 cpm/mℓ) in sheep antimouse Ig serum for 20 hr at 4°C. (B) MAb samples were preincubated with ^{125}I-hGH (10^4 cpm) for 20 hr at 4°C prior to run. Plates were fixed with 0.5% glutaraldehyde in 18% Na_2SO_4. Rinsed and dried plates were exposed to X-ray film.

and QA68 manifested a very different spectrotype composed of 6 to 8 bands of slow mobility (Figure 4a). The latter pattern was confirmed upon recloning and assay of three individual clones of the QA68 hybridoma line. Although various batches of tissue culture media had uniform spectrotypes, slight differences were observed when comparing different ascites/serum batches. Most likely, this variation may be attributed to changes in the net charge of the molecule, resulting from the processing and/or storage of ascites/serum preparations.

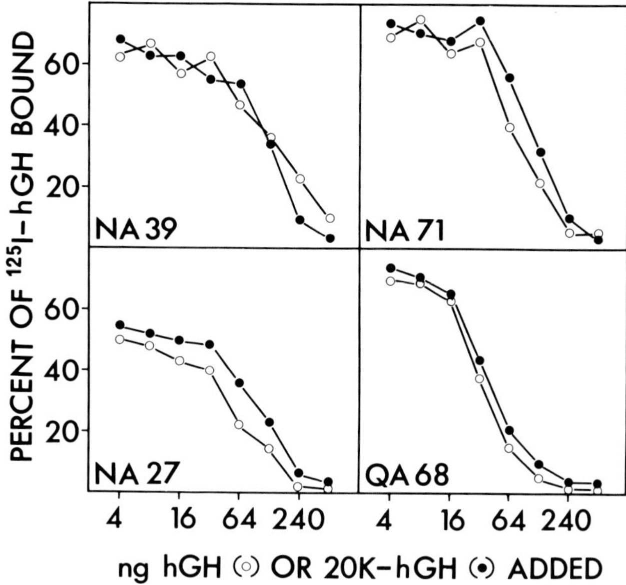

FIGURE 5. Displacement RIA of 20K-hGH. (A purified preparation of 20K-hGH (batch: 305-42-3) was provided for assay by Dr U. J. Lewis, Scripps Clinic and Research Foundation, La Jolla, Calif.)

Since the MAb-hGH immune complexes were soluble in antibody excess, it was of interest to determine their spectrotypes. Good resolution between free ^{125}I-hGH migrating slightly towards the cathode and the immune complexes migrating to the anode was obtained (Figure 4b). In accord with the affinity properties estimated by RIA, most of the radioactivity from nondissociative NA39 and NA71 complexes was distributed in discrete bands along the pH gradient whereas part of QA68 complexes and most of NA27 complexes apparently dissociated when applied into the gel.

VI. ANTIGENICITY OF MOLECULAR VARIANTS OF hGH

Most preparations of hGH and hPRL display various degrees of molecular size heterogeneity. This as been a major problem attended by several authors trying to elucidate whether the multiple biological activities of a particular batch of a hormone are attributable to physiological variants of the hormone, aggregation generated during the isolation procedure, or to impurities (see reviews[1-3]). Several investigators reported also that variable amounts of RIA-reactive hGH, hCS, and hPRL exist in the plasma of individual patients as dimers and oligomers (''big hormones'')[9,14,37] but the relevance of these findings and the question of whether they represent separate biological entities remains open.

A naturally occurring variant of hGH comprising about 15% of the total growth hormone content is present in all human pituitary extracts.[38] The molecular weight of the variant was estimated to be near 20,000 daltons (the major form of hGH has a value of 22,000) because it lacks 15 amino acid residues at the N-terminus at positions 32 to 46 (inclusive) of the polypeptide chain.[39] Although this form of hGH has normal growth promoting activity, it lacks the insulin-like metabolic properties.[40] Since the 20K variant was only about one third as active as a standard preparation of hGH in displacing ^{125}I-hGH from binding to rabbit antibodies it was of interest to ascertain

whether the effect could be selective for any of the epitopes detected by MAbs. The results of radioimmunoassays (Figure 5) suggested that 20K-hGH displaced to a very similar extent the binding of all four tested antibodies to ^{125}I-hGH and that the antigenic activity of the 20K variant was not significantly different from the control "therapeutic grade" preparation of hGH. The obvious conclusion seems to be that neither of the epitopes under study had been altered in their expression as a result of the structural deletion at the NH_2-terminal of hGH.

Fractionation of hGH by preparative electrophoresis revealed four major components differing in molecular net charge.[41] The antigenic potency of these preparations was tested recently and the results showed that fractions B (intact 22K form), D, and E (cleaved at residues 135 to 146 to 150, and of interest because of their enhanced bioactivity) gave virtually identical displacement curves with all four tested anti-hGH MAbs.[42] In another preliminary report the heterogeneity of clinical grades of hGH has been investigated.[43] The preparation was fractionated on Sephadex® G100 into four main peaks corresponding to aggregated, trimeric, dimeric, and monomeric hGH, respectively. Using a conventional rabbit antiserum for RIA, the monomeric and oligomeric fractions were equally active whereas the aggregated fraction had only about 10% of displacing potency. Interestingly, three (NA39, NA27, and QA68) MAbs reacted in a fashion similar to the rabbit antibody, but antibody NA71 was much less reactive with dimeric and trimeric hGH indicating that the site recognized by this antibody could have been masked selectively.[43]

VII. ANTIGENICITY OF PEPTIDES AND MODIFIED OR DIGESTED HORMONES

Several attempts have been made previously to correlate the growth-promoting and lactogenic activities of hGH with its chemical and antigenic structure.[1,2,27] Various chemically modified derivatives and proteolytically degraded preparations were examined. Studies with carbamidomethylated hGH or hCS which retain the native molecular conformation showed full antigenic, biological, and receptor binding activities.[27] Carboxymethylated hGH with native conformation but with poor conformational stability as measured by the rate of tryptic digestion retained 82% of antigenicity, 53% of receptor binding properties, but completely lost its biological activity. The authors suggested that the loss of growth-promoting activity may be attributed to rapid degradation in vivo rather than to a selective alteration of the hormone's "active site".[27,44] Moderate or complete loss of immunoreactivity was observed in derivatives which retained the entire primary structure but had a chemically disrupted tertiary structure. Thus, fragments of hGH or hCS obtained from extensive tryptic or CNBr cleavage were devoid of antigenicity.[27] Besides, fractionation of digests can be complicated by aggregation phenomena which could only be overcome by the use of organic acids at high concentration as dissociating agents.

It was also reported that the antigenic activity of fragments cleaved by CNBr, when tested by hemagglutination and complement fixation methods, was localized in the 73–128 peptide fragment.[45] Subsequently, peptides synthesized by the solid phase method and purified by chromatography and high voltage electrophoresis were tested by RIA. The most active peptide, 98–128, reacted significantly when compared with the other fragments, but nevertheless, the effective concentrations were three orders of magnitude higher than those needed from native hGH.[46] The authors considered that the antigenicity of peptide 98–128 could be sterically concealed by the addition of further residues.

Experiments were set up by Palladini et al.[47] to ascertain whether the active peptides

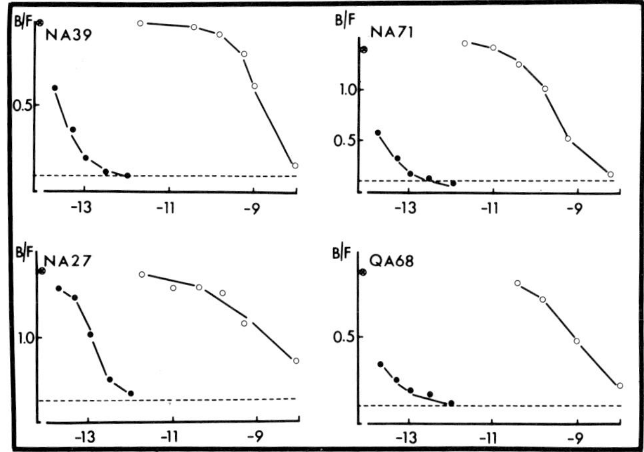

FIGURE 6. Displacement RIA of the synthetic 44–128 peptide. B/F - bound/free ^{125}I-hGH. (Reproduced with permission from Dr A. C. Palladini, Universidad de Buenos Aires, Argentina.[47])

may react selectively with any monoclonal antibodies. The results suggested that peptide 44–128 had a similar displacing activity for all four tested antibodies and that the inhibitory concentrations were four orders of magnitude higher than those needed from native hGH (Figure 6). The lack of specificity of the peptide is difficult to reconcile with the distinct specificities of MAbs when reacting with intact hGH (see following sections). Therefore, it appears that the low affinity binding effect of peptides may not be directly related to the presumably conformational determinants of native hGH.

Recently, Doebber et al.[48] identified a tripeptidyl aminopeptidase (TAP) in pituitary extracts, which cleaves off the first 33 amino acid residues at the N-terminus of rat and bovine growth hormones. The digested hormones lost 70% of their biological activity but retained full antigenicity when tested by RIA. It seemed of interest to determine whether TAP digested hGH (provided for analysis by Dr S. Ellis) would manifest any selective loss of antigenicity when tested by displacement RIA with monoclonal anti-hGH antibodies. The results indicated that both ''precipitate'' and ''supernatant'' fractions of the TAP digest competed to a similar extent with the binding of ^{125}I-hGH with either of the four tested MAbs (Table 4). The loss in displacing activity which is apparent particularly in the precipitate fraction was proportional with all four MAbs and thus resulted probably from a nonspecific loss of antigenicity during incubation. Thus the results with hGH confirmed the previous observations with bovine GH and rabbit antibodies that deletion of the first 33 amino acids at the N-terminus does not alter specifically the antigenic structure.

VIII. COMPETITION ASSAY USING RADIOLABELED ANTIBODIES (LACT)

The failure to obtain evidence for the existence of sequential determinants in hGH indicated that the main if not all of its antigenic structure depends on molecular conformation. Hence, it has become necessary to employ new techniques to determine the combining site, i.e., paratope[49] specificity of monoclonal antibodies while preserving

Table 4
DISPLACEMENT ASSAY OF TRIPEPTIDYL AMINOPEPTIDASE DIGESTED hGH FRACTIONS

	ID_{50} of MAb-^{125}I-hGH binding				
	TAP/P-hGH		TAP/S-hGH		hGH
Antibody	ng	R	ng	R	ng
NA39	160	2.46	80	1.23	65
NA71	90	2.09	52	1.21	43
NA27	135	2.37	65	1.14	57
QA68	88	2.38	47	1.27	37

Note : R = TAP-hGH/hGH ratio.
Tripeptidyl aminopeptidase (TAP), digest precipitate (P), and supernant (S) fraction of hGH were provided for assay by Dr S. Ellis, Ames Research Center, Moffat Field, Calif.

1) Labelled antibody competition test (LACT) :

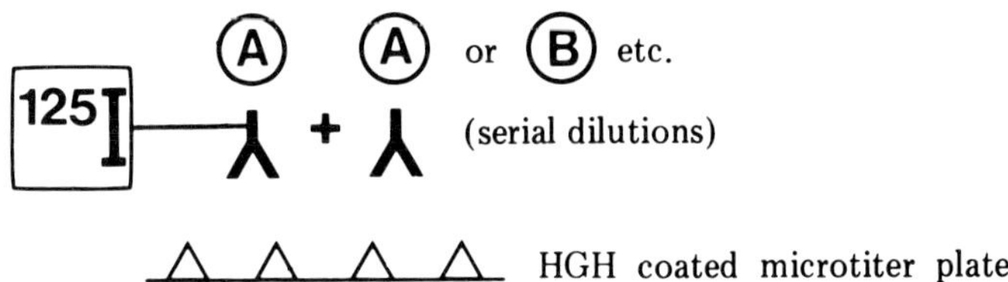

2) Plate antibody competition test (PACT) :

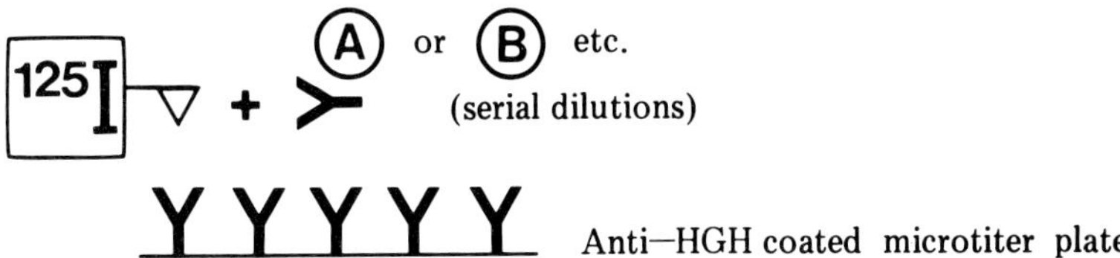

FIGURE 7. Antibody competition techniques. (1) Purified MAbs from culture media were eluted from sheep antimouse Ig/Sepharose 4B columns with glycine-HCℓ pH 2.8 buffer and radioiodinated by the "iodogen" technique[52] (10^6 cpm/μg/10 × ABT_{50}). Wells of polystyrene microtiter plates (Dynatech,® 1-220-24) were coated with hGH (50 μg/mℓ) in 0.05*M* carbonate buffer pH 8.6 for 20 hr at 37°C. Plates were rinsed with PBS and dilutions of competing MAb (in 10% FCS/PBS) added for 4 hr at 4°C. Subsequently ^{125}I-purified MAb (10^4 cpm) was added, plates were mixed, incubated 20 hr at 4°C and rinsed with PBS. Relative binding values of counts bound to wells were calculated. High control: cpm in the presence of NMS instead of competing MAb (1–3 × 10^3 cpm); low control: cpm in human serum albumin (HSA)-coated wells (1000–300 cpm). (2) Microtiter plates were incubated with MAb-ascites/serum diluted to 500 × ABT_{50} in carbonate buffer pH 8.6 for 20 hr at 37°C and rinsed with PBS. Samples of MAbs serially diluted in PBS and mixed with ^{125}I-hGH (in 20% FCS/0.2% Tween-80/PBS) at 4°C were applied to MAb-coated plates within 5 min of mixing; plates were incubated for 20 hr at 4°C and rinsed with cold PBS. Relative values of bound counts were calculated. High control: cpm in the presence of NMS instead of MAb (1–3 × 10^3 cpm): low control: cpm in NMS-coated wells (50–150 cpm).

the intact tertiary molecular structure. This was approached by antibody-antibody competition tests in which two monoclonal antibodies are set to compete for antigen binding (Figure 7). Effective competition between two antibodies would suggest that they bind to the same or overlapping epitopes and conversely, the lack of competition could in-

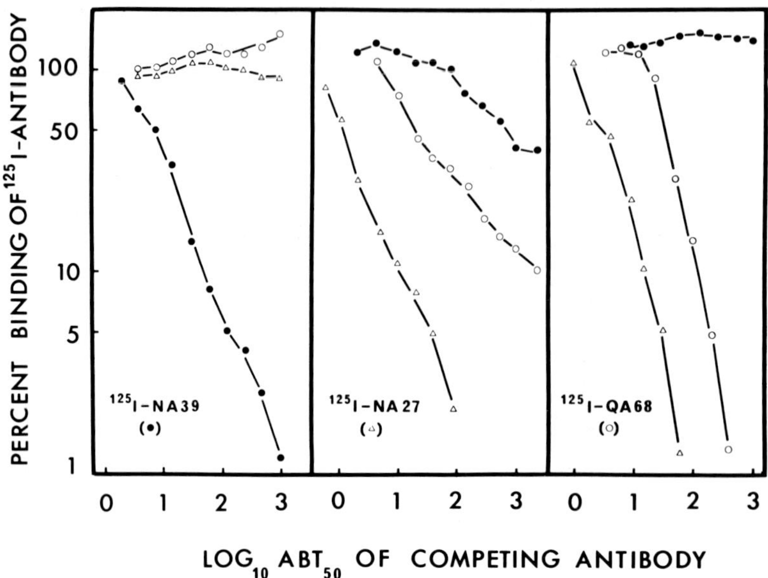

FIGURE 8. LACT analysis of paratope specificities of anti-hGH antibodies hGH-coated plates were incubated with serial dilutions of MAb-ascites/serum and constant amounts of ^{125}I-MAb. The symbol of the competing antibody on each of the three figures is indicated next to its code. LACT technique: see legend to Figure 7.1.

dicate that they combine with separate epitopes which are localized at a sufficient distance to avoid steric hindrance. Furthermore, it was relevant to consider allosteric effects as a possible mechanism of competition; some of these results were reported previously.[50,51]

In the ''labeled antibody competition test'' (LACT), an ^{125}I-labeled antibody is reacted with hGH-coated micrototer plates in the presence of serial dilutions of an unlabeled antibody (Figure 7.1). Successful iodination of NA39, NA27, and QA68 was regularly obtained but so far the binding properties of labeled NA71 have not been satisfactory. The results of the LACT assay presented in Figure 8 showed that NA27 and QA68 antibodies in great excess ($10^3 \times ABT_{50}$) failed to compete with the binding of ^{125}I-NA39 to hGH coated plates. Conversely NA39 antibody did not inhibit the binding of ^{125}I-QA68 and competed at high concentrations only partially with the binding of ^{125}I-NA27. These results are in accord with the distinct differences in the binding MAbs to hCS, i.e., NA39 being the cross-reactive while NA27 and QA68 showing no significant reaction with hCS. The partial effect of high concentrations of NA39 on ^{125}I-NA27 binding may have resulted from steric hindrance or could be attributed to allosteric changes (see also the results of PACT assay in following section).

Antibodies NA27 and QA68 showed reciprocally strong cross-competition, although NA27 was more inhibitory. This seemed surprising, considering the low affinity and strong dissocation characteristics of NA27-hGH complexes.

The interpretation of these results must take into account various technical factors: whereas the affinity measurements were carried out at limiting antibody concentrations (ABT_{60-80}), the LACT assay depends on excess concentrations of the competing antibody. It is not understood whether competition is attributed to simple antigen-antibody binding or whether it entails a change in the steric orientation of the plastic-adsorbed hGH molecules. Although the results do not allow a simple explanation of some of the

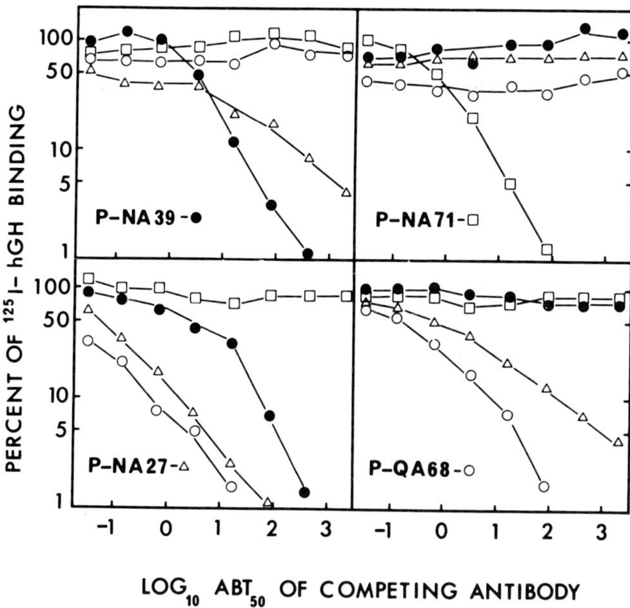

FIGURE 9. PACT analysis of paratope specificities of anti-hGH antibodies. Plates coated with MAbs (P) were incubated with a mixture of ^{125}I-hGH plus serial dilutions of MAb-ascites/serum. The symbol of the competing antibody on each of the four figures is indicated next to its code. (From Ivanyi, J., *Monoclonal Antibodies and T Cell Hybridomas,* Hämmerling, G. J., Hämmerling, U., and Kearney, J. F., Eds., Elsevier/North Holland, Amsterdam, 1981, 349. With permission.)

quantitative aspects of the reaction, it is conceivable that multiple antibody-antigen interactions expected from a low affinity antibody such as NA27 may play a role in the antibody's high competing efficacy.

IX. COMPETITION ASSAY USING PLATE-ADSORBED ANTIBODIES (PACT)

Analysis of antibody paratope specificities by the ''plate antibody competition test'' (PACT) provided data complementary to those described previously. The technique is based on the competition by serial dilutions of unlabeled MAbs with the binding of ^{125}I-hGH to MAb-coated wells (Figure 7.2). This procedure when compared with the LACT technique has the advantage that it does not require purified radiolabeled MAbs and plates coated with relatively high concentrations of the hormone. However, competition in the PACT technique occurs between one antibody forming an immune complex in the fluid phase, with another antibody in solid-phase. Only the LACT technique is applicable for the paratope analysis of mixtures such as conventional antisera.[53] The sensitivity of both techniques was similar as judged by the effective inhibitory concentration of MAb.

The results of competition analysis of four anti-hGH antibodies by the PACT technique are presented in Figure 9. Inhibition of >95% of ^{125}I-hGH binding was detected by the presence of 10 to 100 × ABT_{50} on homologous antibody-coated plates. Antigen-binding to NA71-coated plates was inhibitable only with the homologous antibody and

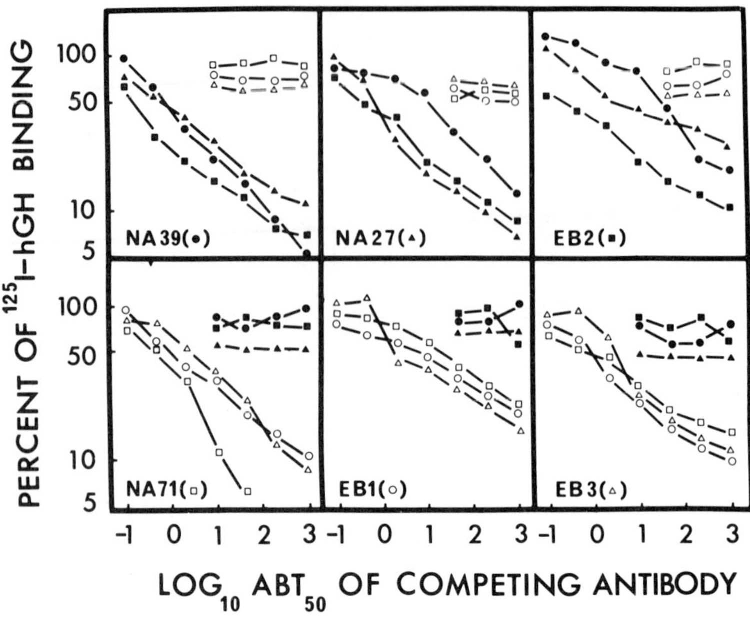

FIGURE 10. PACT analysis of hGH-hCS cross-reactive antibodies. The symbol of the competing antibody is indicated next to its code. PACT technique: see legend to Figure 7.2.

not with any of the other three MAbs up to $10^3 \times ABT_{50}$ concentrations. Conversely, excess amounts of NA71 failed to compete with the binding of ^{125}I-hGH to plates coated with any of the other three MAbs. Antibodies NA27 and QB68 manifested strong reciprocal cross-competition as in the LACT assay suggesting that they react with closely overlapping structures of the hGH-specific (i.e., non-hCS) moiety of the hormone molecule.

An unexpected reciprocal cross-competitive relationship was observed between NA39 and NA27. Each antibody was inhibitory at a 10 to 100 times higher concentration and to a smaller extent on the "heterologous" MAb-coated plate. These cross-competitive reactions between two antibodies binding to the hGH-specific (NA27) or hCS-like (NA39) hormone moieties cannot be interpreted unequivocally. It is unlikely that the results were due to contamination for the following reasons: (1) contamination of NA27 with NA39 was excluded by its failure to bind with ^{125}I-hCS; and (2) contamination of NA39 with NA27 would have produced at least some inhibition on the QA68-coated plate. Since there seems to be a close proximity of NA27 and QA68 epitopes on the hGH molecule, it seems unlikely that NA39 antibody could selectively cause steric hindrance of the NA27-binding epitope without having any effect also on the adjacent QA68-binding epitope. Furthermore, the contrasting reactions of NA39 and NA27 with hCS also indicate that the corresponding epitopes on the hGH molecule are located at a distance from each other.

It is conceivable that interaction of MAbs with the monomeric epitope of a protein antigen could produce an allosteric change in conformation, thus interfering with the presentation of a different epitope of unrelated specificity. A protein such as hGH which has its antigenic structure probably built from conformational rather than structural epitopes would likely be prone to antibody-ligand induced allosteric changes. The poor affinity and high dissociation rate of NA27 from immune complexes may be relevant

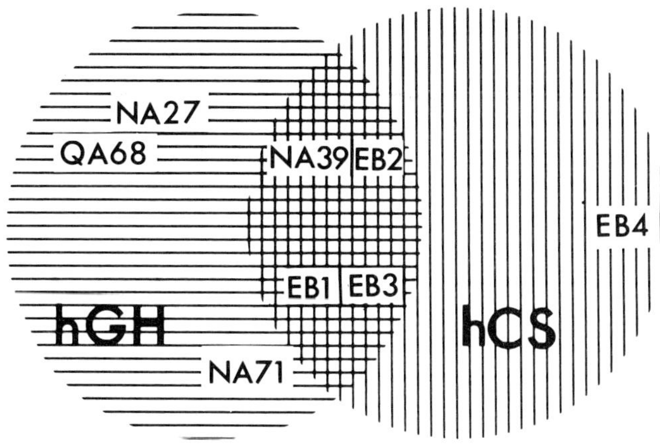

FIGURE 11. Schematic model for the localization of hGH and hCS epitopes recognized by monoclonal antibodies.

for the observed phenomenon. Thus, the inhibition of binding of conformationally altered NA39-hGH complexes could have become apparent on NA27-coated plates rather than on the less dissociative QA68-coated plates. The role of antibody affinity parameters under these circumstances is supported also by the reciprocal data, whereby the inhibitory dose of NA27 was about 100 times higher on the heterologous NA39 plate than on the monologous NA27 plate (Figure 9).

Further analysis by the PACT technique was addressed to antibodies NA39, EB1, EB2, and EB3. (Table 2). The reciprocal competitive activities of these four MAbs directed towards the common determinants of hGH-hCS and of the hGH-specific antibodies NA71 and NA27, were determined using ^{125}I-hGH as antigen. The results showed that, on the basis of cross-competition, the six tested MAbs split into two groups which are represented by NA39, EB2, NA27, and EB1, EB3, NA71, respectively (Figure 10). Within each group, the antibodies competed reciprocally but failed to inhibit significantly the binding to plates coated with MAbs of the other group. These results suggested the existence of at least two nonoverlapping antigenic moieties shared between hGH and hCS (Figure 11). These two determinants appear to be at a distance from each other avoiding steric hindrance when coated with antibodies. Besides, each of the two hGH/hCS determinants is somehow related to another hGH-specific epitope. Namely, NA39 and EB2 competed reciprocally with NA27 whereas EB1 and EB3 cross-reacted with NA71 antibody. The possible mechanisms of this "heterologous" competition have been discussed to some extent in the preceeding paragraph. Although the change in configuration by an allosteric mechanism seems to be the likely explanation, the role of steric hindrance has not been formally excluded. A better understanding of the observed phenomena could be reached only when the underlying conformational determinants are elucidated in further detail.

X. CONCLUSIONS

Previous studies with chemically modified or enzyme digested preparations of hGH and hCS suggested that antigenicity was closely dependent on the integrity of molecular conformation.[27] It has been suggested that beyond the requirement of a polypeptide backbone of certain amino acids, most of the molecular architecture was necessary for the expression of antigenic properties as well as of the hormonal biological functions. This seems to be in contrast to small polypeptide hormones with few secondary or tertiary intramolecular interactions where the distinct antigenic sites are determined by specific amino acid residues.[54]

The failure of monoclonal antibodies to precipitate hGH in double diffusion assays indicated that the corresponding epitopes are nonrepeating monovalent structures. Moreover a mixture of all four tested anti-hGH antibodies still failed to produce a precipitin line[50] probably due to poor lattice formation. Hence, it appears that the epitopes detected by the existing monoclonal antibodies represent only a fraction of the hormone's antigenic repertoire.

The initial demonstration of anti-hGH antibodies with a range of cross-reactivities towards hCS indicated the existence of several epitopes within the antigenic structure of the intact hormone.[32] This assumption was confirmed by the results of antibody-antibody competition assays which provided direct evidence for the presence of distinct antigenic determinants within the structural moieties which are either unique or shared between hGH and hCS. Considering the very close homology between the primary structure of these two hormones, it seems that the difference in a few amino acids can generate pronounced changes in molecular conformation. Since hGH and hCS have almost equal lactogenic effects but hGH is about ten times more potent in somatotropic activity,[1] it is tempting to speculate that the latter biological activity and the hormone-specific epitopes may be structurally related. An answer to this question by modulating the hormone's biological effects or of the hormone's binding to purified specific membrane receptors by monoclonal antibodies is now open to experimental study. Previous studies using reciprocally mixed hGH-hCS recombinant molecules suggested that the hormone-specific antigenic determinants, as well as the sites binding to purified somatotropic and lactogenic receptors resided at the amino-terminal part of the molecule.[55] Considering that the binding of 20K-hGH and TAP-digested hGH (both with deletions at the N-terminus) to either of the monoclonal anti-hGH antibodies was unimpaired, it seems that the antigenically active site must be determined by sequences which are beyond residue 46 from the amino terminal part of the molecule. Further analysis of the antigenic structure of recombinant hormones using monoclonal antibodies would seem to be desirable.

Since the formation of immune complexes seems to result from the binding of antibodies to monovalent antigenic sites, the affinity of interaction is lower than the average avidity of antibodies of different specificities from conventional antisera when reacting with the multideterminant hormone molecule. This represents a disadvantage for the practical application of monoclonal-antibodies for standard displacement radioimmunoassays of hormone levels. This obstacle can be attributed to the general features of the antigenic structure of hormones of this category and it seems unlikely that it could be overcome by a more intensive search for high affinity antibody secreting hybridomas. Nevertheless, the problem may possibly be resolved by the use of reagents prepared by an optimal combination of antibodies of complementary epitope specificity and/or by the application of ''excess-antibody'' radioimmunometric assays.[15,56]

ACKNOWLEDGMENTS

I wish to thank Dr. C. Moreno for his valuable suggestions at various stages of this study. I am grateful also to Drs. D. R. Bangham, G. Bauman, S. Ellis, C. R. Hopkins, B. Hurn, R. Kofler, U. J. Lewis, A. C. Palladini, J. M. Polak, and M. Wallis for their contribution of unpublished data and for providing materials for investigation.

REFERENCES

1. **Wallis, M.,** The chemistry of pituitary growth hormone, prolactin, and related hormones, and its relationship to biological activity, in *Chemistry and Biochemistry of Amino Acids, Peptides and Proteins,* Vol. 5, Weinstein, B., Ed., Marcel Dekker, New York, 1978, 213.
2. **Lewis, U. D., Singh, R. N. P., Tutwiler, G. F., Sigel, M. B., Vanderlaan, E. F., and Vanderlaan, W. P.,** Human growth hormone—a complex of proteins, *Recent Prog. Horm. Res.* 36, 477, 1980.
3. **Friesen, H. G.,** A tale of stature (Raben Lecture), *Endocrine Rev.,* 1, 309. 1980.
4. **Martial, J. A., Hallewell, R., Baxter, J. D., and Goodman, H. M.,** Human growth hormone: complementary DNA cloning and expression in bacteria *Science,* 205, 602, 1979.
5. **Wallis, M.,** The molecular evolution of pituitary growth hormone, prolactin, and placental lactogen: a protein family showing variable rates of evolution, *J. Molec. Evol.* 17, 10, 1981.
6. **Josimovich, J. B. and MacLaren, J. A.,** Presence in the human placenta and term serum of a highly lactogenic substance immunologically related to pituitary growth hormone, *Endocrinology,* 71, 209, 1962.
7. **Sonsken, P. H. and West, T. E. T.,** Growth hormone, in *Hormones in Blood,* Vol. 1, 3rd ed., Gray, C. H. and James, V. H. T., Eds., Academic Press, New York, 1979, 225.
8. **Chard, T.,** Human placental lactogen, in *Hormones in Blood,* Vol. 1, 3rd ed., Gray, C. H. and James, V. H. T., Eds., Academic Press, New York, 1979, 333.
9. **Franks, S.,** Prolactin, in *Hormones in Blood,* Vol. 1, 3rd ed., Gray, C. H. and James, V. H. T., Eds., Academic Press, New York, 1979, 279.
10. **Hall, K. and Fryklund, L.,** Somatomedins, in *Hormones in Blood,* Vol. 1, 3rd ed., Gray, C. H. and James, V. H. T., Eds., Academic Press, New York, 1979, 255.
11. **Waters, M. J. and Friesen, H. G.,** Purification and partial characterization of a nonprimate growth hormone receptor, *J. Biol. Chem.,* 254, 6815, 1979.
12. **Hunter, W. M. and Greenwood, F. C.,** A radio-immunoelectrophoretic assay for human growth hormone, *Biochem. J.,* 91, 43, 1964.
13. **Schalach, D. S. and Parker, M. L.,** A sensitive double antibody immunoassay for human growth hormone in plasma, *Nature (London),* 203, 1141, 1964.
14. **Peake, G. T., Morris, J., and Buckman, M. T.,** Growth hormone, in *Methods of Hormone Radioimmunoassay,* Jaffe, B. M. and Behrman, H. R., Eds., Academic Press, New York, 1979, 223.
15. **Miles, L. E. M. and Hales, C. N.,** Immunoradiometric assay of human growth hormone, *Lancet,* 2, 492, 1968.
16. **Guyda, H. J. and Friesen, H. G.,** The separation of monkey prolactin from monkey growth hormone by affinity chromatography, *Biochem. Biophys. Res. Commun.,* 42, 1068, 1971.
17. **Pasteels, J. L., Gausset, P., Danguy, A., and Ectors, F.,** Immunoflorescent studies on prolactin and the pituitary, in *Prolactin and Carcinogenesis,* Boyns, A. R. and Griffiths, K., Eds., Alpha Omega, Medford, Ore., 1972, 128.
18. **Healy, D. L., Muller, H. K., and Burger, H. G.,** Immunofluorescence shows localisation of prolactin to human amnion, *Nature (London),* 265, 642, 1977.
19. **Hayashida, T.,** Immunochemical and biological studies with antisera to pituitary growth hormones, in *Hormonal Proteins and Peptides,* Vol. 3, Li, C. H., Ed., Academic Press, New York, 1975, 41.
20. **Tashjian, A. H., Levine, L., and Wilhelmi, A. E.,** Immunochemical relatedness of porcine, bovine, ovine, and primate pituitary growth hormones, *Endocrinology,* 77, 563, 1965.
21. **Tashjian, A., Levine, L., Wilhelmi, E., and Parker, M. L.,** Rabbit, guinea pig, rat, and human antibodies to human growth hormone: immunological reactions with human and non-human primate growth hormones, *Endocrinology,* 79, 615, 1966.
22. **Gusdon, J. P., Leake, N. H., van Dyke, A. H., and Atkins, W.,** Immunochemical comparison of human placental lactogen and placental proteins from other species, *Amer. J. Obstet. Gynecol.,* 107, 441, 1970.
23. **Hwang, P., Guyda, H., and Friesen, H.,** A radioimmunoassay for human prolactin, *Proc. Natl. Acad. Sci. U.S.A.,* 68, 1902, 1971.
24. **Jacobs, L. S.,** Prolactin, in *Methods of Hormone Radioimmunoassay,* Jaffe, B. M. and Behrman, H. R., Eds., Academic Press, New York, 1979, 199.
25. **Aubert, M. L., Grumbach, M. M., and Kaplan, S. L.,** Heterologous radioimmunoassay for plasma human prolactin (hPRL): values in normal subjects, puberty, pregnancy, and in pituitary disorders, *Acta Endocrinol., (Copenhagen),* 77, 460, 1974.
26. **Illig, R., Prader, A., Ferrandez, A., and Zachmann, M.,** Hereditary prenatal growth hormone deficiency with increased tendency to growth hormone antibody formation, in *Symp. Dtsch. Ges. Endokrinol.,* 16, 246, 1970.

27. **Aubert, M. L., Bewley, T. A., Grumbach, M. M., and Kaplan, S. L.,** Studies on the relation of molecular conformation of human growth hormone and human chorionic somatomammotropin to activity, in *Advances in Human Growth Hormone Research,* S. Raiti, Ed., Department of Health, Education and Welfare Publ. No. (NIH), 435, 1974.
28. **Murphy, G. and McGarry, E. E.,** Antibodies to porcine growth hormone induced by treatment with human growth hormone, *J. Clin. Endocrinol. Metab.,* 32, 641, 1971.
29. **Biozzi, G., Mouton, D., Sant'Anna, O. A., Passos, H. C., Gennari, M., Reis, M. H., Ferreira, V. C. A., Heumann, A. M., Bouthillier, Y., Ibanez, O. M., Stiffel, C., and Siqueira, M.,** Genetics of immunoresponsiveness to natural antigens in the mouse, *Current Topics in Microbiol. Immunol.,* 85, 31, 1979.
30. **Köhler, G. and Milstein, C.,** Continuous cultures of fused cells secreting antibody of predefined specificity, *Nature (London),* 256, 495, 1975.
31. **Galfre, G., Howe, S. C., Milstein, C., Butcher, G. W., and Howard, J. C.,** Antibodies to major histocompatibility antigens produced by hybrid cell lines, *Nature (London),* 266, 550, 1977.
32. **Ivanyi, J. and Davies, P.,** Monoclonal antibodies against human growth hormone, *Mol. Immunol.,* 17, 287, 1980.
33. **Ivanyi, J. and Davies, P.,** Monoclonal antibodies to human prolactin and chorionic somatomammotropin, in *Proteins and Related Subjects,* Vol. 29, Peters, H., Ed., 1981.
34. **van Noorden, S. and Polak, J. M.,** unpublished data, 1980.
35. **Kofler, R. and Ivanyi, J.,** unpublished data, 1980.
36. **Williamson, A. R.,** Antibody isoelectric spectra. Analysis of the heterogeneity of antibody molecules in serum by isoelectric focusing in gel and specific detection with hapten, *Eur. J. Immunol.,* 1, 390, 1971.
37. **Roy, B. P. and Friesen, H. G.,** Radioimmuno- and radioreceptor assays of placental lactogens, in *Methods of Hormone Radioimmunoassay,* Jaffe, B. M. and Behrman, H. R., Eds., Academic Press, New York, 1979, 831.
38. **Lewis, U. J., Dunn, J. T., Bonewald, L. F., Seavey, B. K., and Vanderlaan, W. P.,** A naturally occurring structural variant of human growth hormone, *J. Biol. Chem.,* 253, 2679, 1978.
39. **Lewis, U. J., Bonewald, L. F., and Lewis, L. J.,** The 20,000 dalton variant of human growth hormone location of the amino acid deletions, *Biochem. Biophys, Res. Commun.,* 92, 511, 1980.
40. **Frigeri, L. G., Peterson, S. M., and Lewis, U. J.,** The 20,000 dalton structural varient of human growth hormone: lack of some early insulin-like effects, *Biochem. Biophys. Res. Commun.,* 91, 778, 1979.
41. **Chrambach, A., Yadley, R. A., Ben-David, M., and Rodbard, D.,** Isohormones of human growth hormone. I. Characterization by electrophoresis and isoelectric focusing in polyacrylamide gel, *Endocrinology,* 93, 848, 1973.
42. **Bauman, G.,** unpublished data, 1980.
43. **Wallis, M., Surowy, T. K., Daniels, M., Hartree, A. S., and Fosten, A.,** An investigation of the heterogeneity of clinical grade human growth hormone, *J. Endocrinol.,* 87, 54, 1980.
44. **Bewley, T. A., Brovetto-Cruz, J., and Li, C. H.,** Human pituitary growth hormone. Physiochemical investigations of the native and reduced-alkylated protein, *Biochemistry,* 8, 4701, 1969.
45. **Poskus, E., Zakin, M. M., Fernandez, H. N., and Paladini, A. C.,** Detection of immunologically active zones in equine growth hormone, *Eur. J. Immunol.,* 6, 409, 1976.
46. **Pena, C., Poskus, E., and Paladini, A. C.,** A relevant antigenic site in human growth hormone localised in sequence, 98–128, *Mol. Immunol.,* 17, 1487, 1980.
47. **Paladini, A. C., Poskus, E., Pena, C., Vita, N., and Perez, E.** unpublished data, 1980.
48. **Doebber, T. W., Divor, A. R., and Ellis, S.,** Identification of a tripeptidyl aminopeptidase in the anterior pituitary gland: effect on the chemical and biological properties of rat and bovine growth hormones, *Endocrinology,* 103, 1794, 1978.
49. **Jerne, N. K.,** Immunological speculations, *Annu. Rev. Microbiol.,* 14, 341, 1960.
50. **Ivanyi, J.,** Competition and affinity assay of monoclonal antibodies against human growth hormone, in *Proteins and Related Subjects,* Vol. 28, Peters, H., Ed., Pergamon Press, Oxford, 1980, 471.
51. **Ivanyi, J.,** Paratope specificity of monoclonal antibodies to human growth hormone, in *Monoclonal Antibodies and T Cell Hybridomas,* Hämmerling, G. J., Hämmerling, U., and Kearney, J. F., Eds., Elsevier/North Holland, Amsterdam, 1981, 349.
52. **Fraker, P. J. and Speck, J. C.,** Protein and cell membrane iodinations with a sparingly soluble chloroamide, 1, 3, 4, 6-tetrachloro-3a, 6a-diphenylglycoluril, *Biochem. Biophys. Res. Comm.,* 80, 849, 1978.
53. **Ivanyi, J.,** Ir-gene control of the murine antibody response to human growth hormone (unpublished results)

54. **Orth, D. N.,** Adrenocorticotropic hormone (ACTH), in *Methods of Hormone Radioimmunoassay,* 2nd ed., Jaffe, B. M. and Behrman, H. R., Eds., Academic Press, New York, 1979, 245.
55. **Burstein, S., Grumbach, M. M., Kaplan, S. L., and Li, C. H.,** Immunoreactivity and receptor binding of mixed recombinants of human growth hormone and chorionic somatomammotropin, *Proc. Natl. Acad. Sci. U.S.A.,* 75, 5391. 1978.
56. **Lader, S. R., Seig, D., and Ivanyi, J.,** Monoclonal antibodies as reagents for radioimmunoassay, in XIth Int. Cong. Clinical Chemistry, Vienna, 1981.

Chapter 3

ANTIBODIES TO ALPHAFETOPROTEIN AND CARCINOEMBRYONIC ANTIGEN PRODUCED BY SOMATIC CELL FUSION

Herbert Z. Kupchik

TABLE OF CONTENTS

I. INTRODUCTION

Carcinoembryonic antigen (CEA) is a glycoprotein of approximately 200,000 daltons described by Gold and Freedman[1,2] as an antigen present exclusively in adenocarcinoma of the human digestive tract and in digestive organs from fetuses of 2 to 6 months gestation. In 1969, a radioimmunoassay for CEA in the serum of patients was described.[3] Circulating levels as low as 2.5 ng/mℓ of serum were reported in 35 of 36 patients with adenocarcinoma of the colon and ''insignificant'' levels were found in the serum of patients with nongastrointestinal malignancies or benign diseases. These findings, plus the disappearance of CEA from the circulation of patients following complete surgical removal of tumor, offered the promise of an early diagnostic procedure for patients with digestive system cancer. Studies from many laboratories have now established that whereas a positive CEA assay may be a good indicator of invasive colonic cancer, and particularly of metastases to the liver, CEA elevation occurs in less than 50% of patients with localized disease (Dukes' Stage A).[4,5] The circulating CEA level apparently depends upon several factors, including the pathological stage and degree of differentiation of the primary tumor, the presence of invasion of lymphatics, blood vessels or perineural spaces, the extent of distant spread of tumor, and the total mass of CEA-producing tumor.[6] The involvement of the liver and its functional status is believed to be of especial importance.[7] Additionally, CEA has been identified and measured in the circulation and body fluids of patients with numerous nongastrointestinal malignancies, patients with gastrointestinal benign diseases, and normal individuals using assays with conventionally produced antisera.[4,8]

This lack of specificity has been attributed both to heterogeneity of purportedly purified CEA and to its variable intramolecular antigenicity.[9] It is also possible that some individual antigenic determinants identified in present CEA assays are associated with CEA molecules synthesized by normal gastrointestinal tissues and only quantitatively distinct in the presence of malignancy.

Although most investigators agree that CEA isolated from gastrointestinal tumors or from plasma of patients with such tumors has a molecular weight of approximately 200,000, the CEA in plasma of patients with other malignancies has been shown to be approximately 370,000.[10,11] The carbohydrate to protein ratio can range from 1:1 in preparations from colonic tissue to 5:1 in those from gastric cancer tissue, and differences have been noted on polyacrylamide gel electrophoresis and on isoelectric focusing of preparations from different sources.[12,13] Numerous studies have confirmed that much of the apparent heterogeneity of CEA is a reflection of differences in the carbohydrate portion of the molecule. The varying sialic acid content probably accounts for a good deal of the heterogeneity seen during gel electrophoresis.

Although protein sequence studies on CEA have been hampered by the high (approximately 50%) carbohydrate content and the relatively large number of amino acids (over 600), recent studies have shown that polypeptide fragments can be obtained by limited proteolysis.[14,15] These studies indicated that the polypeptide chain of CEA is reproducible from preparation to preparation and contains the tumor associated antigenic site recognized by conventional heteroantisera.

Several studies have indicated that the CEA-like antigens identified as nonspecific cross-reacting antigen (NCA), normal glycoprotein (NGP), colonic carcinoembryonic antigen-2, breast carcinoma glycoprotein, colon carcinoma antigen III, and tumor-associated antigen may be identical and that they do not cross-react in radioimmunoassays for CEA performed on perchloric acid extracts.[16] Recent studies of their amino acid sequences suggested that the protein component of CEA and such CEA-like molecules are closely related.[17] These authors proposed that the protein backbone is under control of related genes from a common evolutionary origin.

Antisera obtained from monkeys immunized with CEA were more specific for CEA than those produced by sheep or rabbits.[18] The monkey antisera did not react against the CEA-NCA common site determinants. These authors suggested that monkeys have a normally occurring antigen similar to NCA.

Although most appropriately absorbed anti-CEA antisera prepared against different preparations of CEA to date have been immunochemically indistinguishable, it is apparent that more highly specific antibodies are required.

Alphafetoprotein (AFP) is a glycoprotein of between 65,000 and 70,000 daltons first identified by Bergstrand Czar in 1956 as X-component in human cord blood.[19] In 1963, Abelev et al. demonstrated that this embryonal α-globulin was not only detected in normal pregnant mice and the sera of newborn mice, but also in mice bearing hepatocellular carcinomas.[20] Subsequently, in 1964, Tatarinov identified AFP in the sera of patients with primary liver tumors.[21] It now appears that AFP is first produced in the yolk sac and later in the liver of the embryo. AFP synthesis in the liver subsides or is depressed after birth and can be found in only extremely low amounts in the adult except in the presence of hepatomas or teratomas. Albumin and AFP have similar chemical properties and their concentrations in serum are high and inversely related.[22] This plus the additional evidence that there is a homologous sequence of amino acids in AFP and albumin suggest that these two proteins have a common ancestor.[23] Circulating levels of AFP can be used to diagnose and monitor treatment of patients with primary liver cancers and germ cell tumors. More recently, the measurement of AFP in maternal serum and in amniotic fluid during pregnancy has been useful for the prenatal diagnosis of spina bifida and congenital nephrosis.[24] Although more homogeneous and reproducible than CEA, AFP has been shown to exist as molecular variants which are not distinguishable by conventional antisera.[25] Ruoslahti et al.[25] prepared three different variants of human AFP from fetal serum and amniotic fluid by concanavalin A-Sepharose (ConA) chromatography. Their results suggested that the AFP synthesized by the liver and by the yolk-sac tissue are glycosylated differently. They suggested that methods which could distinguish between such variants might be diagnostically useful in distinguishing between the AFP associated with liver regeneration and that produced by malignant cells. This might be accomplished by the use of monoclonal antibodies to AFP. Such antibodies might also be extremely useful in elucidating factors which regulate AFP production and lead to an understanding of the pathogenesis of AFP producing tumors.

The recent adaptation of cell hybridization techniques to the construction of myeloma-like cell lines producing monoclonal antibodies with desired reactivities has essentially revolutionized the approach to production and utilization of immunospecific reagents.[26] This procedure has been described in detail by Zola and Brooks in Chapter 1. The advantage of this technique in studying antigens as variable as CEA and AFP is that each hybrid clone produces a single species of antibody specific for a single antigenic determinant regardless of the complexity of the antigen. These "hybridomas" can be propagated in culture and/or in pristane primed mice where milligram per milliliter quantities of monoclonal antibody can be obtained from ascitic fluid.

Thus, investigators have begun the search for monoclonal antibodies to both CEA and AFP using somatic cell fusion in order to separate out the heterogeneity seen with these markers and increase the clinical utility of assays for both. The following is an attempt to highlight some of the methods used and the concepts which have become apparent during these studies.

II. METHODS

A. Immunization

Both CEA and AFP are sufficiently good antigens when injected into animals such as goats, rabbits, guinea pigs, sheep, etc., so that after appropriate absorption, antisera of high titer and affinity can be obtained. The same situation appears to prevail in immunizing mice for subsequent somatic cell fusion. Nevertheless, Accolla et al.[14] did report a series of negative results before obtaining hybrids which produced anti-CEA antibodies. The cause of the negative results was not identified.

Table 1 provides a summary of the successful immunization schedules used by various investigators for the production of hybridoma antibodies to AFP and CEA. All used BALB/c mice and gave the initial immunization(s) with purified antigen either intraperitoneally (i.p.) or subcutaneously (s.c.) in complete Freund's adjuvant. The last booster injection was usually given intravenously (i.v.), in buffer or saline, 3 to 4 days prior to removal of the spleen for hybridization. It should also be noted that all of the immunization protocols were performed over a relatively short duration of time (1 to 3 months). An exception to this was the report of Lockhart et al.[32] regarding the successful production of anti-CEA hybridomas using splenic lymphocytes from hyperimmunized mice.

B. Hybridization

The investigators identified in Table 1 reported fairly uniform descriptions of their cell fusion techniques. Each used either the P3×63-Ag8 (×63) or P3NS1/1-AG4 (NS1) plasmacytoma derivatives of the MOPC-21 myeloma cell line. Both of these lines grow in 8-azaguanine and lack the enzyme hypoxanthine guanine phosphoribosyl transferase required for rapid growth in tissue culture medium containing hypoxanthine, aminopterin and thymidine (HAT). The ×63 line secretes its own IgG_1 myeloma protein while the NS1 does not make the IgG heavy chain. All investigators fused approximately 1×10^8 spleen cells with 1 to 3×10^7 myeloma cells in the presence of 30 to 50% polyethylene glycol (PEG) MW 1000 or 1500. Fused cells were diluted and dispensed into 96 or 24 well plates where they were grown in HAT selection medium for the next 2 to 3 weeks. During this time, the growing hybrid cells were tested for antibody activity. Antibody producing cells were passaged and cloned as soon as possible in most instances to avoid overgrowth by nonproducing cells (that is cells producing antibodies of unknown specificities).

C. Antibody Screening Assays

Hybrid cell culture fluids have been assayed for the presence of anti-AFP or anti-CEA antibodies by various techniques. Tsung et al.[29] and Accolla et al.[27] used modifications of the Farr radioimmunoassay (RIA) technique[33] to assay for AFP and CEA respectively. Schröder[28] also used a liquid phase RIA but precipitated antigen-antibody complexes with 12% PEG 6000 in the presence of normal human serum instead of the ammonium sulfate used in the Farr RIA. Uotila et al.[30] used a sensitive enzyme immunoassay sandwich technique. Here, microtiter wells were coated with 10 to 100 ng AFP. Diluted samples of culture media were incubated in the AFP wells (in the presence of Tween 20®) and, after washing, peroxidase conjugated rabbit antibodies to mouse immunoglobulins were incubated in the wells. Enzymatic activity bound to the wells was measured with o-phenylene diamine as chromagen. In this laboratory we also used a microtiter plate sandwich assay; coating the wells with 5 μg CEA and using radiolabeled goat antimouse antibody as the second antibody. Each of these assays was used as a sensitive indicator for the presence of antibodies to AFP or CEA in the culture

Table 1
SUMMARY OF IMMUNIZATION PROTOCOLS FOR ANTI-AFP AND ANTI-CEA ANTIBODY PRODUCING SPLENIC LYMPHOCYTES IN MICE

Antigen	Dose (μg)	Schedule[a]	Ref.
AFP	100.0	4 (i.p.)/6 weeks; 2 (i.v.)/4 weeks	28
AFP	12.5	5 (i.p.)/4 weeks	29
AFP	50.0	3–4 (s.c.)/9–12 weeks; 1 (i.v.)	30
CEA	15.0	1 (i.p.)/2 months; 1 (i.v.)	27
CEA	8.0	1 (i.p.)/1 month; 1 (i.v.)	31

[a]Schedules show the number of doses (route of administration) over a specific time period. Abbreviations: i.p.—intraperitoneal; s.c.—subcutaneous; i.v.—intravenous.

fluid in which hybrid cells were growing as early as possible to select those cells for further passage. In general, the assays described above were not used for the quantitation of antibody nor for determination of relative affinities.

III. RESULTS

A. AlphaFetoprotein

Despite the similarities in immunization and fusion protocols used by various investigators, some differences in the antibodies obtained have become apparent.

Tsung et al.[29] showed that their monoclonal antibody to AFP was of the IgG_1 subclass. Association-dissociation kinetics demonstrated rapid and complete association kinetics as compared to anti-AFP antisera from both an early bleed (10 weeks) and a late bleed (18 months) of a goat immunized with the purified AFP. The monoclonal antibody was also of very high avidity with little dissociation and was comparable to the hyperimmunized goat antiserum in that regard. They suggested that the monoclonal antibody would serve as an ideal reagent in classical RIAs for AFP, immunohistological studies and for localizing AFP producing tumors in patients. No studies on the specificity of the monoclonal antibody were reported.

Uotila et al.[30] reported that the IgG_1 monoclonal anti-AFP antibody they produced was capable of binding the same amount (approximately 90%) of labeled AFP as could conventional antisera and showed that nanogram amounts of unlabeled AFP could inhibit the binding of monoclonal antibody to ^{125}[I]-AFP. In addition, assays based on monoclonal anti-AFP antibody appeared to have a clinical specificity and sensitivity similar to their assay using conventional antisera when normal sera, sera and amniotic fluid from pregnant women, sera from patients with teratocarcinoma or hepatoblastoma patients or international AFP standards were tested.

Schröder studied the characteristics of the IgG_1 anti-AFP antibody produced by one of several clones developed in his laboratory. In his hands, significant inhibition of binding between the monoclonal antibody and ^{125}[I]-AFP required approximately tenfold more purified AFP than necessary when conventional goat antiserum was used in a comparable assay system.[28] However, analyses of serum and amniotic fluid samples for AFP concentrations showed no systematic differences between assays utilizing the two antibodies. He concluded that the monoclonal antibody offered no advantages over conventional antisera in the RIA. Schröder did demonstrate, however, that the monoclonal antibody could be useful for affinity purification of AFP using mild reagents for elution.

B. Carcinoembryonic Antigen

Accolla et al.[27] were able to identify two different monoclonal anti-CEA antibodies (one IgG_1 and the other IgG_2) after screening 400 hybrids from seven fusions. The IgG_1 antibody could bind up to 80% of their purified ^{125}[I]-CEA and 0.4 ng of purified CEA could inhibit this binding. The IgG_2 antibody could bind up to 65% of the labeled antigen but had a sensitivity of 1/70th that seen with the IgG_1 antibody in inhibition studies. Neither antibody showed any significant reactivity with the crossreacting antigen NGP.[34] Verification of the specificity of these two monoclonal antibodies was provided by immunohistochemical localization of CEA on frozen sections of human colon carcinoma and on the surface of colon carcinoma cell lines.[35] Differences in the relative affinities ($1.4 \times 10^8 M^{-1}$ and $1.1 \times 10^7 M^{-1}$, respectively) for these two antibodies were suggested as the reason for differences in sensitivity.

Lindgren and Bång reported the production of four monoclonal anti-CEA antibodies which did not react with NGP and had affinities high enough for RIA.[36] Another four monoclonal antibodies were specific for CEA but had low affinities and two others crossreacted with NGP. Lockhart et al.[37] reported the production of a hybridoma anti-CEA antibody which could bind up to 70% of ^{125}I-labeled CEA and was completely blocked by unlabeled CEA. No additional specificity studies were reported.

We were able to produce a number of hybridoma cell lines which produced anti-CEA antibodies with varying capacities for binding ^{125}[I]-CEA.[31] One of these was cloned and resulted in the production of a monoclonal IgG_1 antibody to CEA which was capable of binding only approximately 70% of the ^{125}[I]-CEA bound by conventional goat anti-CEA antiserum. The monoclonal antibody had a lower relative binding affinity ($1.0 \times 10^8 M^{-1}$) than did conventional goat antiserum ($1.9 \times 10^9 M^{-1}$) in a solid phase RIA and had a sensitivity for unlabeled CEA approximately half that seen with the goat antiserum in inhibition studies. The monoclonal antibody was found useful in immunohistochemical studies for the localization of CEA in tissue sections and colonic cancer cells.

IV. DISCUSSION

The studies presented here demonstrate that monoclonal antibodies to AFP and CEA can be produced by the somatic cell fusion technique.[26] This is important in itself because these are both human tumor markers that have found their way into the clinical testing laboratory. Assays for these markers have been demonstrated as clinically useful in spite of limitations inherent in the heterogeneity of the reagents used. The production of monoclonal antibodies specific for AFP or CEA would appear to present several advantages over conventional antisera.

One of the most obvious advantages would be the potential high specificity. This would be extremely desirable for CEA. Conventional anti-CEA antisera recognize several determinants and frequently require absorption to eliminate reactions with NGP, a normal glycoprotein which crossreacts with CEA and can be found in many normal tissues.[4] It is this heterogeneity of the antisera and purified CEA used in clinical assays that is thought by some to be responsible, at least in part, for the relative lack of diagnostic specificity in a clinical setting. In this regard, although some investigators have described their monoclonal anti-CEA antibodies as specific for CEA, appropriate tests of specificity have not been performed on serum specimens from patients with different cancers or benign diseases responsible for positive results in conventional assays. Similarly, although Uotila et al.[30] have shown in preliminary studies that assays for AFP using their monoclonal antibody exhibit comparable sensitivity and specificity as assays with conventional antisera to AFP, they have not succeeded in distinguishing among molecular variants of AFP which might lead to improved diagnostic applicability.

Another advantage of monoclonal antibodies over conventional antisera is the relatively unlimited supply of antibodies with constant and well characterized specificities, affinities, and titers. After i.p. injection of viable hybridoma cells into mice previously "primed" with pristane, 2 to 6 mg of antibody can frequently be recovered per milliliter of ascites produced (which can amount to 10 to 20 mℓ before the animal succumbs to the tumor innoculum). Obviously this still remains a potential benefit to investigators attempting to develop improved assays for AFP and CEA and could lead to world-wide standardization of reagents and assays.

It has become increasingly apparent that monoclonal antibodies are frequently of not sufficiently high affinity to be immediately introduced into assay systems in which conventional antisera of high affinity have been used. The differences in affinity between conventional antisera and monoclonal antibodies may be due to the availability of several antibodies in an antiserum creating a synergistic effect. The low affinity of monoclonal antibodies may be overcome if monoclonal antibodies for different epitopes on a specific variant of AFP or CEA can be combined in assay systems. An additional utility of combining different monoclonal antibodies in an assay system has been demonstrated by Uotila et al.[38] They were able to develop a sandwich enzyme-linked immunospecific assay in which AFP was bound by one monoclonal antibody immobilized on polystyrene microtiter plates as well as by a second enzyme-labeled monoclonal antibody which recognized a different site on the same AFP molecule. These authors state, "The rapidity, simplicity, and excellent sensitivity of this assay combined with the exquisite specificity associated with the use of two monoclonal antibodies make us believe that assays based on this principle will be useful in the quantitation of substances of medical and biological importance." It would appear that this type of research will be necessary for future effective clinical application of monoclonal antibodies in AFP and/or CEA assays. That is, it is not sufficient to simply substitute a monoclonal antibody for a conventional antiserum in an assay designed for the conventional antiserum.

One must also beware of dependence upon "purified" antigens to which the conventional antisera were prepared. The exquisite specificity of monoclonal antibodies makes it possible to recognize a single determinant on an antigen which may have several determinants identified by a heteroantiserum. Variants of the antigen may appear to be physicochemically and immunochemically identical to each other when using the antiserum for evaluation, but may be defined as "different" by different monoclonal antibodies. For example, our monoclonal antibody could bind only approximately 70% of the radiolabeled purified CEA bound by goat anti-CEA antiserum; thus, it would appear that there are at least two species of CEA in the preparation bound by goat antiserum. Inhibition of the binding of one of these species (the 70%) with purified unlabeled CEA (quantitated as a single pure reagent using goat antiserum) will yield a potentially misleading estimation of the sensitivity of the monoclonal antibody. A similar argument could be made for affinity determinations.

It would be more appropriate to further purify the CEA (both labeled and unlabeled) by immunoadsorption using the monoclonal antibody prior to the use of these reagents in the assay. In this way, inhibition and affinity studies of the monoclonal antibodies would be performed with the antigens recognized by the antibodies rather than potentially heterogeneous mixtures. In addition, the ionic strength and/or pH of the incubation milieu may also require modification to be optimal for monoclonal antibodies. We are in the process of performing such experiments in this laboratory to determine the affinity and sensitivity of our monoclonal antibody for the species of CEA recognized by it.

The use of monoclonal antibodies for the purification of AFP and CEA represents another extremely important development. Schröder pointed out that monoclonal antibodies that recognize a single determinant but have low affinities will have a restricted binding strength and will require only a mild reagent for elution of the antigen from an immunoadsorbent column.[39] He was able to prepare an immunoadsorbent column having a high capacity for AFP per unit volume of gel and achieved 10,000-fold purification following elution with 4.0 *M* Urea in Tris-HCl buffer (pH 7.4).[28]

Other areas in which specific monoclonal antibodies to AFP and CEA may play a role are (1) for therapy and/or localization (using labeled antibody) of tumors in patients—an area currently being explored by numerous investigators using conventional antisera; (2) the use of anti-AFP and/or anti-CEA antibodies of predetermined tissue specificities for immunohistochemical characterization of surgical specimens; and (3) studies to define the biological function of AFP and CEA.

V. SUMMARY

During these early days of the ''hybridoma era'' several monoclonal antibodies to AFP and CEA have already been produced in milligram quantities. Studies to date have shown that these antibodies are neither more sensitive nor specific for AFP and CEA than conventional antisera. However, it is apparent that these antibodies are the forerunners of new and more useful reagents and are already serving to introduce new concepts and potential applications of both AFP and CEA for improved clinical utility.

REFERENCES

1. **Gold, P. and Freedman, S. O.,** Demonstration of tumor specific antigens in human colon carcinoma by immunologic tolerance absorption techniques, *J. Exp. Med.,* 121, 439, 1965.
2. **Gold, P. and Freedman, S. O.,** Specific carcinoembryonic antigens of the human digestive system, *J. Exp. Med.,* 122, 467, 1965.
3. **Thomson, D. M. P., Krupey, J., Freedman, S. O., and Gold, P.,** The radioimmunoassay of circulating carcinoembryonic antigen of the human digestive system, *Proc. Natl. Acad. Sci. USA.,* 64, 161, 1969.
4. **Kupchik, H. Z., Zamcheck, N., and Saravis, C. A.,** Immunochemical studies of carcinoembryonic antigens: methodologic consideration and some clinical implications, in *Aspects of Cancer Research 1971—1978,* National Cancer Institute Monograph No. 52, 1979, 413.
5. **Zamcheck, N., Moore, T. L., Dhar, P., and Kupchik, H. Z.,** Immunologic diagnosis and prognosis of human digestive tract cancer, *N. Engl. J. Med.,* 286, 83, 1972.
6. **Zamcheck, N., Doos, W. G., Prudente, R., Lurie, B. B., and Gottlieb, L. S.,** Prognostic factors in colon carcinoma: correlation of serum carcinoembryonic antigen level and tumor histopathology. *J. Human Pathol.,* 6, 31, 1975.
7. **Loewenstein, M. S. and Zamcheck, N.,** Carcinoembryonic antigen and the liver, *Gastroenterology,* 72, 161, 1977.
8. **Zamcheck, N. and Kupchik, H. A.,** Summary of clinical use and limitations of the carcinoembryonic antigen assay and some methodological considerations, in *Manual of Clinical Immunology,* Rose, N. R. and Friedman, M., Eds., American Cancer Society, Washington, D.C., 1980, 919.
9. **Fuks, A., Banjo, C., Shuster, J., Freedman, S. O., and Gold, P.,** Carcinoembryonic antigen (CEA): molecular biology and clinical significance, *Biochim. Biophys. Acta,* 417, 123, 1974.
10. **Pletsch, Q. and Goldenberg, D. M.,** Molecular size of carcinoembryonic antigen in the plasma of patients with malignant disease, *J. Natl. Cancer Inst.,* 53, 1201, 1974.
11. **Herzog, B., Hendrick, J. C., and Franchimont, P.,** Heterogeneity of carcinoembryonic antigen (CEA) in human serum, *Eur. J. Cancer,* 12, 657, 1976.
12. **Banjo, C., Schuster, J., and Gold, P.,** Intermolecular heterogeneity of the carcinoembryonic antigen, *Cancer Res.,* 34, 2114, 1974.

13. **Rule, A. H. and Golesky-Reilly, C.,** Carcinoembryonic antigen (CEA): separation of CEA-reacting molecules from tumor, fetal gut, meconium, and normal colon, *Immunol. Commun.,* 2, 213, 1973.
14. **Shively, J. E., Todd, C. W., Go, V. L. W., and Egan, M. L.,** Amino-terminal sequence of a carcinoembryonic antigen-like glycoprotein isolated from the colonic lavages of healthy individuals, *Cancer Res.,* 38, 503, 1978.
15. **Ariel, N., Krantz, M., Inoue, S., and Gold, P.,** Examination of CEA structure by biochemical immunological and electron microscopic techniques, *Protides Biol. Fluid Proc. Colloq.,* 27, 37, 1979.
16. **Newman, E. S., Petras, S. W., Georgiadis, A., and Hansen, H. J.,** Interrelationship of carcinoembryonic antigen and colon carcinoma antigen III, *Cancer Res.,* 34, 2125, 1974.
17. **Shively, J. E., Glassman, J. N. S., Engvall, E., and Todd, C. W.,** Aminoacid sequence of CEA and CEA related antigens, in *Carcinoembryonic Proteins,* Vol. 1, Lehman, F. G., Ed. Elsevier/North Holland Biomedical Press, New York, 1979, 9.
18. **Ruoslahti, E., Engvall, E., Vuento, M., and Wigzell, H.,** Monkey antisera with increased specificity to carcinoembryonic antigen (CEA), *Int. J. Cancer,* 17, 358, 1976.
19. **Bergstrand, C. G. and Czar, B.,** Demonstration of a new protein fraction in serum from the human fetus, *Scand. J. Clin. Lab. Invest.,* 8, 174, 1956.
20. **Abelev, G. I., Perova, S. D., Khramkova, N. I., Postnikova, Z. A., and Irlin, I. S.,** Production of embryonal alpha-globulin by transplantable mouse hepatomas, *Transplantation,* 1, 174, 1963.
21. **Tatarinov, Y.,** Detection of embryospecific alpha-globulin in the blood sera of patients with primary liver tumors, *Vopr. Med. Khim.,* 10, 90, 1964.
22. **Kekomäki, M., Seppälä, M., Ehnholm, C., Schwartz, A. L., and Raivio, K.,** Perfusion of isolated human fetal liver: synthesis and release of alphaFetoprotein and albumin, *Int. J. Cancer,* 8, 250, 1971.
23. **Ruoslahti, E. and Terry, W. D.,** AlphaFetoprotein and serum albumin show sequence homology, *Nature (London),* 260, 804, 1976.
24. **Ruoslahti, E., Pekkala, A., Comings, D. E., and Seppälä, M.,** Determination of subfractions of amniotic fluid alpha-fetoprotein. A new test for diagnosis of spina bifida and congenital nephrosis, *Br. Med. J.,* 2, 768, 1979.
25. **Ruoslahti, E., Engvall, E., Pekkala, A., and Seppälä, M.,** Developmental changes in carbohydrate moiety of human alpha-fetoprotein, *Int. J. Cancer,* 22, 575, 1978.
26. **Köhler, G. and Milstein, C.,** Continuous cultures of fused cells secreting antibody of predefined specificity, *Nature (London),* 256, 495, 1975.
27. **Accolla, R. S., Carrel, S., and Mach, J.-P.,** Monoclonal antibodies specific for carcinoembryonic antigen and produced by two hybrid cell lines, *Proc. Natl. Acad. Sci. USA.,* 77, 563, 1980.
28. **Schröder, J.,** personal communication, 1980.
29. **Tsung, Y.-K., Milunsky, A., and Alpert, E.,** Derivation and characterization a monoclonal hybridoma antibody specific for human alpha-fetoprotein, *J. Immunol. Methods.,* 39, 363, 1980.
30. **Uotila, M., Engvall, E., and Ruoslahti, E.,** Monoclonal antibodies to human alphafetoprotein, *Mol. Immunol.,* 17, 791, 1980.
31. **Kupchik, H. Z., Zurawski, V. R., Hurrell, J. G. R., Zamcheck, N., and Black, P. H.,** Monoclonal antibodies to carcinoembryonic antigen produced by somatic cell fusion, *Cancer Res.,* 41, 3306, 1981.
32. **Lockhart, C. G., Stinson, R. S., Magraf, H. W., Parker, C. W., and Philpott, G. W.,** Production of anti-carcinoembryonic antigen (CEA) antibody by somatic cell hybridization, *Fed. Proc.,* 39, 298, 1980.
33. **Farr, R. S.,** A quantitative immunochemical measure of the primary interaction between I*BSA and antibody, *J. Infect. Dis.,* 103, 239, 1958.
34. **Mach, J. P., Pusztaszeri, G.,** Carcinoembryonic antigen (CEA): demonstration of a partial identity between CEA and normal glycoprotein, *Immunochemistry,* 9, 1031, 1972.
35. **Accolla, R. S., Carrel, S., Phan, M., Heumann, D., and Mach, J.-P.,** First report of the production of somatic cell hybrids secreting monoclonal antibodies specific for carcinoembryonic antigen (CEA), *Protides Biol. Fluid Proc. Colloq.,* 27, 31, 1979.
36. **Lindgren, J. and Bång, B.,** Production of monoclonal antibodies to CEA, presented at 8th Meeting of Int. Soc. Oncodev. Biology and Medicine, Tallinn, U.S.S.R., September 15—19, 1980.
37. **Lockhart, C. G., Stinson, R. S., Margraf, H. W., Parker, C. W., and Philpott, G. W.,** Production of anti-carcinoembryonic antigen (CEA) antibody by somatic cell hybridization, *Fed. Proc.,* 39, 928, 1980.
38. **Uotila, M., Ruoslahti, E., and Engvall, E.,** Two-site sandwich enzyme immunoassay with monoclonal antibodies to human alpha-fetoprotein, *J. Immunol. Methods,* 42, 11, 1981.
39. **Schröder, J.,** Monoclonal antibodies: a new tool for research and immunodiagnostics, *Med. Biol.,* 58, 140, 1980.

Chapter 4

MONOCLONAL ANTIBODIES SPECIFIC FOR CARDIAC MYOSIN: IN VIVO AND IN VITRO DIAGNOSTIC TOOLS IN MYOCARDIAL INFARCTION

Edgar Haber, Hugo A. Katus, John G. Hurrell, Gary R. Matsueda, Paul Ehrlich, Vincent Zurawski, Jr., and Ban-An Khaw

TABLE OF CONTENTS

I. INTRODUCTION

The diagnosis of myocardial infarction often does not present a significant challenge to the clinician. Symptoms may be pathognomonic and so-called objective findings unequivocal. Quite often, however, when it is most important to know, associated injury or disease masks symptoms and distorts the results of laboratory tests, none of which are entirely specific. Beyond the question of diagnosis is quantification. There have been many attempts at investigating methods for arresting the progress of infarction and salvaging as much tissue as possible. It is very difficult to evaluate the efficacy of these interventions without an objective measure in vivo of the extent of cardiac tissue necrosis. Up to the present time, quantification of infarct size has only been possible in retrospect.

Other than the venerable electrocardiogram, the approaches to myocardial infarct evaluation have concentrated on the measurement of the plasma concentration of cytoplasmic proteins that leak from the cell as a result of ischemic damage to the cell membrane. Many of the enzymes measured, such as creatine phosphokinase,[1] lactic dehydrogenase,[2] and glutamic oxalacetic transaminase,[3] are shared by many tissues and therefore are not specific to the heart. Myoglobin is common to both skeletal and cardiac muscle.[4] The MB isozyme of creatine phosphokinase is largely found in cardiac tissue, but its specific determination has been difficult.[5] Cardiac myosin and its light chains are, however, unique structural proteins of cardiac tissue. They may be differentiated antigenically from cardiac- and smooth-muscle myosins and thus offer an opportunity for specifically identifying and quantifying cardiac muscle damage.

We have taken two approaches to myocardial infarct diagnosis, each identifying necrotic tissue by virtue of increased membrane permeability. The first method is akin to the measurement of the release of serum enzymes or myoglobin, but utilizes a more specific marker, cardiac-myosin light chains.[6] The second approach employs radionuclide scintigraphy to visualize the size and extent of the intracardiac lesion. The carrier for the radionuclide is an antibody specific for cardiac myosin. Only those cells that have lost their membrane integrity admit the antibody and allow it to bind to its intracellular antigen.[7]

These methods were first developed utilizing conventionally elicited myosin and myosin-(light chain) antibodies. Because of problems inherent in the lack of specificity of conventional antibodies, as well as significant limitation in supply when extensive clinical applications are contemplated, we turned to monoclonal antibodies produced by the technique of somatic cell fusion.[8]

II. MONOCLONAL ANTIBODIES IN IMMUNOASSAY

The advent of cell fusion methods for selecting and propagating clones of plasma cells that secrete antibodies characterized by molecular homogeneity[8] permits substantial refinement in immunoassay. Antibodies may now be obtained that recognize a single epitope on a protein molecule, which should make it possible to differentiate among antigens that share some common structural features. Since antisera produced by conventional immunization always contain a mixture of many antibodies of varying affinity and specificity, cross reactivity of varying degrees is always observed among antigens that share epitopes. We have encountered this problem in the differentiation between canine[6] and human[9] cardiac- and skeletal-muscle light chains. Each molecule has a unique amino acid sequence,[10] yet there are many structural features in common. The differentiation between cardiac- and skeletal-myosin light chains is of clinical importance because cardiac-myosin light chains are released after myocardial necrosis, and

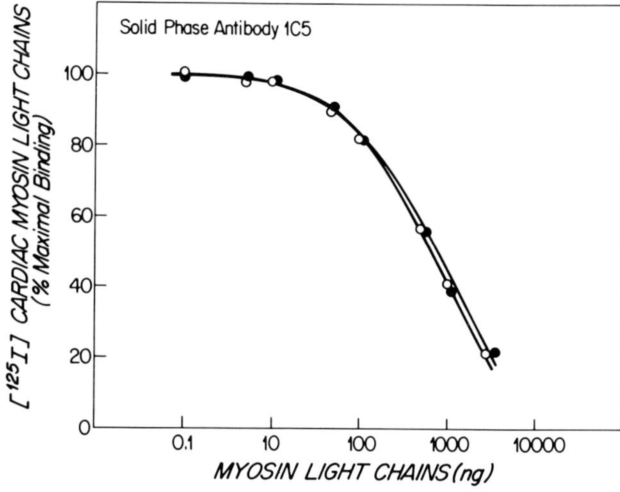

A

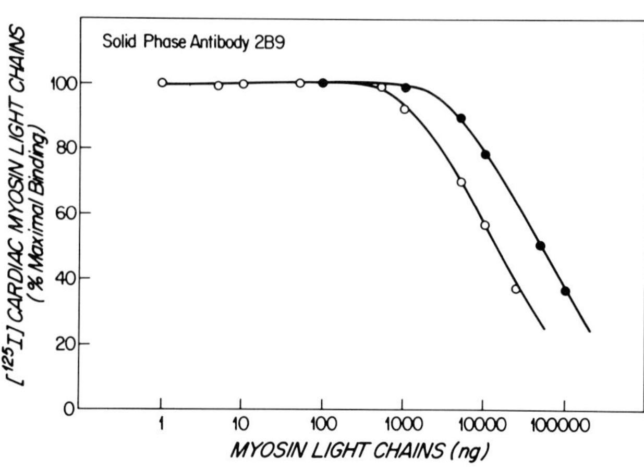

B

FIGURE 1. Binding of ^{125}I cardiac-myosin light chains to monoclonal antibodies immobilized on Sepharose in the presence of increasing concentrations of unlabeled cardiac- or skeletal-muscle myosin light chains (●——●), unlabeled skeletal muscle light chains added (○——○), unlabeled cardiac-muscle light chains added. (A), antibody 1C5; (B), antibody 2B9; (C), antibody 4F10. (unpublished data)

the detection of circulating myosin light chains by radioimmunoassay is useful in the specific diagnosis of myocardial infarction.[6,9,11] If there is not complete differentiation between skeletal and cardiac light chains, false-positive results are likely to occur when there has been damage to skeletal muscle. This is of considerable importance when the diagnosis of myocardial infarction must be made after surgery or following a traumatic accident.

As an example of the problems encountered, the sera of 25 rabbits immunized with human cardiac-myosin light chains were examined at varying times after immunization.

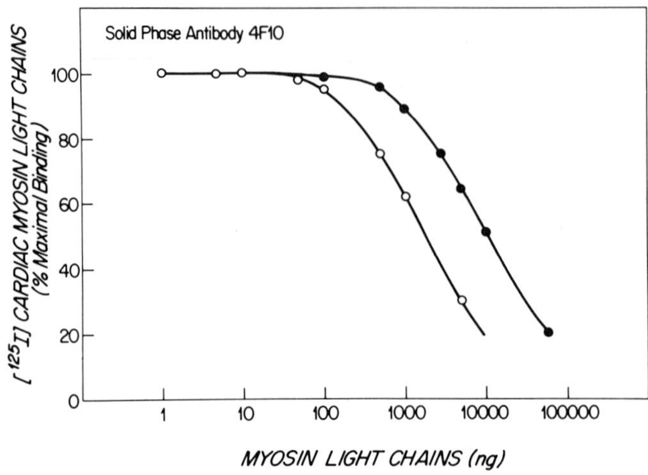

FIGURE 1C

Cross reactivity between cardiac- and skeletal-muscle light chains varied between 10 and 100%. An antiserum could not be found that would provide the requisite specificity useful in clinical assay. The solution to this problem entailed the use of monoclonal antibodies that recognize two different epitopes on the same antigen and thus markedly enhances the resolution possible in immunoassay.

III. THE BIDETERMINANT ASSAY

A. Preparation of Monoclonal Antibodies Specific for Myosin Light Chains

Human cardiac and skeletal myosin were isolated from ventricular myocardium or psoas muscle obtained at necropsy. Myosin light chains were separated from myosin heavy chains[12] and their homogeneity assessed by SDS gel electrophoresis. Somatic-cell fusion was performed according to the general method of Köhler and Milstein.[8] BALB/c mice were hyperimmunized with several injections of human cardiac-myosin light chains in complete Freund's adjuvant injected intraperitoneally, followed two months later by an intravenous booster injection. The spleens were excised 3 days thereafter and spleen cells fused with 10^7 PS-NS1/1-Ag4-1 (NS1) cells[13] in 30% polyethyleneglycol. The cells were seeded in four culture plates (Costar, Cambridge, MA). Of a total of 229 wells, 89.5% showed growth in selective medium.[14] To screen for antibody in the culture medium, a solid-phase assay was employed[15] utilizing myosin light chains immobilized on plastic and iodinated goat-(anti-mouse) $F(ab')_2$ as second antibody. In 35% of the wells showing cell growth, antimyosin light chain antibody could be detected. There were four cell lines selected for further characterization which were subcloned three times to assure monoclonality, utilizing limiting dilution computed to yield one cell per well. The cell culture was propagated in vivo utilizing BALB/c mice primed with Pristane. Antibody-enriched ascites could be collected 7 to 14 days after tumor cell injection by paracentesis. Isotypic analysis showed IgG_2 antibodies in all four cell lines.

B. Development of Myosin Light Chain Radioimmunoassay

Either the mixed proteins from ascites fluid or a DEAE cellulose-purified IgG fraction was coupled to cyanogen bromide-activated Sepharose 4B[10] using 2 to 3 mg protein per

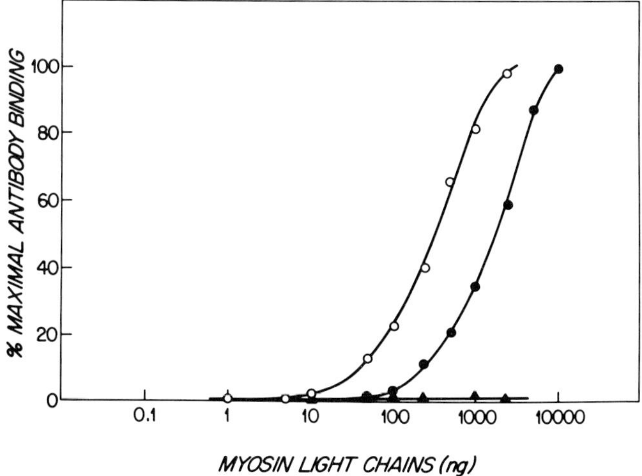

A

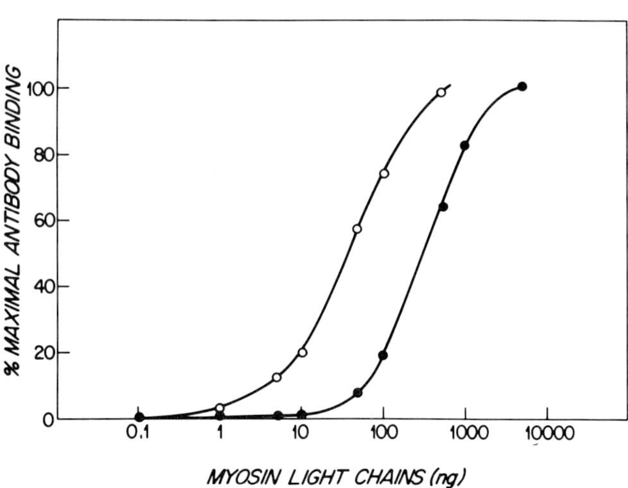

B

FIGURE 2. Binding of ^{125}I-labeled second antibody to antigen that had first been bound to Sepharose-immobilized antibody. Percent maximal labeled-antibody binding in antigen excess if plotted against the amount of cardiac- or skeletal-muscle light chain added. (A), skeletal-muscle light chains (●——●), cardiac-muscle light chains (○——○) measured with antibody 2B9 immobilized on Sepharose and antibody 1C5 labeled. Cardiac-muscle light chains ▲——▲ measured with antibody 2B9 immobilized on Sepharose and antibody 2B9 labeled. (B), cardiac-muscle light chains (○——○), skeletal-muscle light chains (●——●) measured with antibody 4F10 immobilized on Sepharose and antibody 1C5 labeled. (C), cardiac-muscle light chains (○——○), skeletal-muscle light chains (●——●) measured with antibody 4F10 immobilized on Sepharose and antibody 2B9 labeled. (unpublished data)

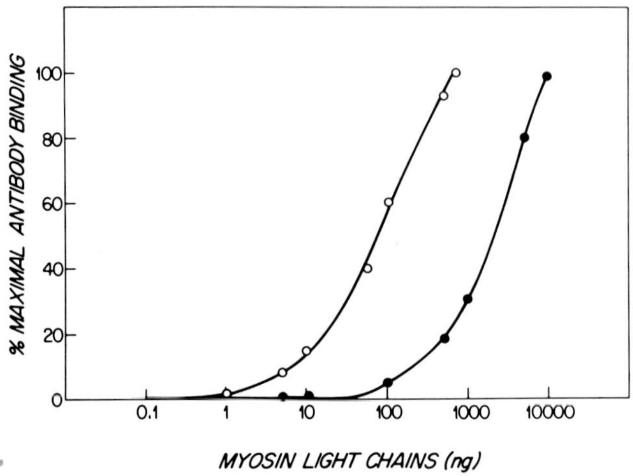

FIGURE 2C

milliliter of Sepharose. Purified antimyosin (light chain) antibody and human heart-myosin light chains were iodinated with 1 mCi ^{125}I, using the lactoperoxidase method[17] to a specific activity of 10 μCi/ug. Goat-(anti-mouse) $F(ab')_2$ was iodinated with 1 mCi ^{125}I using chloramine T as oxidant.[18] The antibody-binding capacity of Sepharose-substituted antibody was examined by measuring the binding of ^{125}I-myosin light chains. The quantity of antibody substituted onto Sepharose was determined by the binding of ^{125}I-goat-(anti-mouse) $F(ab')_2$. The capacity of ^{125}I-substituted antibodies to bind myosin light chains was examined in a similar manner utilizing Sepharose 4B to which myosin light chains had been bound. The sandwich assay was carried out utilizing Sepharose-antibody, myosin light chains, and ^{125}I-antibody.

C. Results of the Bideterminant Assay

Three monoclonal antibodies that exhibited varying degrees of cross reactivity between cardiac- and skeletal-myosin light chains were selected for study. When immobilized on Sepharose, each bound ^{125}I-cardiac-myosin light chains effectively, allowing ready determination of cross reactivity with skeletal-muscle light chains utilizing a solid-phase competitive radioimmunoassay (Figure 1). Increasing concentrations of either unlabeled cardiac or skeletal light chains resulted in decreased binding of ^{125}I-cardiac light chains. Antibody 1C5 proved to be fully cross reactive (Figure 1A), 2B9 was 17.5% cross reactive (Figure 1B), and 4F10 was 25% cross reactive (Figure 1C). The antibodies appear to possess varying affinities of myosin light chains, the most cross-reactive antibody, 1C5, provided the greatest sensitivity in measurement.

Figure 2 demonstrates the enhanced specificity that is inherent in an assay where two epitopes are independently measured. One monoclonal antibody is immobilized by covalent linkage of Sepharose. When exposed to an antigen mixture, only those components recognized by that antibody will adhere. A second antibody labeled with ^{125}I is then added. It will bind only to those antigen molecules that are both immobilized on the column and possess the epitope for which it is specific; thus, immobilized radioactivity represents the recognition of two different epitopes on the antigen molecule.

In Figure 2A a fully cross-reactive antibody is combined with a partially cross-reactive one, resulting in apparent cross reactivity that reflects only the discrimination

Table 1
COMPETITIVE ASSAY UTILIZING LABELED ANTIGEN

Antibody	Measured fractional cross-reactivity
1C5	1.00
2B9	0.17
4F10	0.25

Table 2
BIDETERMINANT ASSAY UTILIZING LABELED SECOND ANTIBODY

Antibodies	Calculated cross-reactivity	Measured cross-reactivity
1C5 and 2B9	0.17	0.17
1C5 and 4F10	0.25	0.25
2B9 and 4F10	0.037	0.043

of the partially cross-reactive antibody (Tables 1 and 2). In Figures 2B and 2C enhanced resolution is afforded by combining two partially cross-reactive antibodies (Table 1). A logical consequence of the last argument is that the use of the same antibody, both immobilized to Sepharose and labeled, should result in no apparent binding of the label. This is demonstrated in Figure 2A. When antibody 2B9 is both immobilized on the support and labeled, no radioactivity remains on the solid support after washing.

Why should a bideterminant assay be necessary when monoclonal antibodies recognize a single antigenic determinant? One should be able to select an antibody specific for the epitope that defines the difference between two very similar molecules. Yet it appears that cross reactivity is often seen. With monoclonal antibodies this is probably a manifestation of the sharing of parts of an epitope by two antigens. A method that entailed the combination of two antibodies that recognize different epitopes on the same molecule should enhance specificity markedly (Figure 3). The differentiation between cardiac- and skeletal-muscle myosin appears to offer a good test case. The molecules are different structurally, yet elicited antibodies (mixtures) and the monoclonal antibodies we have tested utilizing a conventional solid-phase radioimmunoassay (Figure 1 and Table 1) exhibit varying degrees of cross reactivity. When the assay is constructed so that two different monoclonal antibodies must bind to the same antigen, the resultant cross reactivity observed corresponds as might be expected from theoretical considerations to approximately the product of the two fractional cross reactivities (Table 1).

It is likely that the two epitopes selected must be sufficiently far from one another on the molecule's surface so that steric hindrance between the two monoclonal antibodies does not occur. We have not as yet seen an example of this problem, but Figure 1A clearly demonstrates that it is impossible to bind two antibody molecules to the same epitope.

An additional feature of interest in this assay is its capability of measuring a very large range of antigen concentrations. Unlike the conventional competitive radioimmunoassay, which is dependent on the establishment of an equilibrium between labeled antigen and antibody and thus is practically limited to a range of measurement 10 times

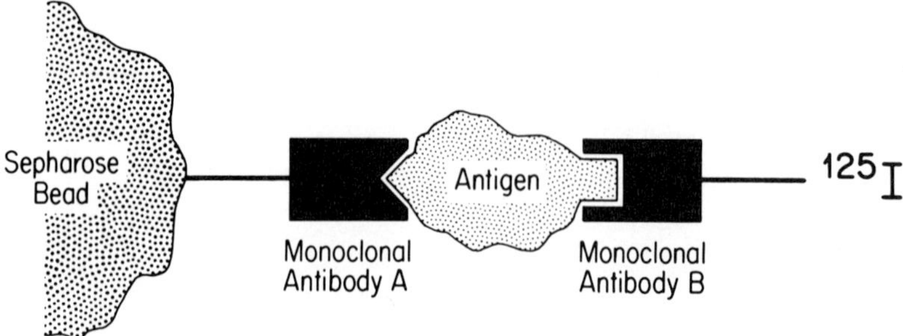

FIGURE 3. Schematic representation of the bideterminant immunoassay utilizing two monoclonal antibodies. (From Haber, E., Donahoe, P., Ehrlich, P., Hurrell, J., Katus, H., Khaw, B. A., Margolies, M. N., Mudgett-Hunter, M., and Zurawski, V. R., *Monoclonal Antibodies in Endocrine Research,* Fellows, R. E. and Eisenbarth, G., Eds., Raven Press, New York, 1981: With permission.)

the lowest antigen concentration detectable, the dual antibody method does not suffer from this limitation. The quantity of immobilized first antibody is in great excess and may bind antigen (unlabeled) over a wide range. Each bound antigen molecule then binds a labeled second antibody, which forms the basis for measurement. The range is only limited by the number of first antibody binding sites immobilized on the column. For example, the concentration of skeletal-muscle light chains is measured over a range of 1000 in Figure 2B.

IV. MONOCLONAL MYOSIN-SPECIFIC ANTIBODIES IN MYOCARDIAL INFARCT IMAGING

While the concept of imaging of specific target organs dates to 1948,[19] there has been increasing interest in this technique recently.[7,20–25] We have demonstrated the feasibility of using radiolabeled, affinity column-purified, anticanine cardiac myosin antibody fragments administered intravenously for localization and visualization of necrotic regions of infarcted myocardium in vivo.[7,26] When cell death occurs, the intracellular protein, myosin, is exposed to extracellular fluid. It is then available to react with labeled antibodies or antibody fragments. Myosin is very insoluble in physiological fluids so that membrane breakdown does not result in antigen loss. This allows for in vivo infarct detection utilizing affinity column-purified antibodies labeled with various radioisotopes such as ^{125}I-Ab(Fab')$_2$,[19] ^{131}I-Ab(Fab')$_2$,[27] ^{111}In-DTPA-Ab Fab,[28] ^{67}Ga-DTPA Fab,[29] and ^{99m}Tc-DTPA-Ab Fab.[30]

The technique of labeling biologically active macromolecules with ^{99m}Technetium developed in our laboratory has enhanced the application of antibodies to the imaging of specific target organs. The labeling procedure involves derivatization of antibodies with diethylene triamine pentaacetic acid (DTPA) by the procedure of Krejcarek and Tucker[31] followed by reaction with dithionite-reduced pertechnetate.[30] The procedure is very mild and results in minimal denaturation of antibody.

The antibodies used in these studies were conventionally elicited antibodies obtained in rabbits. Myocardial-infarct imaging is a particularly effective application because the relative concentration of antibody Fab in the lesion in comparison to normal tissue is in the range of 10 to 50:1. This permits imaging to be done directly with a gamma camera. The various attempts at tumor imaging discussed in the references cited are more difficult and require subtractive imaging methods because of limited relative concentration of antibody in the tumor (about 2:1).

While elicited antibodies have been very useful in pilot studies, they present major impediments in wide-scale clinical application of myocardial-infarct imaging. Elicited antibodies are intrinsically heterogeneous. As a consequence, different batches of serum even from the same donor animal are likely to present a different spectrum of antigenic specificities. Antibodies must be affinity purified from serum since a monospecific antibody preparation is required in imaging studies. An admixture of radiolabeled proteins that are not antibodies to the antigen to be imaged results not only in an increased radiation dose to the patient but also unnecessary background radioactivity. Both affinity purification and repeated immunization require large amounts of scarce antigens. In myocardial-infarct imaging, the antigen in question is human cardiac myosin, a material obviously in limited supply.

The hybridoma method of antibody production[8] provides a solution to all these problems. Antibodies from monoclonal cell cultures are homogeneous and reproducible in industrial quantities. Since the major product of the cell line is a specific antibody (especially when nonsecreting myeloma cell lines are used in the initial cell fusion), affinity chromatography is often unnecessary, and the antibody may be isolated by simple ion-exchange chromatography. Finally, antigen requirements are minimal. Initial immunization is generally carried out in mice, each animal requiring only a few micrograms of antigen. Once a desired cell line is obtained, further immunization is not needed. An additional dividend inherent in the selection of desirable clones, and a keystone of this technique, is that highly purified antigen is not needed. If a mixture of antigens is used in the initial immunization, only those clones of hybrid cells that secrete antibody to the desired antigen need to be propagated.

A. Preparation of Monoclonal Antibodies Specific for Myosin

BALB/c mice were immunized with human cardiac myosin purified from left ventricular myocardium obtained at necropsy utilizing the same method as previously described for canine myosin.[7] A similar schedule of immunization was utilized as described above for cardiac light chain, the cell-fusion procedure was carried out in an identical manner, and screening for antibody in the culture medium was performed utilizing a solid-phase assay as above. Antimyosin antibody activity could be detected in 75% of wells showing cell growth in selective media. The cell line, WM-2, the product of which was utilized in the imaging experiments described here, was subcloned three times utilizing limiting dilution to one cell per well to assure monoclonality. This antibody reacted with both canine and human cardiac myosin and thus could be used for imaging experimental canine myocardial infarcts. It was labeled with ^{99m}Technetium using the technique described above.

B. The Canine Myocardial Infarct

Dogs were anesthetized by intravenous pentobarbitol; left thoracotomy was performed under sterile conditions, and the left anterior descending (LAD) coronary artery was occluded with a silk suture approximately two thirds the distance from the apex to the base in order to produce approximately 30% left-ventricular-wall cyanosis.[19,27] Ligature was removed and 5 mCi of ^{99m}Technetium-labeled antimyosin hybridoma WM-2 was injected into the LAD coronary artery 4 hr following LAD occlusion. A scintigraphic image (left lateral and anteroposterior views) was obtained 18 hr later (Figure 4) that demonstrated the localization of the labeled antibody in the anteroapical region of the heart.

The power of specific antibody as a vehicle for imaging specific antigens in vivo has been amply demonstrated. The availability of monoclonal antibodies as well as better radioactive labeling techniques will allow wider application of this approach to the de-

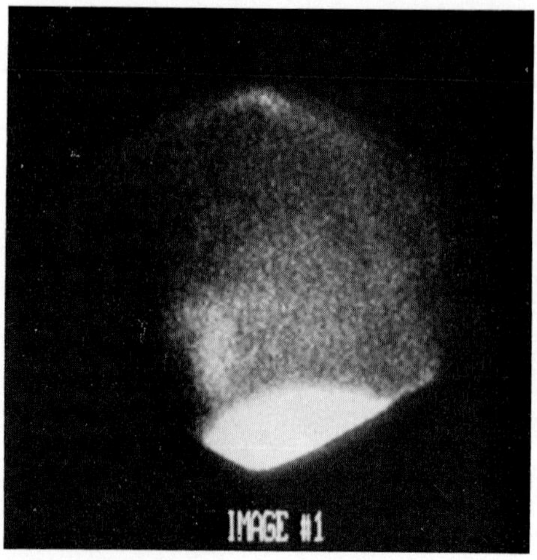

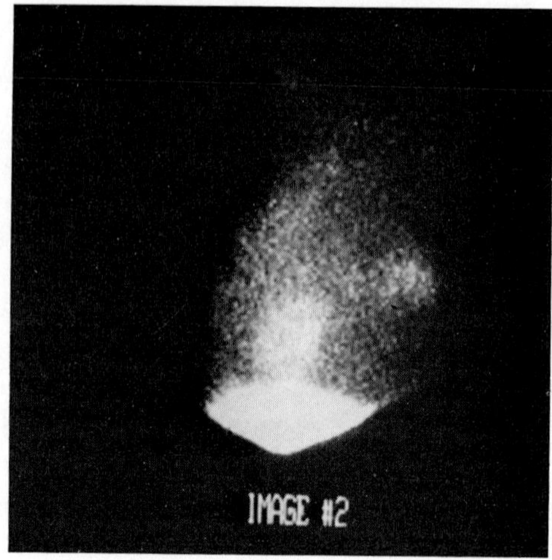

FIGURE 4. Left lateral (IMAGE #1) and anteroposterior (IMAGE #2) scintigrams showing localization of ^{99m}Tc-labeled monoclonal DTPA-antimyosin (WM-2) Fab fragments 18 h post intracoronary administration in a canine experimental myocardial infarction. The lower central activity is also due to liver activity. (From Khaw, B. A. and Haber, E., *Monoclonal Antibodies and T Cell Hybridomas,* Hämmerling, G., Hämmerling, U., and Kearney, J. F., Eds., Elsevier/North-Holland, New York, 1981. With permission.)

tection of antigens that are rare and difficult to purify. Candidates for imaging include specific tumor antigen, intracellular antigens for detection of necrotic tissue, as well as organ- or tissue-specific antigens.

Two major properties inherent in monoclonal antibodies, selectivity, and availability in essentially limitless quantities, have effected a potential solution to significant problems in myocardial infarct diagnosis.

REFERENCES

1. **Shell, W. E., Kjekshus, J. K., and Shell, B. E.,** Quantitative assessment of the extent of myocardial infarction in the conscious dog by means of analysis of serial changes in serum creatine phosphokinase activity, *J. Clin. Invest.,* 50, 2614, 1971.
2. **Sobel, B. E. and Shell, W. E.,** Serum enzyme determinations in the diagnosis and assessment of myocardial infarction, *Circulation,* 45, 471, 1972.
3. **Mydick, I., Wroblewski, F., and LaDue, J. S.,** Evidence for increased serum glutamic oxalacetic transaminase (SGO-T) activity following graded myocardial infarcts in dogs, *Circulation,* 12, 161, 1955.
4. **Stone, M. J., Willerson, J. T., Gomez-Sanchez, C. E., and Waterman, M. R.,** Radioimmunoassay of myoglobin in human serum: results in patients with acute myocardial infarction, *J. Clin. Invest.,* 56, 1334, 1975.
5. **Roberts, R., Sobel, B. E., and Parker, C. W.,** Radioimmunoassay for creatine kinase isoenzymes, *Science,* 194, 855, 1976.
6. **Khaw, B. A., Gold, H. K., Fallon, J. T., and Haber, E.,** Detection of serum cardiac myosin light chains in acute experimental myocardial infarction: radioimmunoassay of cardiac myosin light chains, *Circulation,* 58, 1130, 1978.
7. **Khaw, B. A., Beller, G. A., Haber, E., and Smith, T. W.,** Localization of cardiac myosin-specific antibody in experimental myocardial infarction, *J. Clin. Invest.,* 58, 439, 1976.
8. **Köhler, G. and Milstein, C.,** Continuous cultures of fused cells secreting antibody of predefined specificity, *Nature (London),* 256, 495, 1975.

9. **Katus, H. A., Khaw, B. A., Mizusawa, E., Gold, H., and Haber, E.,** Circulating cardiac myosin light chains in myocardial infarction: detection by radioimmunoassay, *Circulation,* 59—60(II), 139, 1979.
10. **Leger, J. J. and Elzinga, M.,** Studies on cardiac myosin light chains: comparison of the sequences of cardiac and skeletal myosin LC-2, *Biochem. Biophys. Res. Commun.,* 74, 1390, 1977.
11. **Trahern, C. A., Gere, J. B., Krauth, G., II, and Bigham, D. A.,** Clinical assessment of serum myosin light chains in the diagnosis of acute myocardial infarction, *Am. J. Cardiol.,* 4, 541, 1978.
12. **Perrie, W. T. and Perry, S. V.,** An electrophoretic study of the low-molecular-weight components of myosin, *Biochem. J.,* 119, 31, 1970.
13. **Köhler, G. and Milstein, C.,** Derivation of specific antibody-producing-tissue culture and tumor lines by cell fusion, *Eur. J. Immunol.,* 6, 511, 1976.
14. **Littlefield, J. W.,** Selection of hybrids from matings of fibroblasts in vitro and their presumed recombinants, *Science,* 145, 709, 1964.
15. **Rosenthal, J. D., Hayashi, K., and Notkins, A. L.,** Comparison of direct and indirect solid-phase microradioimmunoassays for the detection of viral antigens and antiviral antibody, *Appl. Microbiol.,* 25, 567, 1973.
16. **Cuatrecasas, P., and Anfinsen, C. B.,** Affinity chromatography, in *Methods in Enzymology,* Vol. 22, Jakoby, W. B., Ed., Academic Press, New York, 1971, chap. 31.
17. **Marchalonis, J. J.,** An enzymatic method for the trace iodination of immunoglobulins and other proteins, *Biochem. J.,* 113, 299, 1969.
18. **Greenwood, F. C. and Hunter, W. M.,** The preparation of ^{131}I-labelled human growth hormone of high specific radioactivity, *Biochem. J.,* 89, 114, 1963.
19. **Pressman, D. and Keighley, G.,** Zone of activity of antibodies as determined by use of radioactive tracers; zone of activity of nephritoxic antikidney serum, *J. Immunol.,* 59, 141, 1948.
20. **Hoffer, P. B., Lathrop, K., Bekermen, C., Fang, V. S., and Refetoffs, S. J.,** Use of 131-I-CEA antibody as a tumor scanning agent, *Nucl. Med.,* 15, 323, 1974.
21. **Spar, I. L., Bale, W. F., Goodland, R. L., Casarett, G. W., and Michaelson, S. M.,** Distribution of injected I^{131}-labeled antibody to dog fibrin in tumor-bearing dogs, *Cancer Res.,* 20, 1501, 1960.
22. **Izzo, M. J., Buchsbaum, D. J., and Bale, W. J.,** Localization of an ^{125}I-labeled rat transplantation antibody in tumors carrying the corresponding antigen (36326), *Proc. Soc. Exp. Biol. Med.,* 139, 1185, 1972.
23. **Goldenberg, D. M., Preston, D. F., Primus, F. J., and Hansen, H. J.,** Photoscan localization of GW-39 tumors in hamsters using radiolabeled anticarcinoembryonic antigen immunoglobulin G, *Cancer Res.,* 34, 1, 1974.
24. **Belitsky, P., Ghose, T., Aquino, J., Norvell, S. T., and Blair, A. H.,** Radionuclide imaging of primary renal-cell carcinoma by I-131-labeled antitumor antibody, *J. Nucl. Med.,* 19, 427, 1978.
25. **Willerson, J. T., Kulkarni, P., Stone, M., Lewis, S. E., Eigenbrodt, E., Bonte, F. J., Parkey, R. W., and Buja, L. M.,** Localization of anti-mitochondrial antibody in experimental canine myocardial infarction, *Proc. Natl. Acad. Sci. USA.,* 77, 6856, 1980.
26. **Khaw, B. A., Fallon, J. T., Beller, G. A., and Haber, E.,** Specificity of localization of myosin specific antibody fragments in experimental myocardial infarction: histologic, histochemical, autoradiographic and scintigraphic studies, *Circulation,* 60, 1527, 1979.
27. **Khaw, B. A., Beller, G. A., and Haber, E.,** Experimental myocardial infarct imaging following administration of Iodine-131 labeled antibody $(Fab')_2$ fragments specific for cardiac myosin, *Circulation,* 57, 743, 1978.
28. **Khaw, B. A., Fallon, J. T., Strauss, H. W., and Haber, E.,** Myocardial infarct imaging with Indium-111-diethylene triamine pentaacetic acid-anticanine cardiac myosin antibodies, *Science,* 209, 295, 1980.
29. **Khaw, B. A., Fallon, J. T., Katus, H., Elmaleh, D., Strauss, H. W., Locke, E., Pohost, G. M., and Haber, E.,** Positron imaging of experimental myocardial infarction with ^{68}Ga-DTPA-antimyosin antibody, *Circulation,* 59—60(II), 135, 1979.
30. **Khaw, B. A., Strauss, H. W., Carvalho, A., Gold, H., Locke, E., and Haber, E.,** in preparation.
31. **Krejcarek, G. E. and Tucker, K. L.,** Covalent attachment of chelating groups to macromolecules, *Biochem. Biophys. Res. Commun.,* 77, 581, 1977.

Chapter 5

THE USE OF MONOCLONAL ANTIBODIES TO INVESTIGATE ANTIGENIC DRIFT IN INFLUENZA VIRUS

W. G. Laver

TABLE OF CONTENTS

I. INTRODUCTION

A. Two Kinds of Antigenic Variation in Influenza Virus

Influenza type A viruses undergo two quite distinct kinds of antigenic variation, antigenic drift and major antigenic shifts. In the latter kind of variation, "new" viruses suddenly appear in the human population with surface antigens totally unrelated to the virus circulating before the new virus appeared. The origin of these new viruses and the way in which they suddenly arise in the human population is not known. First, they may be viruses which caused epidemics in man many years previously and have remained hidden and unchanged in some unknown place ever since. More and more evidence that this does happen is being obtained. The strain of "Russian flu" (H1N1) which appeared in Anshan in northern China on May 4, 1977 and subsequently spread to the rest of the world, seems to be identical, in all respects, to the virus which caused an influenza epidemic in 1950.[1,2] Where was this virus for 27 years? An influenza virus isolated from a 3-year old child in Adelaide in 1979 was the same as one of the first Hong Kong (H3N2) influenza viruses isolated in 1968.[3] Where has this virus been for 11 years? We have no answer to these questions at the moment.

Second, the "new" viruses may be derived from animal or avian viruses. These normally do not have the capacity to infect and spread in man but may acquire this by recombination (reassortment) of their genes. One strain of human influenza has been shown to be such a recombinant. The Hong Kong (H3N2) virus contains the neuraminidase (and other) genes from an Asian (H2N2) strain of human influenza and the hemagglutinin gene of some other virus. Which one? Hong Kong hemagglutinin is closely related to that of Duck/Ukraine and Equi-2 viruses but we have no idea if it was an animal or bird virus which donated the hemagglutinin gene during the recombinational event which led to the formation of the Hong Kong strain. It could just as well have been a virus left over from a much earlier human influenza epidemic and maintained unchanged in the same way as was "Russian Flu." Antibodies in the sera of people who were born around 1900 suggest that a virus with a hemagglutinin similar to that of the Hong Kong virus was causing influenza at that time.

The third way in which "new" viruses could appear in the human population is by direct mutation of an animal or bird virus to give a virus with the capacity to cause epidemic influenza in man. We do not fully understand why a virus will infect one host and not another, but this "host specificity" may be associated with one of the large "P" genes and mutations here may have a profound effect on the kind of host the virus is able to infect.

Between the major shifts in antigenic structure which define the beginning and end of each pandemic era, the virus undergoes a series of smaller changes. As the human population becomes immune to infection by extant strains of influenza virus, so the pressure rises to select variants which, by displaying small but significant changes in antigenicity, can evade the immune response. This process is known as antigenic drift.

The changes which are responsible for antigenic drift accumulate with time, and field strains isolated several years apart from within a single pandemic era show considerable antigenic differences in their surface antigens.[4]

B. Properties of the Surface Antigens

There are two antigens on the surface of the influenza virus particle, the hemagglutinin (HA) and the neuraminidase (NA). Antibody to the HA neutralizes the infectivity of the virus and therefore variation in the HA is of greater importance than variation in the NA.

1. The Hemagglutinin

Influenza virus HA is a triangular, rod-shaped glycoprotein molecule composed of three pairs of disulfide-linked polypeptide chains, HA1 and HA2.[5] These are coded by one of the 8 single-stranded RNA segments (segment 4) in the influenza virus genome. The complete amino acid sequence of HA1 and HA2 is known for strains within three different subtypes of type A influenza, fowl plague (Hav1N1) virus,[6] Asian (H2N2) influenza virus[7] and Hong Kong (H3N2) influenza virus.[8–12] The N-terminal sequences of HA1 (up to 90 amino acids) has been determined for 32 other virus strains, including representatives of each of the 12 known HA subtypes of type A influenza.[41] Incomplete, bromelain-released HA molecules of Hong Kong (H3N2) influenza virus have been crystallized[13] and the three-dimensional structure has been determined by X-ray diffraction methods.[14,15]

Before the development of monoclonal antibodies to the HA, variant influenza viruses were characterized using heterogeneous ferret, mouse, chicken, goat, or rabbit antisera in hemagglutination-inhibition or double immunodiffusion tests. There were two groups of antigenic determinants, strain-specific and common or cross-reacting, that could be distinguished on the hemagglutinin[16,17] but the heterogeneity of the antisera used prevented further dissection of the antigenic structure of the HA molecule. Individual animals were found to differ greatly in their antibody response to the two groups of determinants, some animals giving a stronger response to the ''common'' determinants than to the ''strain-specific'', whereas in others the reverse was the case. This diversity of the antibody response to the HA made it difficult to accurately characterize antigenic variants of influenza virus as they arose in nature.

2. The Neuraminidase

The other surface antigen on the influenza virus particle is the enzyme, neuraminidase (NA). Pure intact neuraminidase molecules can be isolated from some influenza viruses after disruption of the virus particles with detergents. Electron microscopy showed these molecules to consist of a square box-like head with a long thin tail. In the absence of detergent these molecules aggregate by the hydrophobic tips of their tails, which serve to attach the molecules to the lipid of the virus envelope.

Proteolytic digestion of virus particles releases neuraminidase molecules which have lost their hydrophobic regions. It is thought that protease treatment digests the fiber portion of the neuraminidase, which appears to be responsible for the attachment of the neuraminidase to the lipid layer of the virus, releasing the ''head'' of the neuraminidase molecule from the virus particle. These heads retain full enzymatic activity and all the antigenic properties of the intact neuraminidase molecule. Neuraminidase heads isolated from influenza B virus by trypsin treatment have been studied in some detail.[18] These heads, measuring 80 Å × 80 Å × 80 Å, appeared to be made of four coplanar and roughly spherical subunits each about 40 Å in diameter. Examination of the neuraminidase heads by polyacrylamide gel electrophoresis showed that these contained a single polypeptide chain with a molecular weight of about 48,000, whereas intact neuraminidase molecules isolated from detergent-disrupted influenza B virus particles contained a single species of polypeptide of about 60,000 mol wt.

The function of the neuraminidase is probably to effect the release of virus from the infected cells. Antibody to the neuraminidase does not neutralize the infectivity of the virus directly, but does slow down release of virus from infected cells and helps combat infection this way. Antigenic drift occurs in the neuraminidase as well as in the hemagglutinin of influenza virus and a large number of antigenically distinct neuraminidase molecules exist in influenza viruses infecting man, lower mammals, and birds.

Partially degraded neuraminidase molecules (heads) from a number of strains of type A influenza virus have been crystallized[19] and the heads from one strain (A/Tokyo/3/67, H2N2) formed large crystals suitable for X-ray diffraction studies.[20,21]

When purified preparations of HA or NA are injected into animals the resulting sera contain antibodies directed against a large number of different antigenic sites on these molecules. Each individual animal will produce different amounts of antibody to each site, so that no two sera will give the same cross-reactions between variants. As mentioned above, a crude fractionation of sera to the HA gave antibodies directed against two groups of determinants, but further fractionation of the sera to give antibodies against individual sites on the HA could not be done.

II. MONOCLONAL HYBRIDOMA ANTIBODIES TO INFLUENZA ANTIGENS

The development of monoclonal hybridoma antibodies to influenza HA and NA (and to the matrix and nucleoprotein antigens) has however changed all this and the precise analysis of antigenic variants of influenza viruses is now possible.

Monoclonal antibodies to influenza virus antigens were used first by Walter Gerhard and his colleagues at the Wistar Institute to delineate the antigenic determinants on the hemagglutinin of A/PR/8/34 and other type A influenza viruses. This work has been covered in two excellent reviews by Gerhard and his colleagues.[22,23]

A. Use of Monoclonal Antibodies to Select Antigenic Variants of Influenza Viruses

Antigenic variants of the A/PR8 (H1N1) and A/Hong Kong/68 (H3N2) strains of influenza virus were isolated after a single passage of these viruses in the presence of monoclonal hybridoma antibodies to the hemagglutinin. The properties of the PR8 variants are described in the above Reviews[22,23] and those of the Hong Kong variants are described below.

1. Frequency of Isolation of Variants

By determining the reactivity patterns (in hemagglutination-inhibition tests) of 30 different monoclonal antibodies, it was established that at least three nonoverlapping antigenic areas existed on the hemagglutinin molecule of A/Mem/1/71 (H3N2) influenza virus.[24] Variants which grew in the presence of monoclonal antibodies from each of these reactivity groups (used singly) existed in the wild-type stock at a frequency of about 1 in 10^5. Variants selected with one monoclonal antibody were not recognized by the other two monoclonal antibodies as being different from wild-type virus, confirming that the three antibodies bound to different sites on the surface of the hemagglutinin molecules. No variants grew in the presence of a mixture of monoclonal antibodies from two or more reactivity groups, which was to be expected since the infectivity titer of the wild-type virus was of the order of 10^7 to 10^8 EID_{50} and the expected frequency of variants with changes in two independent sites was 1 in 10^{10}. The frequency of antigenic variants in preparations of influenza B virus, on the other hand, was surprisingly low.[25]

The frequency of antigenic variants in cloned preparations of influenza B/HK/8/73 with most monoclonal antibodies was less than 1 in 10^8. This figure is 2 to 3 orders of magnitude below that found with influenza A viruses,[26] suggesting that the hemagglutinins of influenza B viruses are less variable than influenza A virus hemagglutinins. As in the case of type A influenza, each variant was not inhibited in HI tests by the monoclonal antibodies used in its selection. One explanation for the low levels of antigenic variants in influenza B preparations was that the antibody preparations were not monoclonal but contained mixtures of antibodies to different nonoverlapping antigenic areas.

However, this possibility was ruled out by recloning the antibody secreting hybridoma cells and retesting the frequency of variation; the results did not change. Another possible explanation was that different cloned preparations of influenza B/HK/8/73 showed significant differences in the frequency of antigenic variants. There were four different cloned preparations of B/HK/8/73, therefore, examined and were found to give similar results. It is unlikely that the mutation frequency in the RNA coding for the influenza B hemagglutinin is less than in influenza A viruses and some other explanation for the ease with which variants of Type A influenza can be isolated must be sought.

It is interesting that similar frequencies of antigenic variants were found in Sendai, vesicular stomatitis, and influenza A viruses, although variants of VSV or Sendai are relatively rare in nature.[27]

Monoclonal antibodies to the hemagglutinin of Sendai virus, the surface glycoprotein molecule of vesicular stomatitis virus (VSV), and the hemagglutinin of influenza A virus were prepared and used to analyze the frequencies of antigenic variants in cloned virus populations. The frequencies of antigenic variants detected with monoclonal antibodies directed toward different antigenic sites were approximately the same, namely, $10^{-4.5}$ to $10^{-4.7}$ for the three different viruses; thus the marked degree of antigenic variation of influenza A viruses cannot be explained by an enhanced capacity to produce mutant virions.

B. Sequence Changes in the HA of Variants Selected with Monoclonal Antibodies

Hyperimmune rabbit antisera reacted (in hemagglutination-inhibition tests) to high titer with both wild-type and variant viruses, but the monoclonal antibodies, which reacted with the wild-type virus to titers of the order of $1/10^5$ did not react at all (or to very low titer) with the variants that they selected.

This suggests that the changes occurring in the monoclonal variants are restricted to a single antigenic site out of many on the hemagglutinin molecule.

Amino acid analysis of the soluble tryptic peptides from the hemagglutinin "spikes" of wild-type and variant viruses showed that the dramatic loss in the ability of the variants to bind the monoclonal antibody used in their selection was associated with a single change in the amino acid sequence of the large hemagglutinin polypeptide, HA1.

For PR8 virus, eight out of ten variants selected with one monoclonal antibody showed the same sequence change of serine to leucine at position 157[42] in the HA1 polypeptide. The change in the other two variants was not determined.[28]

In 10 variants of Hong Kong (H3N2) influenza virus selected with monoclonal antibodies of reactivity group II, the proline at position 143 in HA1 changed to serine, threonine, leucine, or histidine. In other variants, asparagine 133 changed to lysine, glycine 144 to aspartic acid, and serine 145 to lysine.[29] All these changes are possible by single base changes in the RNA except the last, which requires a double base change. Residues 142 to 146 also changed in field strains of Hong Kong influenza isolated between 1968 and 1977.[30] The single amino acid sequence changes in HA1 of the monoclonal variants were detected by comparing the compositions of the soluble tryptic peptides from the variants with the known sequences of these peptides from wild-type virus. In the HA1 molecule, two insoluble tryptic peptides, comprising residues 110–140 and 230–255, were not examined and it is not known if additional changes occurred in these regions.

In variants of Hong Kong virus selected with monoclonal antibodies in reactivity

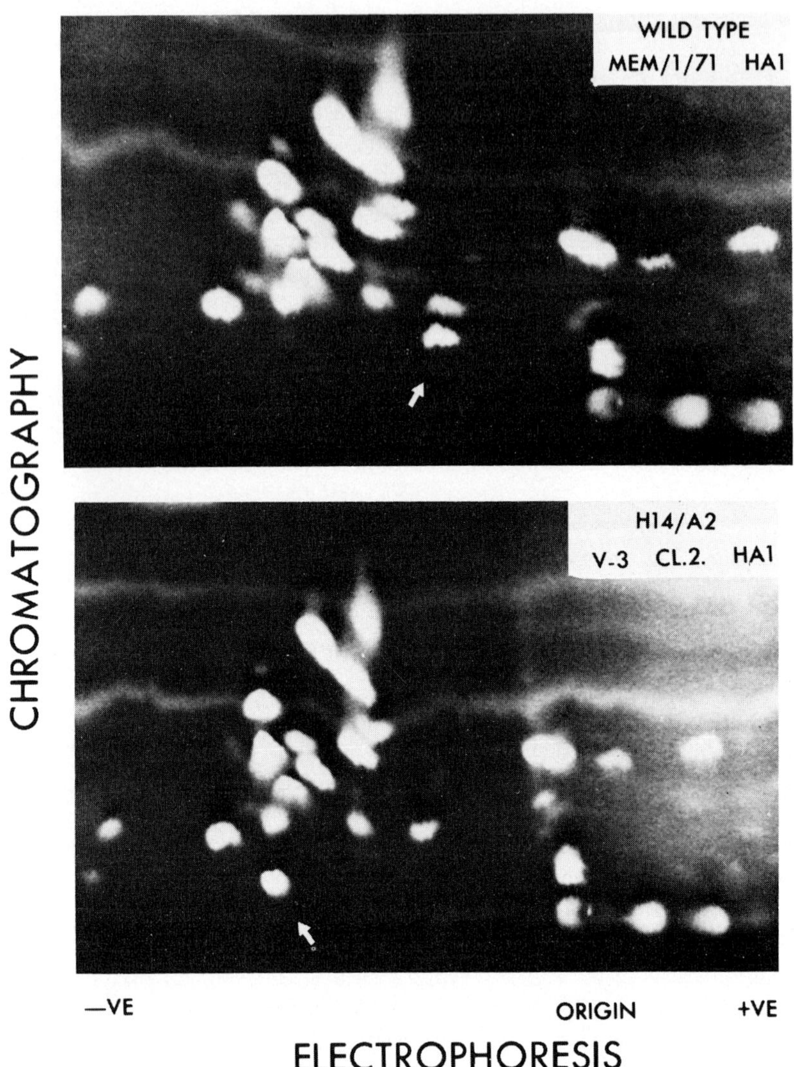

FIGURE 1. Maps of the tryptic peptides (soluble at pH 6.5) from S-carboxymethylated HA1 of wild-type Mem/71 virus and one of the four variants selected with H14/A2 monoclonal hybridoma antibody. The maps were stained with fluorescamine. A single peptide difference (arrow) was seen on the maps. This peptide comprised residues 51–57 in HA1 from wild-type Mem/71 virus.[8] The asparagine residue at position 53 was replaced by lysine in the variant. No differences were found in any of the other peptides.

group I, the asparagine at position 53 in HA1 was replaced by lysine. This resulted in a marked change in the map of the tryptic peptides (Figure 1).

The composition of the altered peptide (peptide 11)[31] is shown in Table 1. The sequence of peptide 11 in wild-type Hong Kong virus is

51 57
-ILE-CYS-ASN-ASN-PRO-HIS-ARG-

It was originally thought[31] that the asparagine at position 54 was the residue which

Table 1
NUMBER OF RESIDUES OF EACH AMINO ACID FOUND IN PEPTIDE 11 FROM WILD-TYPE VIRUS AND THE HI4/A2 MONOCLONAL VARIANT

	Wild-type	Variant
Lysine	0.0	1.0
Histidine	1.0	0.9
Arginine	1.1	1.0
S-Carboxymethyl Cysteine	0.8	0.3
Aspartic acid	2.1	1.1
Proline	1.1	1.2
Isoleucine	0.8	0.8

lysine replaced (since the next residue was proline, making the peptide stable to tryptic digestion) but nucleotide sequence analysis (Figure 2) showed that ASN 53 had been replaced. The proximity of S-carboxymethylated cysteine presumably prevented cleavage of the peptide by trypsin. These experiments illustrate how RNA sequence data can complement protein sequence data where each on its own may show ambiguity.

In variants of Hong Kong virus selected with monoclonal antibodies in reactivity group III, the serine at position 205 in HA1 was replaced by tyrosine. Other variants in this group had changes in one of the large tryptic peptides (number 4) or showed no change at all (these were probably in the two insoluble peptides which could not be examined) and therefore the changes in these variants have not yet been precisely located.[31]

C. Location of the Sequence Changes in the Three-Dimensional Structure of the HA

Bromelain-released HA from A/Hong Kong/68 (H3N2) virus (closely related to A/Mem/1/71 virus) has been crystallized and the three-dimensional structure determined at 3 Å resolution.[13–15]

The amino acids which changed during the selection of variants with the monoclonal antibodies have been located on the surface of the molecule.[15] The areas in which these changes occurred have tentatively been identified as antibody binding sites (four such sites appear to exist), but it is not certain whether the variable residues are "contact" amino acids or whether, on changing, they induce conformational changes in the rest of the HA molecule and so change the true "binding site" which may be located elsewhere.

D. Sequence Changes During Natural Antigenic Drift

Hemagglutinin molecules from nine strains of A/Hong Kong/68 (H3N2) influenza virus, isolated between 1968 and 1977, were examined for changes in amino acid sequences.[30] At least 18 changes, 9 of which were located precisely, occurred in the soluble tryptic peptides of the large hemagglutinin polypeptide (HA1) during this period. These peptides contained 262 residues (82% of HA1). In HA2, only two changes in 129 residues (58% of HA2) were detected.

The nucleotide sequence of the hemagglutinin gene and the deduced amino acid sequence of the protein of the Aichi/68 and Victoria/75 strains have also been com-

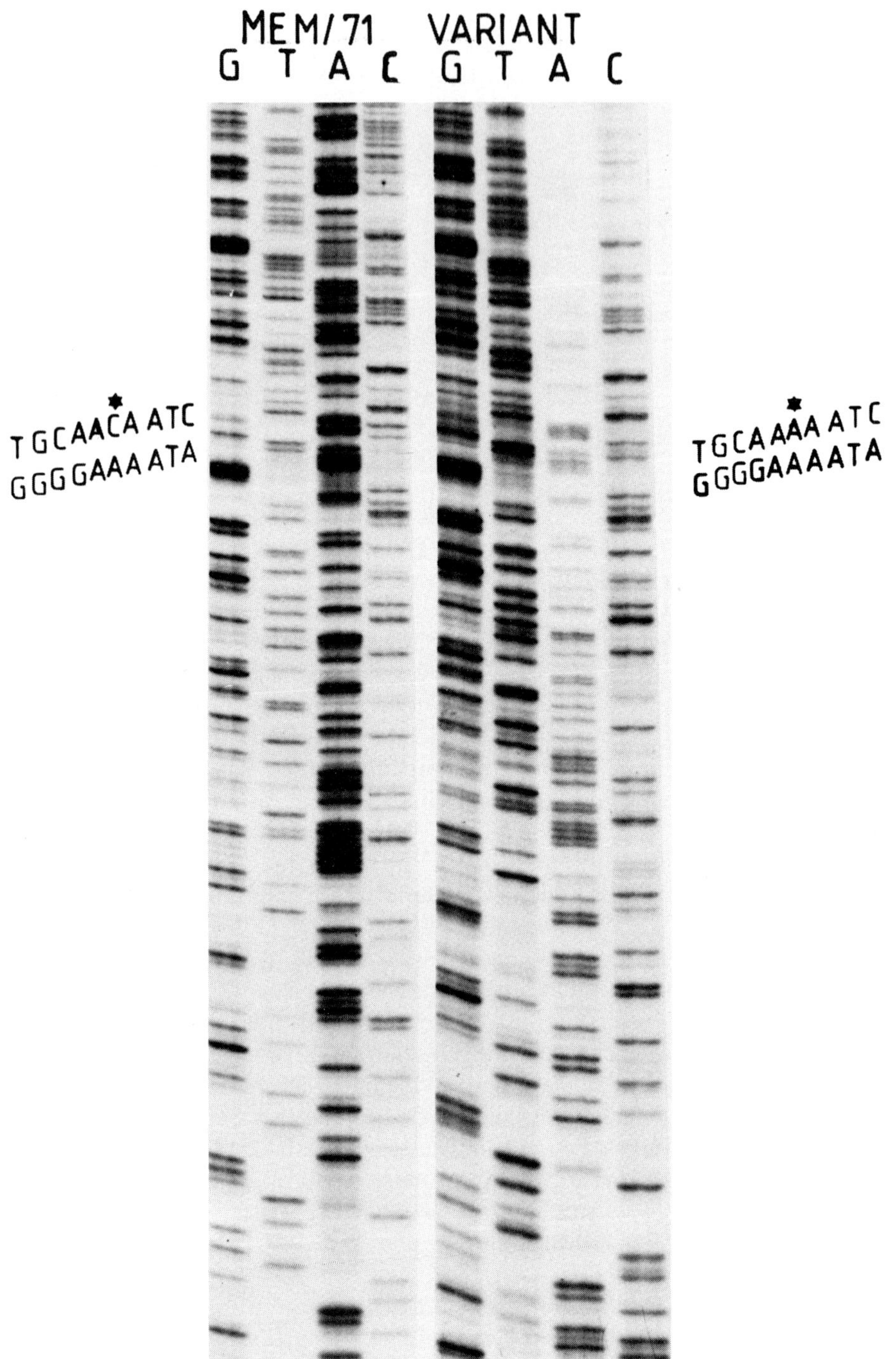

FIGURE 2. Autoradioagraph of 8% polyacrylamide gels showing the sequence from nucleotide 105 of the cDNA transcribed from RNA segment 4 (HA gene) of A/MEM/1/71 virus and the H14/M2 monoclonal variant. Part of the sequence is lettered, and the nucleotide difference is indicated by an asterisk.[45]

pared.[10] There were 67 nucleotide differences (3.8%): an insertion in the Victoria gene of three nucleotides close to the NH_2 terminus of the HA1 (coding for an extra asparagine residue) and 64 nucleotide substitutions. Of these latter changes, 63 occurred in the coding region: 34 were silent nucleotide substitutions and the other 29 changes caused 28 amino acid differences (there is one case, at position 155 of the HA1, of two nucleotide changes resulting in a single amino acid change); thus, in total there are 29 amino acid differences (including one insertion) or a 5.1% amino acid divergence accumulated over a 7-year period (1968–1975).

Another conclusion was that once a residue had changed, it did not change again in the later variants, except for a few apparent reversions to the original amino acid (apparent because there is no reason to believe that prototypes of successive epidemics as isolated from nature form a direct genealogical lineage). The same observations are made when the complete amino acid sequence of the three H3 hemagglutinin molecules, Victoria/75, Memphis/72, and Aichi/68, are compared. Again, a likely explanation for the apparent reversions is that, for example, the Memphis strain is not the parent of the Victoria strain. Also, at the level of silent mutation, the same phenomenon of an occasional apparent reversion is observed; however, the analysis of amino acid sequence changes in natural influenza variants may not necessarily indicate which portions of the sequences make up the antigenic determinants. Some of the changes observed may be unrelated to the antigenic differences between the various HAs.

Consequently we do not know which of the changes in sequence found to occur between 1968 and 1977 were responsible for the changes in antigenicity which occurred in the Hong Kong virus during this period.

E. Sequential Selection of Variants

As mentioned above, when natural variants of Hong Kong virus (field strains) were examined, sequential changes at a particular locus in HA1 were not found. Once an amino acid changed, it did not change again in any subsequent variant examined.

It has been proposed[32–36] that the hemagglutinin molecules of influenza viruses possess a single antigenic site and that antigenic drift occurs by the sequential substitution of increasingly bulky hydrophobic amino acids at a unique locus; however, no direct experimental evidence for this theory has ever been presented.

In order to determine whether sequential changes at the same position occurred during antigenic drift, antibody was prepared against the new antigenic site on the variants in which proline 143 changed to histidine or threonine.

Since the Hong Kong HA molecule appears to possess a large number of overlapping antigenic sites[24] it was thought it would be difficult to prepare monoclonal hybridoma antibodies which bound specifically to the new site. Hyperimmune antisera to the variant HA molecules were therefore absorbed with purified concentrated wild-type virus until the hemagglutinin-inhibition titers of the sera for the wild-type virus reached undetectable levels. The absorbed sera were then tested in HI tests, against the variant viruses.

High levels of HI activity to the variants remained after all HI activity to the wild-type virus had been removed. This antibody to the variants was not removed after repeated absorption of the sera with wild-type virus and therefore must have been directed against a single new antigenic site on the variant HA. In this respect it behaved like "monoclonal" antibody.[29]

This absorbed antiserum was used to select second generation variants of the variants in which PRO (143) had changed to HIS or THR. In the first case, the glycine residue (144) next to the histidine changed to aspartic acid and in the second, the threonine at position 143 reverted to proline and the virus regained the antigenicity of wild-type.[29]

Table 2
SEQUENCE CHANGES FOUND IN THE HA1 POLYPEPTIDES FROM VARIANTS OF TYPE A INFLUENZA VIRUS SELECTED WITH THE MONOCLONAL ANTIBODIES LISTED

Virus	Monoclonal antibody used in the selection	Variant number	Sequence change
A/PR/8/34 (H1N1)	PEG—1	V11[a]	(157) Serine → Leucine
A/MEM/1/71 (H3N2)	Mem 212/1	V1	(143) Proline → Serine
	Mem/212/1	V2	(143) Proline → Threonine
	Mem 212/1	V3	(143) Proline → Leucine
	Mem 212/1	V7	(143) Proline → Histidine
	Mem 27/2	V5	(143) Proline → Serine
	Mem 27/2	V9	(143) Proline → Threonine
	Mem 123/4	V1	(143) Proline → Histidine
	Mem 123/4	V3	(143) Proline → Histidine
	Mem 123/4	V10	(144) Glycine → Aspartic acid
	H14/A20	V1	(133) Asparagine → Lysine
	H14/A20	V2	(143) Proline → Serine
	H14/A20	V3	(143) Proline → Leucine
	H14/A2	V1	(53) Asparagine → Lysine
	H14/A2	V2	(53) Asparagine → Lysine
	H14/A2	V3	(53) Asparagine → Lysine
	H14/A2	V4	(53) Asparagine → Lysine
	H14/A21	V1	(205) Serine → Tyrosine
	H14/A20[b]	V1	(145) Serine → Lysine
	HK 30/2	V12	Glutamine → Histidine[c]

[a]Nine other variants selected with PEG-1 probably had the same sequence change.
[b]The third selection in a triple-step selection. The first selection was with H14/A2 and the second with H14/A21.
[c]Between residues 158 and 201 in HA1. Exact position unknown.

The latter experiment provides the best indication that the monoclonal variants have only single changes in the amino sequence of the HA. Had more than one sequence change been involved in the alteration of antigenic reactivity in the first selection, reversions at the other (unknown) positions must also have occurred in the second selection, which seems unlikely.

F. Antigenic Properties of the Monoclonal Variants

The antigenic variants of A/Mem/1/71 virus selected with monoclonal antibodies for which the sequence changes are known, are listed in Table 2. It can be seen that in some cases, the same monoclonal antibody selected variants with different sequence changes, and that in others, different monoclonal antibodies selected variants which have the same sequence changes.

It is not known how substitution of a single amino acid in the HA sequence totally abolishes the ability of the monoclonal antibody used to select the variant to bind to the HA (reduction in HI titers were of the order of 50,000-fold); nor is it known how other monoclonal antibodies to A/Mem/1/71 hemagglutinin were able to discriminate

Table 3
CROSS-REACTIONS OF THE ANTIGENIC VARIANTS WITH A PANEL OF MONOCLONAL ANTIBODIES TO A/MEM/1/71 HEMAGGLUTININ

Monoclonal antibody preparation	Wild-type	HI titers with the following variants[a]					
		Selected with H14/A20			Selected with H14/A21		
		V1	V2	V3	V1	V2	V3
Mem 93/1	4.1	<[b]	<	<	+[c]	+	+
Mem 27/2	5.0	5.0	<	<	+	+	+
Mem 212/1	5.1	5.1	2.6	<	+	+	+
Mem 123/4	4.6	4.6	2.5	3.6	+	+	+
H14/B18	4.0	+	+	+	2.5	<	2.5
Mem 200/2	5.0	+	+	+	4.4	3.2	4.4
HK 30/2	4.8	+	+	+	4.4	4.4	4.4
12 Other monoclonal antibody preparations	+	+	+	+	+	+	+

[a]HI titers expressed as $\log_{10}$.
[b]Less than 1.7.
[c]Titers for wild-type and variants were identical.

between some of the variants selected with the same monoclonal antibody (Table 3). This may be because a conformational change induced by an amino acid substitution affecting one antigenic site can also affect others, or because some amino acids may be part of two (or more) sites.

This suggests that not all of the antigenic sites on the hemagglutinin are discrete but that considerable overlapping of some sites may occur.

When heterogeneous antisera (rabbit, mouse, or ferret) were used in the tests most of the monoclonal variants could not be distinguished, antigenically, from wild-type virus. This would fit in with the concept of a very large number (40 to 50) of overlapping antigenic determinants on the hemagglutinin molecule, each of which is capable of inducing a particular monoclonal antibody. These appear in greater or smaller amounts in the sera of infected or vaccinated animals. However, some monoclonal variants were distinguishable from wild-type virus in hemagglutination-inhibition and immuno-double-diffusion tests using heterogeneous hyperimmune rabbit antisera or postinfection ferret sera. These were variants showing a change at position 144 in HA1 of glycine to aspartic acid, the third variant obtained in the multistep selection experiment which showed a change at position 145 in HA1 of serine to lysine, and the second-generation variant of the PRO (143) → HIS variant which had a change at position 144 of glycine to aspartic acid.

Moss et al.[38] also found a change at position 144 in HA1 of glycine to aspartic acid in an antigenically distinguishable (with heterogeneous sera) mutant (29C) of Hong Kong influenza virus selected with the most avid fraction of homologous antibody.[35]

These findings suggest that sequence changes in the region comprising residues 142 to 146 of HA1 affect an important antigenic site on the hemagglutinin molecule, but whether this region forms an actual part of the site or how the sequence changes affect the antigenic properties are not yet known.

G. Use of Monoclonal Antibodies to Investigate Antigenic Drift in the Nucleocapsid Antigen (NP)

Direct evidence for antigenic variation in the NP was first reported by Schild et al.[39] Using immune sera to purified NP in double immunodiffusion tests, they found that the NP of the PR/8/34 (H1N1) strain differed antigenically from the NP of the H3N2 strains. Although their results indicated that antigenic variation in the NP of human strains occurred during the period from 1934 to 1968, interpretation of their data were limited by the source of antibody used and the low sensitivity of the serological assay employed. Because immune serum is a heterogeneous mixture of antibodies, small changes in the NP would not be detected in serological tests with such antisera. Furthermore, immunodiffusion tests are insensitive and detect only antibodies which form visible precipitates; minor subpopulations of antibodies to different determinants are not detectable.

To examine antigenic variation in NP more precisely, homogeneous monoclonal antibodies to NP were tested in enzyme-linked immunosorbent assays (ELISA) with human and "animal" influenza strains isolated between 1933 and 1979.[40]

It was found that the nucleoprotein molecule of the WSN/33 strain possessed at least five different determinants. Viruses of other influenza A virus subtypes showed antigenic variation in these nucleoprotein determinants, although changes in only one determinant were detected in H1N1 and animal strains. The nucleoprotein of human strains isolated from 1933 through 1979 could be divided into six groups, based on their reactivities with monoclonal antibodies, these groups did not correlate with any particular hemagglutinin or neuraminidase subtype. The results indicated that antigenic variation in the nucleoproteins of influenza A viruses proceeded independently of changes in the viral surface antigens.

H. Variants Selected with Monoclonal Antibodies to the Neuraminidase

Monoclonal, hybridoma antibodies have been prepared which bind to the neuraminidase of A/Tokyo/67 (H2N2) virus and inhibit its enzymatic activity.

Variants of the recombinant virus A/NWS_H−$Tokyo/67_N$ (H1N2) have been selected with these monoclonal antibodies to the neuraminidase.[43] The neuraminidase of the variant does not bind (and is not inhibited by) the monoclonal antibody used in the selection. The sequence changes in these variants are being determined.

Tokyo/67 neuraminidase "heads" (released from the virus partially by pronase digestion) have been crystallized[19,21] and the three-dimensional structure is being determined.[20] Isomorphous crystals of NA heads from one of the variants selected with monoclonal antibody to the NA are also being examined as well as crystals of Fab from the monoclonal antibody used in the selection.[44]

These experiments should provide information about the structure of an antigenic site on the neuraminidase and the complementary binding site on the antibody molecule.

III. SUMMARY AND CONCLUSIONS

Monoclonal antibodies provide a tool for the precise antigenic analysis of influenza virus variants. Monoclonal antibodies have also been used to select antigenic variants of influenza type A virus in which changes in antigenicity have been found to be associated with single sequence changes in the hemagglutinin molecule. The location of these changes in the 3-dimensional structure of the HA is known, and the way in which the changes alter the sites which bind neutralizing antibody is currently under investigation.

ACKNOWLEDGMENTS

The work of the author was supported in part by Research Grant number AI 15343 from the National Institute of Allergy and Infectious Diseases.

REFERENCES

1. **Nakajima, K., Desselberger, U., and Palese, P.,** Recent human influenza A (H1N1) viruses are closely related genetically to strains isolated in 1950, *Nature (London)*, 274, 334, 1978.
2. **Kendal, A. P., Noble, G. R., Skehel, J. J., and Dowdle, W. R.,** Antigenic similarity of influenza A (H1N1) viruses from epidemics in 1977—1978 to "Scandinavian" strains isolated in epidemics of 1950—1951, *Virology*, 89, 632, 1978.
3. **Moore, B. W., Webster, R. G., Bean, W. J., van Wyke, K. L., Laver, W. G., Evered, M. G., and Downie, J. C.,** Reappearance in 1979 of a1968 Hong Kong-like influenza virus, *Virology*, 109, 219, 1981.
4. **Pereira, M. S.,** Global surveillance of influenza, *Br. Med. Bull.*, 35(1), 9, 1979.
5. **Wiley, D. C., Skehel, J. J., and Waterfield, M.,** Evidence from studies with a cross-linking reagent that the hemagglutinin of influenza virus is a trimer, *Virology*, 79, 446, 1977.
6. **Porter, A. G., Barber, C., Carey, N. H., Hallewell, R. A., Threlfall, G., and Emtage, J. S.,** Complete nucleotide sequence of an influenza virus hemagglutinin gene from cloned DNA, *Nature (London)*, 282, 471, 1979.
7. **Gething, M. J., Bye, J., Skehel, J., and Waterfield, M.,** Cloning and DNA sequence of double-stranded copies of hemagglutinin genes from H2 and H3 strains elucidates antigenic shift and drift in human influenza virus, *Nature (London)*, 287, 301, 1980.
8. **Ward, C. W. and Dopheide, T. A.,** Developments in cell biology 5. The Hong Kong (H3) hemagglutinin. Complete amino acid sequence and oligosaccharide distribution for the heavy chain of A/Memphis/102/72, in *Structure and Variation in Influenza Virus*, Laver, W. G. and Air, G. M., Eds., Elsevier, New York, 1980, 27.
9. **Sleigh, M. J., Both, G. W., Brownlee, G. G., Bender, V. J., and Moss, B. A.,** Developments in cell biology 5. The hemagglutinin gene of influenza A virus: nucleotide sequence analysis of cloned DNA copies, in *Structure and Variation in Influenza Virus*, Laver, W. G. and Air, G. M. Eds., Elsevier, New York, 1980, 69.
10. **Verhoeyen, M., Fang, R., Min Jou, W., Devos, R., Huylebroeck, D., Saman, E., and Fiers, W.,** Antigenic drift between the hemagglutinin of the Hong Kong influenza strains A/Aichi/2/68 and A/Victoria/3/75, *Nature (London)*, 286, 771, 1980.
11. **Threlfall, G., Barber, C., Carey, N., and Emtage, S.,** Developments in cell biology 5. Nucleotide sequence of the HA2 region of the A/Victoria/3/75 hemagglutinin gene determined from a cloned DNA transcript, in *Structure and Variation in Influenza Virus*, Laver, W. G. and Air, G. M., Eds., Elsevier, New York, 1980, 51.
12. **Min Jou, W., Verhoeyen, M., Devos, R., Saman, E., Fang, R., Huylebroeck, D., Fiers, W., Threlfall, G., Barber, C., Carey, N., and Emtage, S.,** Complete structure of the hemagglutinin gene from the human influenza A/Victoria/3/75 (H3N2) strain as determined from cloned DNA, *Cell*, 19, 683, 1980.
13. **Wiley, D. C. and Skehel, J. J.,** Crystallization and X-ray diffraction studies on the hemagglutinin glycoprotein from the membrane of influenza virus, *J. Mol. Biol.*, 112, 343, 1977.
14. **Wilson, I. A., Skehel, J. J., Wiley, D. C.,** Structure of the hemagglutinin membrane glycoprotein of influenza virus at 3 Å resolution, *Nature (London)*, 289, 366, 1981.
15. **Wiley, D. C., Wilson, I. A., and Skehel, J. J.,** Structural identification of the antibody-binding sites of Hong Kong influenza haemagglutinin and their involvement in antigenic variation, *Nature (London)*, 289, 373, 1981.
16. **Laver, W. G., Downie, J. C., and Webster, R. G.,** Studies on antigenic variation in influenza virus. Evidence for multiple antigenic determinants on the hemagglutinin subunits of A/Hong Kong/68 (H3N2) virus and the A/England/72 strains, *Virology*, 59, 230, 1974.

17. **Virelizier, J. L., Allison, A. C., and Schild, G. C.,** Antibody responses to antigenic determinants of influenza virus hemagglutinin. II. Original antigenic sin: a bone marrow-derived lymphocyte memory phenomenon modulated by thymus-derived lymphocytes, *J. Exp. Med.*, 140, 1571, 1974.
18. **Wrigley, N. G., Skehel, J. J., Charlwood, P. A., and Brand, C. M.,** The size and shape of influenza virus neuraminidase, *Virology*, 51, 525, 1973.
19. **Laver, W. G.,** Crystallization and peptide maps of neuraminidase "heads" from H2N2 and H3N2 influenza virus strains, *Virology*, 86, 78, 1978.
20. **Colman, P. M., Tulloch, P. A., and Laver, W. G.,** Preliminary structural studies on two influenza virus neuraminidases, developments in cell biology 5, in *Structure and Variation in Influenza Virus*, Laver, W. G. and Air, G. M., Eds., Elsevier, New York, 1980, 351.
21. **Wright, C. E. and Laver, W. G.,** Preliminary crystallographic data for influenza virus neuraminidase "heads", *J. Mol. Biol.*, 120, 133, 1978.
22. **Gerhard, W., Yewdell, J., Frankel, M. E., Lopes, D. A., and Staudt, L.,** Monoclonal antibodies against influenza virus, in *Monoclonal Antibodies*, Kennett, R. H., McKean, T. J., and Bechtol, K. B., Eds., Plenum, 1980, 317.
23. **Yewdell, J. W. and Gerhard, W.,** Antigenic characterization of viruses by monoclonal antibodies, *Annu. Rev. Microbiol.*, 35, 185, 1981.
24. **Webster, R. G. and Laver, W. G.,** Determination of the number of nonoverlapping antigenic areas on Hong Kong (H3N2) influenza virus haemagglutinin with monoclonal antibodies and the selection of variants with potential epidemiological significance, *Virology*, 104, 139, 1980.
25. **Webster, R. G. and Berton, M. T.,** Analysis of antigenic drift in the hemagglutinin molecules of influenza B virus with monoclonal antibodies, *J. Gen. Virol.*, 54, 243, 1981.
26. **Yewdell, J. W., Webster, R. G., Gerhard, W. U.,** Antigenic variation in three distinct determinants of an influenza type A haemagglutinin molecule, *Nature (London)*, 279, 246, 1979.
27. **Portner, A., Webster, R. G., and Bean, J. W.,** Similar frequencies of antigenic variants in Sendai, vesicular stomatitis, and influenza A viruses, *Virology*, 104, 235, 1980.
28. **Laver, W. G., Gerhard, W., Webster, R. G., Frankel, M. E., and Air, G. M.,** Antigenic drift in type A influenza virus: peptide mapping and antigenic analysis of A/PR/8/34 (H0N1) variants selected with monoclonal antibodies, *Proc. Natl. Acad. Sci., U.S.A.*, 76, 1425, 1979.
29. **Laver, W. G., Air, G. M., and Webster, R. G.,** Mechanism of antigenic drift in influenza virus. Amino acid sequence changes in an antigenically active region of Hong Kong (H3N2) influenza virus hemagglutinin, *J. Mol. Biol.*, 145, 339, 1981.
30. **Laver, W. G., Air, G. M., Dopheide, T. A., and Ward, C. W.,** Amino acid sequence changes in the haemagglutinin of A/Hong Kong (H3N2) influenza virus during the period 1968—77, *Nature (London)*, 283, 454, 1980.
31. **Laver, W. G., Air, G. M., Webster, R. G., Gerhard, W., Ward, C. W., and Dopheide, T. A.,** Antigenic drift in type A influenza virus: sequence differences in the hemagglutinin of Hong Kong (H3N2) variants selected with monoclonal hybridoma antibodies, *Virology*, 98, 226, 1979.
32. **Fazekas de St. Groth, S.,** New criteria for the selection of influenza vaccine strains, *Bull. W.H.O.*, 41, 651, 1969.
33. **Fazekas de St. Groth, S.,** Evolution and hierachy of influenza viruses, *Arch. Environ. Health*, 21, 293, 1970.
34. **Fazekas de St. Groth, S.,** The phylogeny of influenza, in *Negative Strand Viruses: Proceedings*, Vol. 2, Mahy, B. W. and Barry, R. D., Eds., 1973, 741.
35. **Fazekas de St. Groth, S.,** Antigenic, adaptive and adsorptive variants of the influenza A hemagglutinin, *Top. Infect. Dis.*, 3, 25, 1978.
36. **Underwood, P. A.,** Serology and energetics of cross-reactions among the H3 antigens of influenza viruses, *Infect. Immun.*, 27, 397, 1980.
37. **Gerhard, W.,** The delineation of antigenic determinants of the hemagglutinin of influenza A viruses by means of monoclonal antibodies, *Top. Infect. Dis.*, 3, 15, 1978.
38. **Moss, B. A., Underwood, P. A., Bender, V. J., and Whittaker, R. G.,** Antigenic drift in the haemagglutinin from various strains of influenza virus A/Hong Kong/68 (H3N2), developments in cell biology 5, in *Structure and Variation in Influenza Virus*, Laver, W. G. and Air, G. M., Eds., Elsevier, New York, 1980, 329.
39. **Schild, G. C., Oxford, J. S., and Newman, R. W.,** Evidence for antigenic variation in influenza A nucleoproteins, *Virology*, 93, 569, 1979.
40. **van Wyke, K. L., Hinshaw, V. S., Bean, W. J., and Webster, R. G.,** Antigenic variation of influenza A virus nucleoprotein detected with monoclonal antibodies, *J. Virol.*, 35, 24, 1980.
41. **Air, G. M.,** Sequence relationships between the hemagglutinin genes of twelve subtypes of influenza A virus, *Proc. Natl. Acad. Sci. U.S.A.*, in press.

42. **Winter, G., Fields, S., and Brownlee, G. G.,** Nucleotide sequence of the haemagglutinin gene of a human influenza virus H1 subtype, *Nature* (*London*), 292, 72, 1981.
43. **Webster, R. G., Hinshaw, V. S., and Laver, W. G.,** Selection and analysis of antigenic variants of the neuraminidase of N2 viruses with monoclonal antibodies, *Virology,* in press.
44. **Colman, P. M., Gough, K. H., Lilley, G. G., Blagrove, R. J., Webster, R. G., and Laver, W. G.,** A crystalline monoclonal FAB fragment with specificity towards an influenza virus neuraminidase, *J. Molec. Biol.,* in press.
45. **Air, G. M.,** (unpublished data), 1981.

Chapter 6

MONOCLONAL ANTIBODIES TO HERPES SIMPLEX VIRUSES 1 AND 2

Lenore Pereira

TABLE OF CONTENTS

I. INTRODUCTION

This chapter describes hybridomas to herpes simplex viruses 1 and 2 (HSV-1, HSV-2) and the use of monoclonal antibodies as serologic reagents to study antigenic determinants of the viral glycoproteins. HSV-1 and HSV-2 have a linear double-stranded DNA genome with a molecular weight of 100 million, an icosahedral capsid consisting of 162 capsomeres, and an envelope acquired by budding of capsids through infected cell membranes.[1] HSV virions consist of four morphologically distinct structures. Innermost is the DNA core around which is the capsid having a well-defined protein composition. An amorphous layer of protein, designated the tegument, surrounds the capsid. The third layer is the virion envelope, a trilaminar membrane comprised of virus specific glycoproteins. HSV is subdivided into types 1 and 2 on the basis of neutralization tests with immune sera.[2,3] Studies of the immunologic specificity of the viral glycoproteins are complicated by the fact that conventional antisera produced against one serotype cross react with the heterologous serotype. Many laboratories have shown that HSV-1 and HSV-2 share biologic properties, including the structural organization of their genomes.[4,5] They were found, however, to differ in restriction enzyme cleavage sites in their DNAs, in the electrophoretic properties of the virus specific polypeptides, and in immunologic specificity of some of the viral proteins.[5–9] In order to better characterize the antigenic determinants of HSV glycoproteins, monoclonal antibodies were prepared to use as immunologic probes for cross reacting and type specific sites. We produced hybridomas and selected for antibody with neutralizing and nonneutralizing activity to HSV-1 and HSV-2.[10] During the process of characterizing hybridoma monoclonal antibodies we found that our result confirmed and extended studies done with monospecific antisera in other laboratories. On this basis, a brief summary of the current understanding of HSV glycoprotein structure, synthesis, function, and immunology will be presented prior to a discussion of monoclonal antibodies to HSV.

II. HSV GLYCOPROTEINS

A. Structure and Synthesis of Viral Glycoproteins

The HSV glycoproteins have been designated as gC, gB, gA, gE, and gD in order of their descreasing apparent molecular weights in polyacrylamide gels.[11–13] These fully glycosylated proteins correspond to virion proteins VP8, VP7, VP8.5, VP12.6, and VP18 respectively and are located in the virion envelope.[14,15] HSV protein synthesis is coordinately regulated and sequentially ordered to form at least three groups, designated α, β, and γ.[16] Most, if not all, of the major glycoproteins and structural proteins fall largely into the γ group.[17] Glycosylation of HSV proteins occurs in several discrete steps which produce partially glycosylated polypeptides.[11,18–20] Fully glycosylated proteins have a decreased mobility and higher apparent molecular weight than their glycosylated precursors. Pulse-chase experiments where a short interval of radioactive labeling was followed by a chase period in unlabeled media have shown that gC, gA, gB, gD, and gE are glycosylated in a stepwise fashion and that gA and gB glycoproteins are synthesized from a common precursor polypeptide.[11,12,19,20] It is known that 2-deoxyglucose or tunicamycin reduces glycosylation of viral glycoproteins; however, the structure of the nonglycosylated precursors has not been fully established.[21,22] Moreover, it is not clear whether glycosylation is dependent upon cellular enzymes or whether the virus specifies one or several glycosyltransferases. The conformation of glycoproteins gA, gC, and gD is monomeric, whereas gB appears to exist in a dimer form.[23] Viral glycoproteins bound to intracellular membranes and inserted into the plasma membrane of infected cells share antigenic determinants with glycoproteins in the virion envelope.[24–26] Cell surface immunofluorescence, antibody-dependent cell-mediated cytotoxicity tests and complement-dependent cytolytic tests show that antisera with neutralizing activity react with viral antigens at the surface of HSV infected cells.[27–30]

B. Glycoprotein Functions

Glycoproteins in the virion envelope are presumed to function in adsorption and penetration of the virion into uninfected cells. Those at the surface of infected cells moderate the interaction of cells in culture. Most HSV strains isolated thus far form large aggregates of rounded infected cells; however, strains which fuse cells into large polykaryocytes or syncytium have been selected.[31] Properties which result in polykaryocyte formation are genetically determined and expressed at the cell surface; mutants which fail to synthesize or accumulate certain glycoproteins have been isolated based on syncytial plaque morphology.[31] HSV-1(MP) strain, deficient in glycoprotein gC, causes fusion of infected cells; it is clear that the glycoprotein is not necessary for infectivity since gC deficient virions are infectious. Many other polykaryocyte forming mutants do synthesize all viral glycoproteins, which suggests that the *syn* phenotype is induced by different mutations.[32] HSV-1 mutant tsB5 which fails to accumulate glycoprotein gB at the nonpermissive temperature appears to be capable of adsorption, but not penetration.[33] Studies with a recombinant produced by a genetic cross between a mutant strain lacking glycoprotein gC and a strain temperature sensitive for glycoprotein gB indicated that the glycoproteins interact during infection.[34] Since fusion occured only at the permissive temperature, when gB was produced, the data suggest that glycoprotein gB functions to promote cell fusion, whereas glycoprotein gC is a fusion inhibitor. HSV infected cells acquire a new Fc-binding receptor on their surface.[35,36] Purification of the Fc-receptor showed that it is a viral glycoprotein which has been designated gE[12]. The function of glycoprotein gD is unknown; however, this glycoprotein is made in relatively large amounts and appears to be a powerful inducer of neutralizing antibody.[37]

C. Glycoprotein Gene Templates

Studies mapping the location of HSV glycoprotein genes showed that they are not contiguous on the physical map of HSV DNA.[32] There have been two methods used to map the gene template of HSV polypeptides. The first technique was based on the observation that the location of restriction endonuclease cleavage sites of HSV-1 and HSV-2 DNAs is different, and that some infected cell polypeptides and glycoproteins have different electrophoretic properties.[6,32] Analysis of HSV-1 × HSV-2 recombinants with respect to their DNA sequences and the glycoproteins they specify indicated that gA and gB map between 0.30 and 0.42 map units, whereas gD maps between 0.90 and 0.945 map units on the physical map of HSV DNA.[32] Genes specifying glycoprotein gC do not appear to be colinear in HSV-1 and HSV-2 DNAs, and intertypic recombinants specifying gC with the electrophoretic mobilities of both serotypes have been isolated. Glycoprotein gC of HSV-1 maps between 0.530 and 0.645, whereas the HSV-2 gene maps between 0.645 and 0.690. The second method used for mapping involved marker rescue of mutants with fragments of HSV-1 and HSV-2 DNA.[32] This technique confirmed the map position of the glycoprotein gB gene obtained by the first analysis.

The observation that some strains of HSV cause fusion of human and animal cell lines, whereas other strains fuse only some cell lines (e.g., Vero cells but not HEp-2 cells), was the basis for studies mapping genes involved in fusion. Three genetic loci, designated *syn 1*, *syn 2*, and *syn 3*, each mapping within a different physical region of the DNA, appear to determine cell fusion.[32] It is of interest to note that the *syn 3* locus is within the region of the map specifying glycoprotein gA and gB genes. The *syn 1* and *syn 2* genes which map to the right of the glycoprotein gC gene do not code for viral glycoproteins; however, some proteins in the virion envelope may be nonglycosylated. There is an additional genetic locus designated *Cr* which appears to control the synthesis of glycoprotein gC. It is conceivable that under certain physiological conditions expression of the *Cr* locus is modified and synthesis of gC is suppressed, permitting virus to spread from cell to cell without first being released. In view of the fact that fusion is induced by mutations in different genetic loci, it may be concluded that membrane proteins specified by HSV-1 are highly interactive and that mutations in one gene product may change the conformation and function of the others.

D. Antisera to Viral Glycoproteins

1. gC Glycoprotein

Antisera to HSV-1 glycoprotein gC (apparent molecular weight 130,000) have been produced in three ways: (1) the method used by Spear involved extensive adsorption of polyspecific serum to wild-type HSV-1 virions with cells infected with HSV-1(MP), a mutant which lacks the ability to produce gC,[11] (2) other investigators immunized with denatured HSV-1 gC polypeptides from polyacrylamide gels,[38,39] and (3) Vestergaard and Norrild immunized with a protein from agarose gels (Ag-6) immunoprecipitated from nonionic detergent-extracted HSV-1 antigens.[40] Although the antisera were produced by different methods, they have similar reactivities. Antisera produced by adsorption precipitated glycoprotein gC and its precursor pgC from HSV-1 infected cell extracts. The denatured gC glycoprotein retained many type specific determinants since antisera produced in this way discriminated between HSV-1 and HSV-2 in neutralization tests and reacted by immunofluorescence and agglutination only with homologous virus. Antisera produced against Ag-6 reacted with glycoproteins gC and pgC in immune precipitation tests.

2. gD Glycoprotein

Different methods have been used to produce antisera to HSV-1 glycoprotein gD (apparent molecular weight 62,000). Powell and Watson immunized with denatured polypeptides from polyacrylamide gels.[41] Sim and Watson immunized with immunoprecipitates from antigen ''band II''.[42] Vestergaard and Norrild immunized with immune precipitates of an antigen (Ag-8) from crossed immunoelectrophoresis.[40] Cohen et al.[43] immunized with a purified protein (CP-1) from affinity chromatography of soluble infected cell extracts. Concerning their reactivities, antisera to gD prepared against the denatured polypeptide failed to neutralize virions. In contrast, cross reacting and type specific neutralization of HSV-1 was obtained with antisera to ''band II'' antigen, suggesting that gD specifies type specific and type common determinants. Antisera produced against Ag-8 and CP-1 proteins neutralized both HSV-1 and HSV-2 and precipitated glycoprotein gD and its precursor pgD from HSV-1 infected cell extracts.

3. gE Glycoprotein

Taking advantage of the Fc-binding activity of glycoprotein gE, Bauke and Spear used affinity chromatography with BSA/anti-BSA coupled columns to purify gE.[12] Antisera to gE precipitated glycoprotein gE (apparent molecular weight 66,000 and its precursor pgE (apparent molecular weight 64,000) from HSV-1 infected cell extracts. In the presence of complement, cross-neutralizing activity was found with antisera to gE. It should be noted that HSV-1 was neutralized more efficiently than was HSV-2, suggesting that gE contains type specific and type common determinants. Para et al.[44]

showed that Fc-binding receptors were transferred to the cell surface presumably by fusion of the virion envelope with the plasma membrane during infection.

4. gA and gB Glycoproteins

Antisera to gA and gB glycoproteins of HSV-1 have been produced by Vestergaard and Norrild with immunoprecipitated Ag-11 and by Eberle and Courtney using denatured polypeptides from polyacrylamide gels.[20,40] In both instances the antisera did not differentiate the glycoproteins and immunoprecipitated both gA (apparent molecular weight 119,000) and gB (apparent molecular weight 126,000) from infected cell extracts; thus, gA and gB glycoproteins are antigenically similar and appear to be two different forms of the same polypeptide. Antisera to gA and gB cross react and neutralize viral infectivity in the presence or absence of complement.[20]

III. MONOCLONAL ANTIBODY TO HSV-1 AND HSV-2

A. Production of Hybridomas to HSV

To produce hybridomas secreting antibody to HSV we used the method described by Oi and Herzenberg for somatic cell hybridization and cloning of hybrid cells.[10,45] One month after infection of BALB/c mice with HSV-1(F) or HSV-2(G) the mice were immunized with nonionic detergent-treated infected cell extracts in complete Freund adjuvant. Prior to fusion the mice were injected with an aqueous extract of infected cells. The spleen cells were fused with an equal number of NS-1 cells using polyethylene glycol, and hybrids were selected in culture medium containing hypoxanthine, aminopterin, and thymidine (see Chapter 1).

Three series of experiments were done as described below to characterize the specificity of antibody produced by the hybridomas: indirect immunofluorescence tests, plaque reduction assays, and immune precipitation reactions. The initial step in selection required screening large numbers of clones for antibody reactive with HSV antigens. For this series of experiments immunofluorescence tests were done with homologous and heterologous virus-infected cells. In the secondary characterizations, hybridoma fluids positive by immunofluorescence were tested for neutralizing activity to HSV-1 and HSV-2 in plaque reduction assays. In this way hybridomas which produced type specific and cross reacting antibody to viral glycoproteins were selected. To characterize the reactivity of both neutralizing and nonneutralizing antibody for HSV proteins, immune precipitation reactions were done with radiolabeled infected cell extracts, and the precipitates were analyzed in polyacrylamide gels. By these procedures 200 clones were selected, approximately 15% of which produced neutralizing antibody and precipitated glycoproteins gC, gA, gB, and gD of HSV-1 and glycoproteins gA, gB, and gD of HSV-2. Immunologic characteristics of hybridoma antibodies reactive with the viral glycoproteins are shown in Table 1.

B. Screening for Antibody to HSV

In the first series of experiments indirect immunofluorescence tests were done to select hybridomas producing antibody reactive with cells infected with homologous and heterologous serotypes. Hybridoma supernatant fluids were reacted with artificial mixtures of HSV-1(F) or HSV(G) infected and uninfected HEp-2 cells. Typical patterns of immunofluorescence obtained with hybridomas which produced neutralizing antibody to viral glycoproteins are shown in the photomicrographs in Figure 1. Hybridoma antibody HC1 to glycoprotein gC of HSV-1 fluoresced strongly with antigen in the membranes of infected cells (panel a). Hybridoma antibody H368 reacted with glycoproteins gA and gB in HSV-2 infected cells (panel b). Hybridoma antibodies H233

Table 1
REACTIVITY OF HYBRIDOMAS TO HSV-1(F) AND HSV-2(G)

Classes of hybridomas	Hybridoma clones	Immunofluorescence reaction		Neutralizing activity		Glycoprotein immunoprecipitated	
		HSV-1	HSV-2	HSV-1	HSV-2	HSV-1	HSV-2
1	HC1, HC2	+	—	+[a]	0	gC	—
2	HD1, HD2, 66, 128, 132, 136, 147, 162, 170, 181, 183, 192, 193, 238, 286, 329, 350, 351, 357, 387	+	+	+	+	gD	gD
3	HD3	+	+	+	0	gD	gD
4	120, 144, 146, 157, 172, 194, 233, 307, B7	+	+	+	+	gA,gB	gA,gB
5	154	—	+	0	+	—	gD
6	368	—	+	0	+	—	gA,gB
7	113, 115, 116, 123, 134, 179, 182, 195, 209, 211, 247, 277, 330, 358	+	+	0	0	gD	gD
8	356, 369	—	+	0	0	—	gD
9	112, 121, 126, 131, 167, 189, 309, 336, 343, 352, 367	+	+	0	0	gA,gB	gA,gB
10	110	—	+	0	0	—	gA,gB

[a]Failed to neutralize HSV-1(MP), a mutant strain deficient in gC glycoprotein.

and H157 reacted with glycoproteins gA and gB of both serotypes (panels c and d), as did H193 and HD1 reactive with glycoprotein gD heavily concentrated in the membranes of infected cells (panels e and f).

C. Characteristics of Monoclonal Antibody to HSV

1. Neutralizing Activity

In this series of experiments hybridomas which produced antibody to HSV detectable in immunofluorescence tests were assayed for neutralizing activity in plaque reduction assays against homologous and heterologous virus. Extracellular fluids from microwells were diluted serially and mixed with 30 to 50 plaque-forming units of HSV-1(F) or of HSV-2(G), incubated at 37°C for 30 min and plated on Vero cell monolayers.

To date, we have produced monoclonal antibodies to HSV-1 glycoproteins gC, gA, gB, and gD, and to HSV-2 glycoproteins gA, gB, and gD (Table 1). All hybridomas produced to glycoprotein gC of type 1 are type specific and neutralizing, in the sense that they precipitate only glycoprotein gC and its precursors and neutralize only HSV-1. The hybridoma antibodies to glycoproteins gA and gB of HSV-2 fall into four groups: (1) hybridomas which neutralize both HSV-1 and HSV-2 and precipitate glycoproteins gA and gB of both serotypes; (2) hybridomas which precipitate gA and gB of HSV-1 and HSV-2 but do not neutralize either virus; (3) hybridomas which neutralize HSV-2 and precipitate homologous glycoproteins gA and gB but are totally unreactive with HSV-1 virus or glycoproteins; and (4) hybridomas which precipitate gA and gB of HSV-2 but are nonneutralizing. Characterization of hybridoma antibodies to glycoproteins gA and gB of HSV-1 are in progress. The hybridoma antibodies to glycoprotein gD of HSV-2 fall into four groups: (1) hybridomas which precipitate glycoprotein gD of both HSV-1 and HSV-2 and neutralize both viruses; (2) hybridomas which precipitate

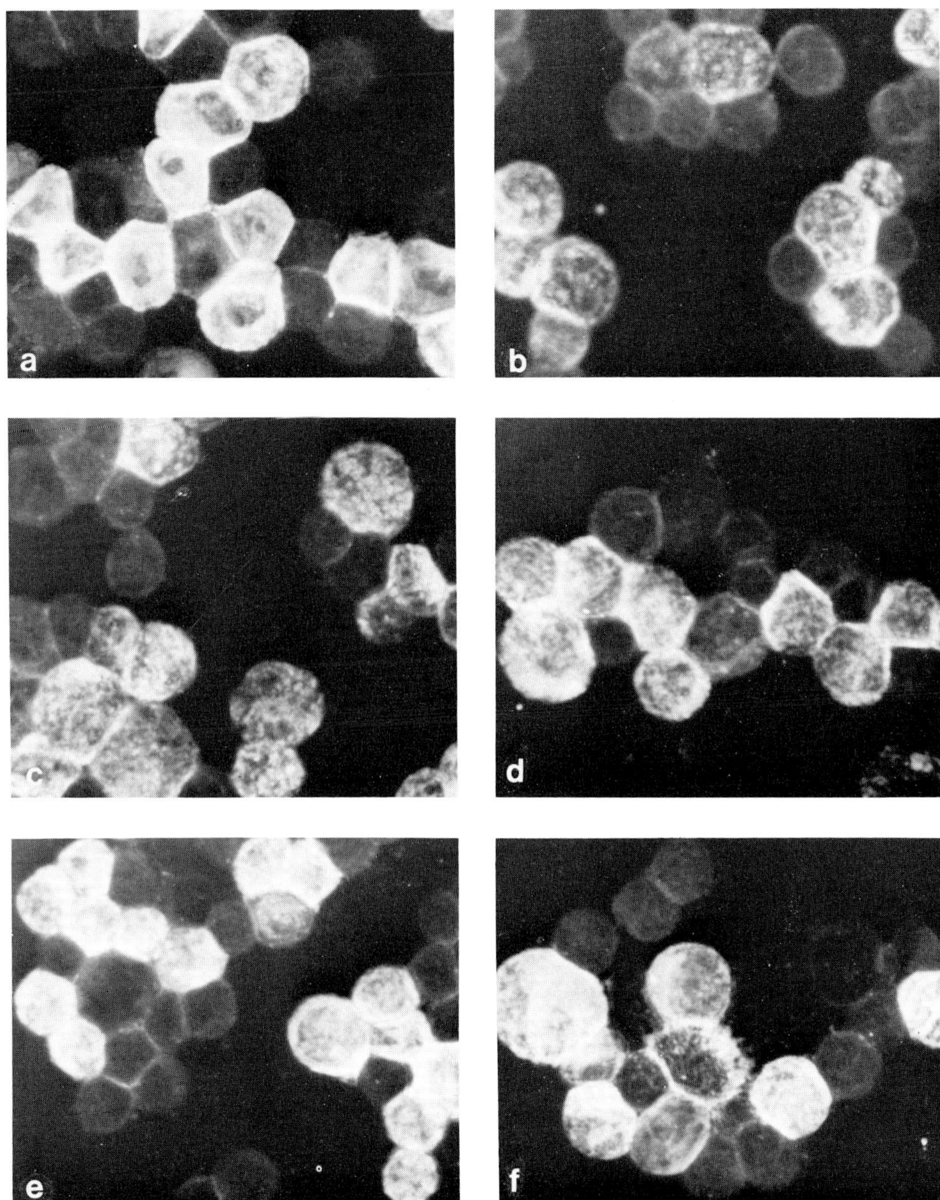

FIGURE 1. Photomicrographs of acetone-fixed HSV infected HEp-2 cells in indirect immunofluorescence tests with monoclonal antibody. Panel a: HSV-1(F) with hybridoma HC1. Panels b through h show HSV-2(G) infected cells with hybridomas (b) H368, (c) H233, (d) H157, (e) H193, (f) HD1. Magnification, X937.

both HSV-1 and HSV-2 gD but do not neutralize the virus; (3) hybridomas which neutralize HSV-2 only and precipitate glycoprotein gD of HSV-2 only; and (4) hybridomas which precipitate HSV-2 gD but are nonneutralizing. The hybridoma antibodies to glycoprotein gD of HSV-1 fall into two groups: (1) hybridomas which precipitate gD of both serotypes and neutralize both serotypes; and (2) hybridomas which precipitate gD of both serotypes but neutralize only HSV-1.

2. Reactivity with Antigens of the Surface of Infected Cells

Immunofluorescence reactions of hybridoma antibodies against unfixed HSV infected cells were done to determine whether antibody with neutralizing activity reacted with viral antigens in the plasma membranes of intact cells. Photomicrographs in Figure 2 compare the reactions of conventional immune antisera with HSV-1(F) and HSV-2(G) infected HEp-2 cells (panels a and b) with the reactions of monoclonal antibodies. Hybridoma antibody HC1 to HSV-1 glycoprotein gC showed immunofluorescence with HSV-1(F), but not with HSV-2(G) and HSV-1(MP) infected cells (MP is a mutant which fails to make glycoprotein gC) (panels c, d, and g). Hybridoma antibody HD1 to glycoprotein gD of both serotypes reacted by immunofluorescence with cells infected with all these strains (e, f, and h). One interesting finding which emerged from this study concerned the pattern of immunofluorescence. The immune sera produced a diffuse immunofluorescence on the surfaces of HSV-1 and HSV-2 infected cells, whereas the monoclonal antibody produced discrete foci of immunofluorescence on the surfaces of the infected cells with which it reacted. The punctate nature of the immunofluorescence produced by the monoclonal antibody suggests either that the individual glycoproteins aggregate on the plasma membrane or that they become aggregated following reaction with antibody.

3. Reactivity with HSV Glycoproteins

Immune precipitation tests were done to characterize the reactivity of monoclonal antibody to HSV glycoproteins. Cells were infected and labeled from 6 to 16 hr post infection with ^{35}S-methionine or ^{14}C-glucosamine. Radiolabeled antigens were prepared by treating the cells with nonionic detergents and centrifuging the extracts at 25,000 rpm at 4°C for 60 min to remove any insoluble protein complexes. For immunoprecipitation reactions the extracts were mixed with 1 to 10 $\mu\ell$ of mouse ascites fluid containing monoclonal antibody. The immune precipitates were adsorbed to protein A-Sepharose, washed and disrupted in sodium dodecyl sulfate and β-mercaptoethanol for electrophoresis in polyacrylamide gels. Comparisons of the immune precipitates of polyvalent antisera and of monoclonal antibodies HC1 and HD1 are shown in Figure 3. Antisera to HSV-1 reacted with glycoprotein gC of HSV-1 and gD of both serotypes. Glycoproteins gA and gB of HSV-1 were also precipitated and were present in trace amounts in immune precipitates of HSV-2 infected cells. Immune sera reacted with glycoprotein gD and its precursor, but predominantly with the fully glycosylated form of HSV-1 glycoprotein gC, whereas hybridoma antibody HC1 precipitated both precursor and fully glycosylated product. Antibody from this clone produced no detectable precipitates with extracts from HSV-1(MP) (a mutant which lacks gC) or HSV-2 infected cells (Figure 4). Antibody produced by hybridoma HD1 precipitated both the precursor and product forms of glycoprotein gD from HSV-1(F), HSV-1(MP), and HSV-2(G) infected cells (Figures 3 and 4). Evidence that the two bands precipitated by hybridoma antibodies HC1 and HD1 are related as precursor and product was shown by pulse-chase experiments. Based on the fact that the electrophoretic mobility of fully glycosylated proteins and their partially glycosylated precursors are different, the experiments were designed to show that precursors are processed into fully glycosylated products. Duplicate cultures were infected and radiolabeled for a short interval, after which one was terminated (pulse) and the other incubated without radiolabel for 10 hr (chase). The tests showed that only the slower migrating form of glycoproteins gC and gD was precipitated by hybridoma antibodies HC1 and HD1 (Figure 5).

With one exception, type specific and type common hybridoma antibodies with neutralizing activity precipitated similar glycoproteins. Polypeptides immunoprecipitated by three type specific hybridoma antibodies are compared with those precipitated by

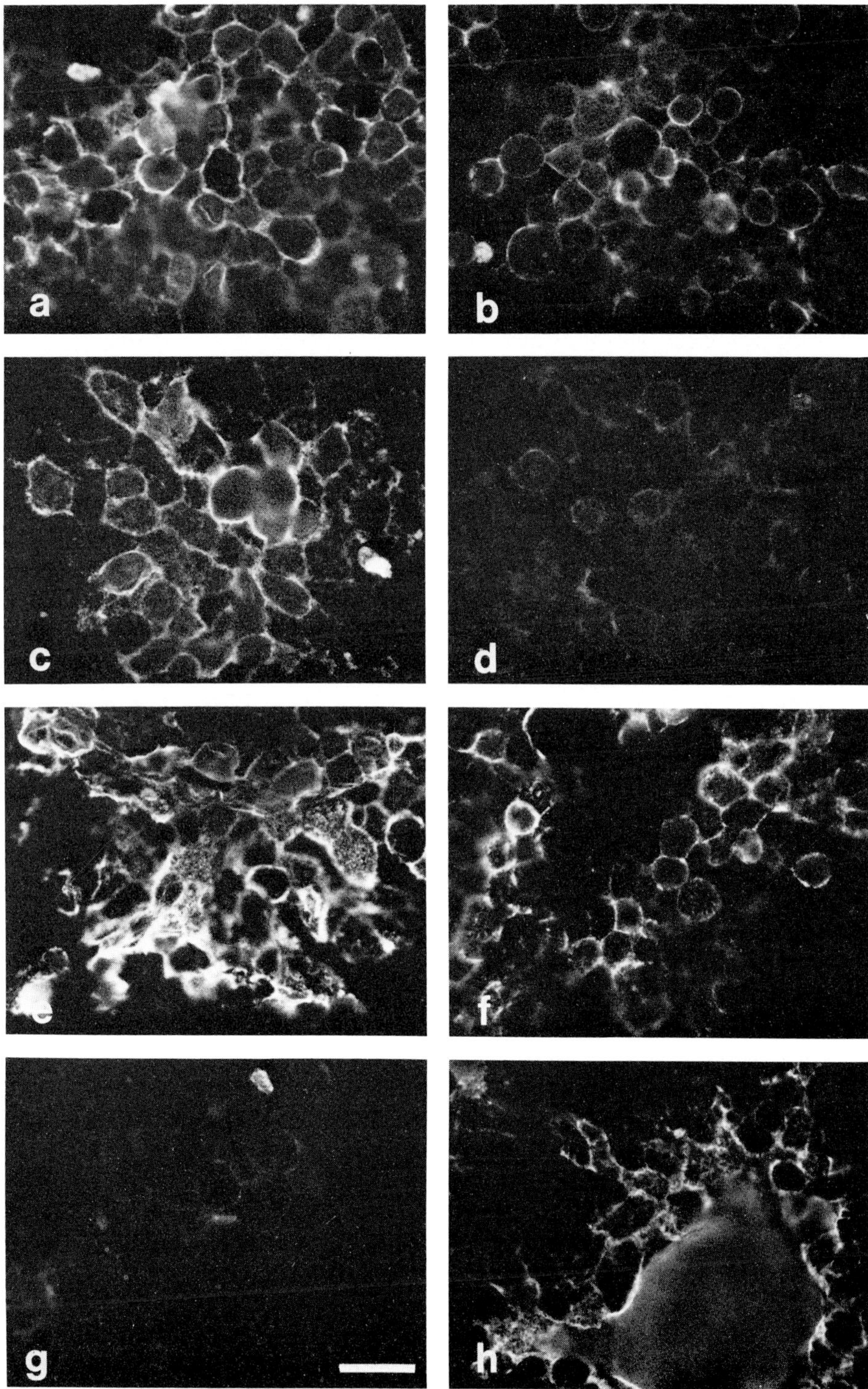

FIGURE 2. Photomicrographs of unfixed HSV-1 and HSV-2 infected HEp-2 cells in immunofluorescence reactions with immune sera and monoclonal antibodies. Panels a, HSV-1(F) and b, HSV-2(G) with HSV-1 immune serum; c, HSV-1(F) and d, HSV-2(G) with hybridoma HC1; e, HSV-1(F) and f, HSV-2(G) with hybridoma HD1; HSV-1(MP) with hybridoma HC1 (g) and hybridoma HD1 (h). The bar represents 24 μ.

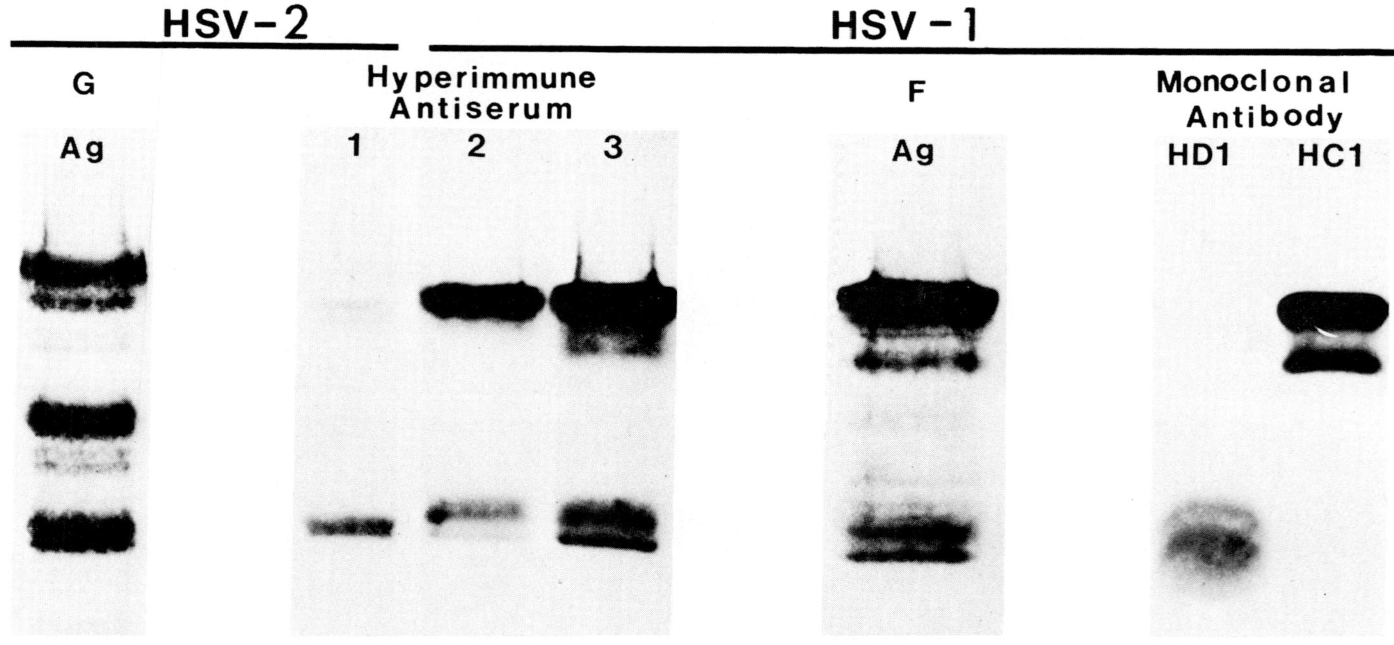

FIGURE 3. Autoradiograms of electrophoretically separated ^{14}C-glucosamine labeled immune precipitates of HSV-1(F) and HSV-2(G) infected HEp-2 cell extracts with immune sera and monoclonal antibody. Immune precipitates with antisera were done with HSV-2(G) infected cells radiolabeled from 5 to 24 hr pulse-labeled and chased HSV-1(F), and 5 to 24 hr labeled HSV-1(F) antigen. Immune precipitates of radiolabeled HSV-1(F) antigen with hybridomas HD1 and HC1 are shown in the right panel.

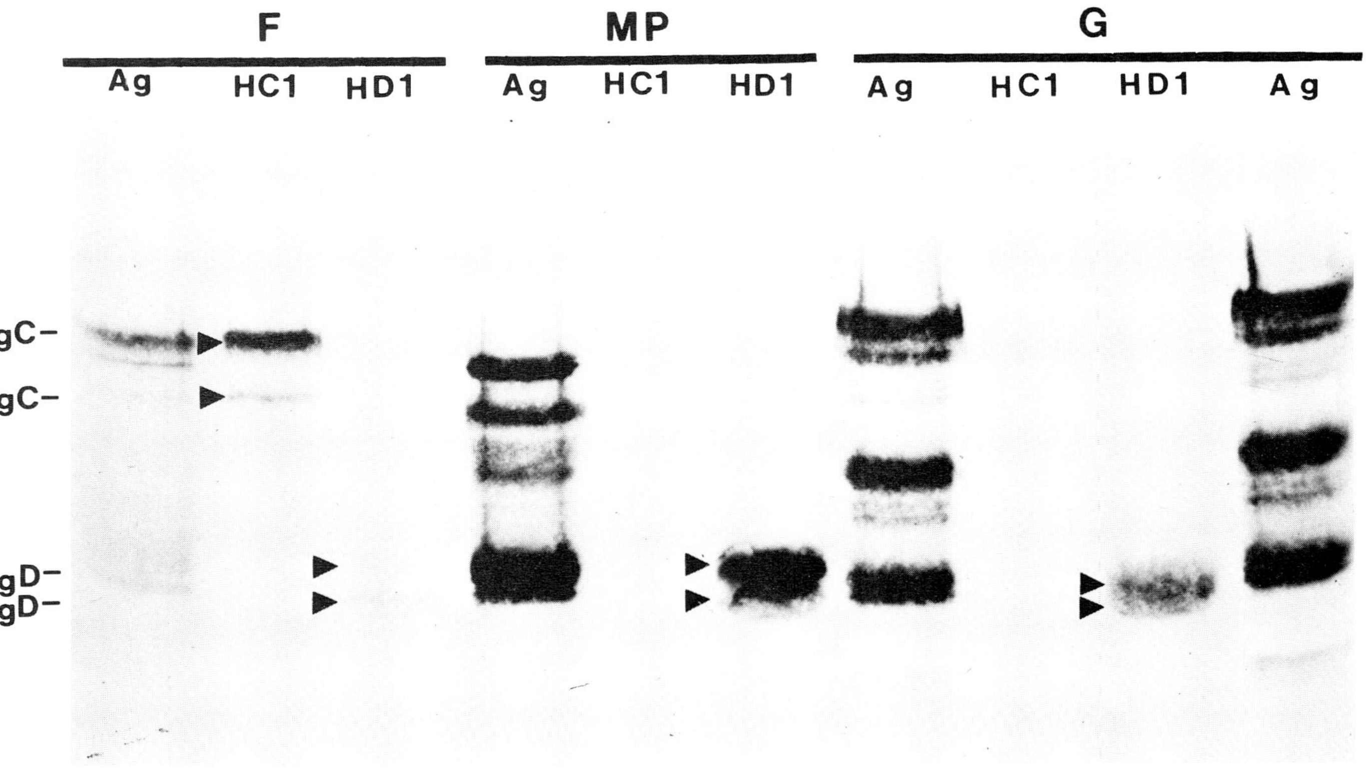

FIGURE 4. Autoradiograms of ^{14}C-glucosamine labeled antigen and immune precipitates of HSV-1(F), HSV-1(MP), and HSV-2(G) with hybridoma antibodies HC1 and HD1.

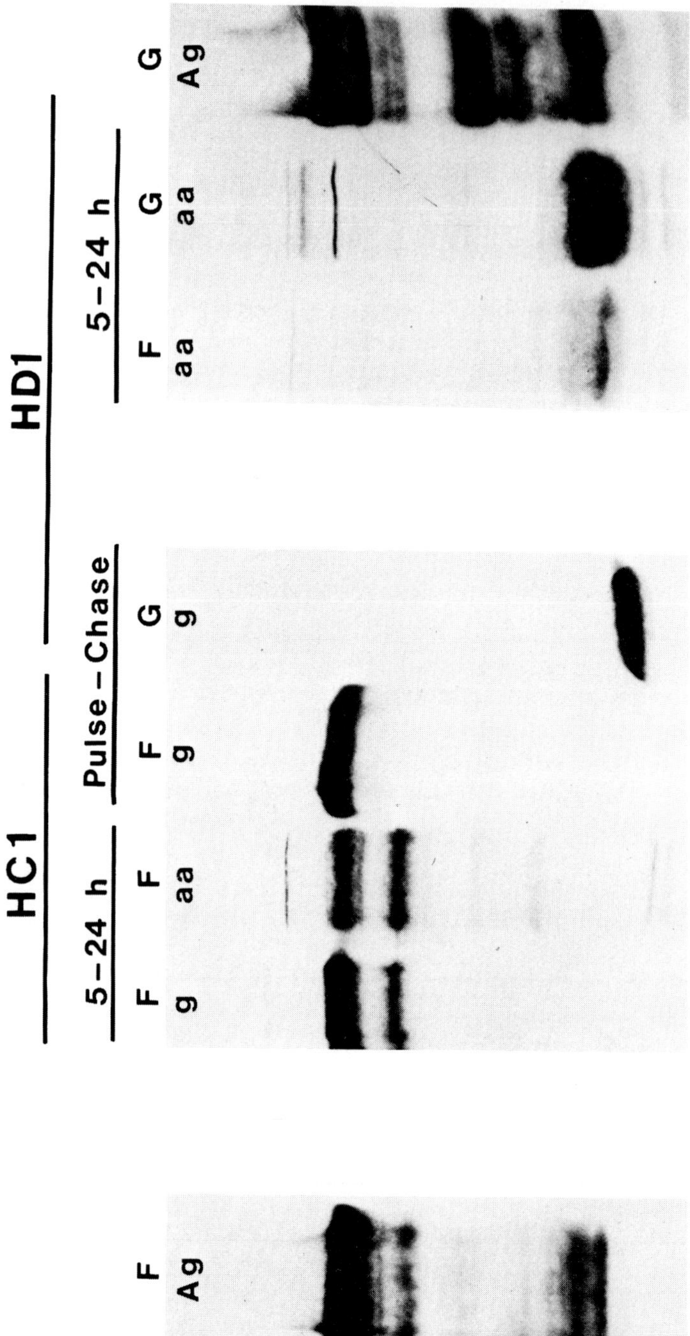

FIGURE 5. Autoradiograms of HSV-1(F) and HSV-2(G) antigen and immune precipitates from reaction with hybridomas HC1 and HD1. Infected cell extracts were radiolabeled with ^{14}C-glucosamine (g) or ^{14}C-amino acids (aa) from 5 to 24 hr post infection or for a 15 min interval at 6 hr post infection (pulse) and incubated in media without radioisotopes for 19 hr (chase).

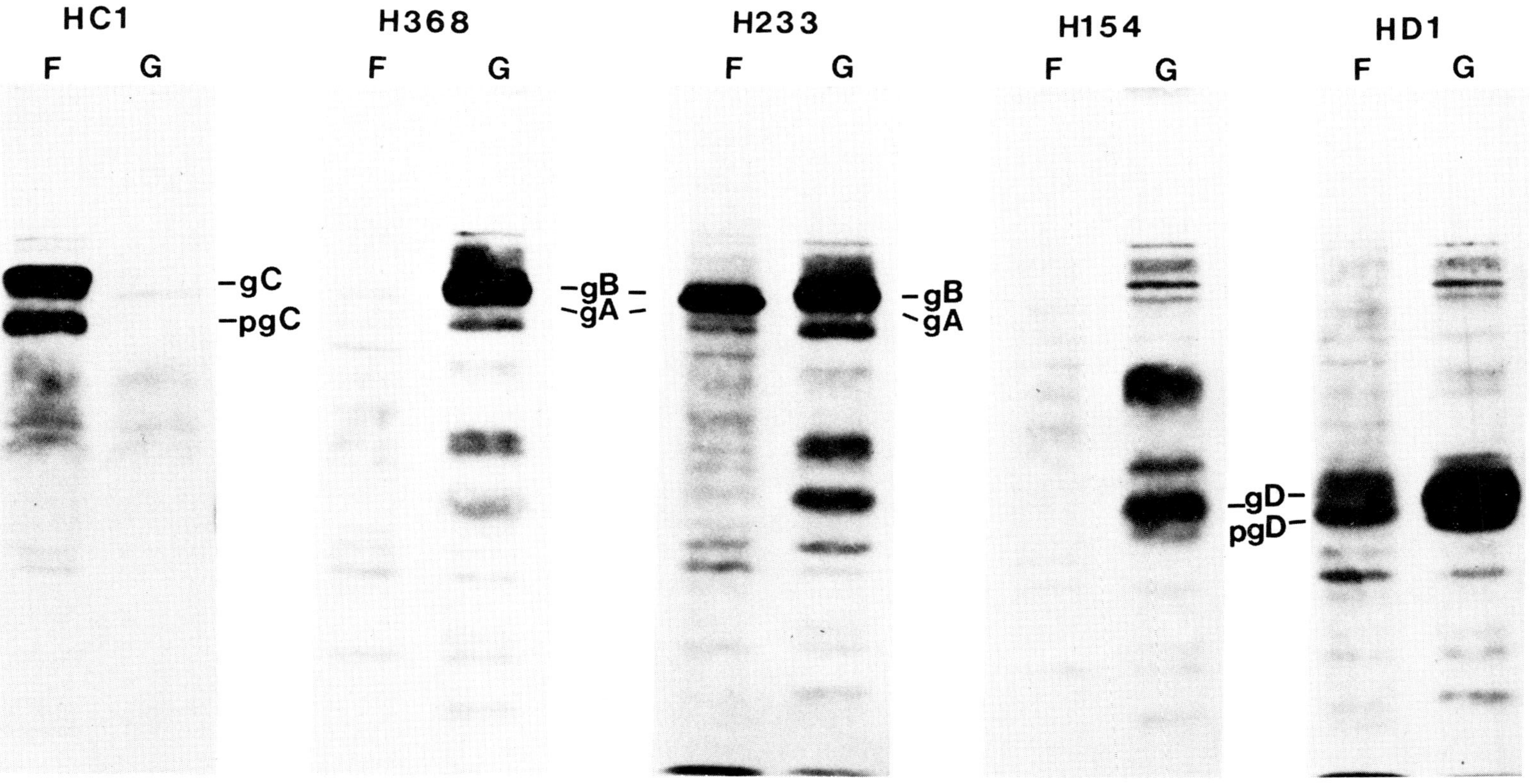

FIGURE 6. Autoradiograms of electrophoretically separated ^{35}S-methionine labeled polypeptides from immune precipitates of HSV-1(F) and HSV-2(G) with type specific hybridomas HC1, H368, H154, and cross reacting hybridoma antibodies H233, HD1.

type common hybridoma antibodies in Figure 6. Hybridoma antibody HC1 precipitated glycoprotein gC and its precursor from HSV-1 infected cell extracts. No antigenically homologous glycoprotein was precipitated from HSV-2(G) infected cells. Hybridoma antibody H368 precipitated glycoproteins gA and gB and hybridoma antibody H154 precipitated glycoprotein gD only from homologous HSV-2 infected cells. Hybridoma antibody H233 precipitated glycoproteins gA and gB and hybridoma antibody HD1 precipitated glycoprotein gD from cells infected with both serotypes.

4. Immunologic Specificity of HSV Glycoproteins

By correlating neutralizing activity, type specificity and reactivity of hybridoma antibodies with viral glycoproteins, four important points emerged:

1. In accord with previous conclusions that determinants on glycoprotein gC are not shared between HSV-1 and HSV-2, only type specific hybridomas precipitated glycoprotein gC.
2. Reactions of type specific and cross reacting hybridomas with glycoprotein gD showed that gD contains type specific and type common determinants. It should be noted that hybridoma antibody HD3 neutralized HSV-1 and precipitated glycoprotein gD of both serotypes, which suggests that the site is specified by gD of HSV-2 but is not available for reaction with antibody. Failure of HD3 to neutralize HSV-2 virions indicates that the glycoprotein may have a different conformation in the virion envelope.
3. All of the hybridoma antibodies to gA and gB precipitated both glycoproteins, which shows that they are immunologically related. Reactions of type specific and type common monoclonal antibodies to glycoproteins gA and gB of HSV-2 demonstrated that they contain both type specific and cross reacting sites.
4. Generation of a large number of hybridoma antibodies without neutralizing activity to gA, gB and gD glycoproteins suggests that determinants which bind neutralizing antibody may be different from those which bind nonneutralizing antibodies. It is possible that some domains of the glycoproteins are exposed at the surface of the virion envelope and elicit neutralizing antibody, whereas others, buried in the membrane, are not readily accessible to recognition by the immune system. This might be verified by topological mapping of the antigenic domains contained in the viral glycoproteins.

IV. STUDIES WITH HYBRIDOMAS TO HERPES SIMPLEX VIRUS

A. Antigenic Variation Among HSV Strains Detected by Serological Analysis with Monoclonal Antibodies

Serotyping HSV isolates presents a major problem in immunologic tests because polyvalent antisera produced against one serotype cross react with the heterologous serotype. Previous studies by Pereira et al.[46] showed that HSV-1 strains vary among themselves in the electrophoretic properties of their structural polypeptides, and by Buchman et al.[47,48] showed that restriction endonuclease cleavage patterns of the DNAs of epidemiologically unrelated HSV strains are different. In the course of testing type specific and type common monoclonal antibodies as reagents for serologic typing of HSV isolates, we found that some naturally occurring strains of each serotype varied in their antigenic determinants.[56] Variants were identified by failing to react with monoclonal antibody to a specific antigenic domain, as shown in similar types of studies with other viruses.[49–51] Currently we are analyzing strains with a panel of monoclonal antibodies to the viral glycoproteins. Preliminary results of serological analysis of 86 strains showed the hybridoma antibody HC1 reactive with glycoprotein gC of HSV-1 failed to react with 2% of the strains typed as HSV-1 with polyvalent antisera. Fully 30% of the strains typed as HSV-2 failed to react with hybridoma antibody H368 to glycoproteins gA and gB of HSV-2, however they did react with hybridoma antibody H233 to gA and gB of both serotypes. All of the strains in this study reacted with type common hybridoma antibody HD1 to glycoprotein gD. Two important points emerged from these studies: (1) HSV strains vary intratypically in the immunologic determinants specified by their glycoproteins and naturally occurring variants nonreactive with monoclonal antibodies can be selected, and (2) determinants on viral glycoproteins are not specified by all strains of a serotype; thus, the most useful reagents for serologic tests will consist of mixtures of type specific monoclonal antibodies.

B. Electrophoretic and Immunologic Properties of HSV Glycoproteins Produced in Different Cell Lines

In the course of characterizing the hybridoma antibodies to HSV we observed three interesting phenomena which suggested that viral glycoproteins are processed differently in different cell lines.[52] The first observation relates to the electrophoretic mobility of glycoproteins gA, gB, and gD made in infected HEp-2 (human epidermoid carcinoma No. 2) and Vero (African green monkey kidney) cells. Immune precipitates of HSV-1 and HSV-2 infected cells with hybridoma antibodies H233 and HD1 are shown in Figure 7. The electrophoretic mobility of the fully glycosylated proteins in HEp-2 cells was significantly slower than that of the corresponding glycoproteins produced in Vero cells. The second oberservation is that the HSV-2 infected Vero cell lysates contained three additional polypeptides with electrophoretic mobilities greater than glycoprotein gD which react with hybridoma antibodies to glycoproteins gA and gB. Lysates of infected HEp-2 cells did not contain such polypeptides. For purposes of identification we have designated these polypeptides as gA and gB reactive (A + B)r antigens. Other investigators with monoclonal antibodies to HSV capsid proteins have found that antigenically related proteins with different electrophoretic and structural properties are also precipitated.[53] The third observation concerns the reactivity of hybridoma antibody H368 to gA and gB of HSV-2, which reacts only with the glycoprotein of the homologous type (Figure 8). Hybridoma antibody H368 reacted only with the glycoproteins gA and gB made in HEp-2 cells but not with those made in Vero cells. This observation suggests that viral glycoproteins are processed differently in different cell lines; that the glycoprotein products made in some lines may not react with a specific hybridoma antibody either because the antigenic determinant site is cleaved off or that it is in some fashion masked. Furthermore, because (A + B)r antigens present in HSV-1(F) infected Vero cells differ in electrophoretic mobility from those present in HSV-2(G) infected Vero cells, and because they accumulate in Vero and not HEp-2 cells, it may be that they represent cleavage products of gA and gB that are host cell specific. Studies are now in progress to determine the basis for the differences observed and the origin of the (A + B)r antigens.

C. Studies on Fine-Mapping of Glycoproteins gA and gB

We took advantage of the type specific electrophoretic and immunologic properties of glycoproteins gA and gB to more precisely determine the map location of their genes by serological analysis of recombinants with monoclonal antibodies. Studies by Ruyechen et al.[32] showed that the genes for glycoproteins gA and gB are located between 0.03 and 0.42 map units on the HSV genome. Recently, Conley et al.[57] described

FIGURE 7. Autoradiograms of electrophoretically separated polypeptides labeled with ^{35}S-methionine and immunoprecipitated from HSV-1(F) and HSV-2(G) infected Vero and HEp-2 cells with hybridoma antibodies HC1, H233, and HD1.

intertypic recombinants from marker rescue with HSV-2 DNA digests of an HSV-1 temperature sensitive mutant. Several recombinants have crossover sites within the 10 million fragment region coding for gA and gB genes.

Preliminary results of a collaborative study in which we analyzed the intertypic recombinants with monoclonal antibodies are summarized. There were two kinds of experiments done. In the first series of experiments, cross reacting monoclonal antibody H157 was used to characterize the electrophoretic properties of glycoproteins gA and gB produced by the recombinants. Preliminary results of these experiments showed the three recombinants specified gA and gB with the electrophoretic mobility of HSV-2

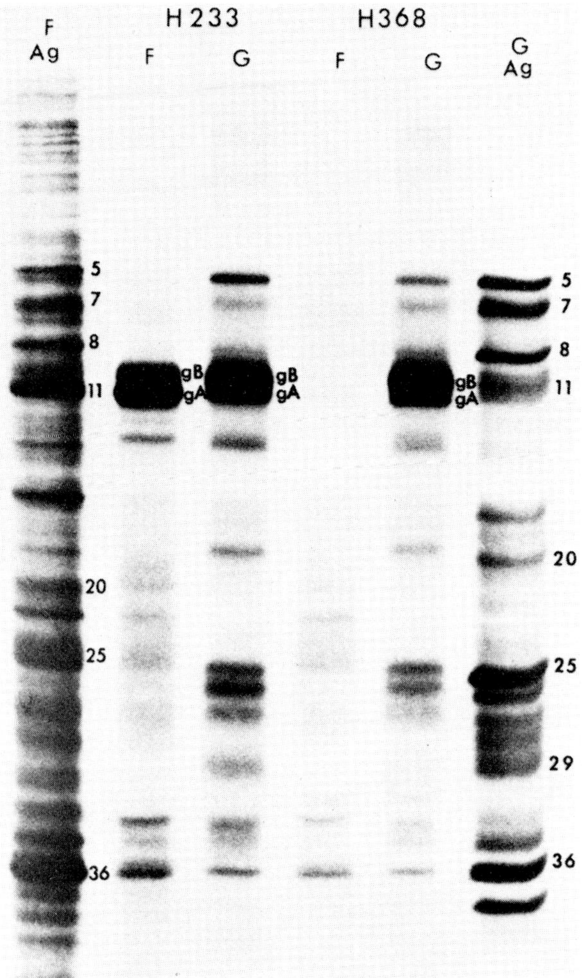

FIGURE 8. Autoradiograms of electrophoretically separated polypeptides labeled with ^{35}S-methionine and immunoprecipitated with hybridoma antibodies H233 and H368.

glycoproteins, whereas one recombinant specified glycoproteins which comigrated with the HSV-1 parent strain. We compared the electrophoretic properties of the glycoproteins with the HSV-1 or HSV-2 sequences present in the DNAs of recombinants to more closely define the boundaries of gA and gB genes. The data showed that the gene templates lie within a one million segment of DNA between 0.38 and 0.39 map units. In the second series of experiments, monoclonal antibody from HSV-2 specific hybridoma H368 was used to analyze the immunologic specificity of gA and gB glycoproteins produced by the recombinants. Preliminary analysis with immunofluorescence, neutralization, and immunoprecipitation tests corresponded with the electrophoretic properties of the glycoproteins. Recombinants identified as producing glycoproteins gA and gB with electrophoretic properties of HSV-2 reacted with hybridoma antibody H368, whereas the recombinant which failed to react produced gA and gB of HSV-1.

These experiments illustrated that monoclonal antibodies can be used as site specific immunologic probes in reaction with intertypic recombinants for localizing map positions of viral glycoprotein genes on HSV DNA, and that the genes can be mapped on the basis of the immunologic and electrophoretic properties of their gene products.

D. Effect of Monoclonal Antibody on HSV-Induced Neurological Disease

In a collaborative study reported by Dix et al.,[54] we tested the effect of monoclonal antibody to viral glycoproteins on acute HSV-induced neurological disease in mice. A murine model system was used in which onset of illness and mortality due to HSV-induced neurologic disease was proportional to the number of plaque forming units of virus inoculated into the footpad.[55] Monoclonal antibody HC1 to glycoprotein gC of HSV-1 and antibody from the cross reacting clone HD1 to glycoprotein gD were injected intraperitoneally prior to infection or at different times after infection. Results of these experiments correlated with the specificity of the antibody but differed for HSV-1 and HSV-2. When monoclonal antibody HC1 or HD1 was administered 2 hours prior to infection or up to 48 hours afterward 100% survival was obtained; however, monoclonal antibody HC1 did not limit HSV-2 infection regardless of the time antibody was administered. Monoclonal antibody HD1 was protective when injected up to 6 hr after HSV-2 infection, but failed to be effective at subsequent times.

These studies demonstrated for the first time the protective role of monoclonal antibody in an animal model system for acute HSV neurologic disease. Studies are in progress to test the effect of monoclonal antibody to other viral glycoproteins and the possible role of neutralizing antibody in mediating latent HSV infection.

V. CONCLUDING REMARKS

In our experience monoclonal antibodies proved to be powerful site specific probes for type specific and type common determinants on HSV glycoproteins. With a repertoire of hybridomas it will be feasible to conduct topological mapping studies of antigenic domains contained in the viral glycoproteins to determine their conformation in the virion envelope. The ultimate goal of these studies is to characterize the structure of the viral glycoproteins as it relates to their function in infection and the immune response to these viruses.

REFERENCES

1. **Roizman, B. and Furlong, D.,** The replication of herpesviruses, in *Comprehensive Virology,* Vol. 3., Fraenkel-Conrat, H. and Wagner, R. R., Eds., Plenum Press, New York, 1974, 229.
2. **Nahmias, A. J. and Dowdle, W. R.,** Antigenic and biologic differences in herpesvirus hominis, *Prog. Med. Virol.,* 10, 110, 1968.
3. **Rawls, W. E., Laurel, D., Melnick, J., Glickman, M., and Kaufman, R.,** A search for viruses in smegma, premalignant and early malignant tissues. The isolation of herpesviruses with distinct antigenic properties, *Am. J. Epidemiol.,* 87, 647, 1968.
4. **Nahmias, A. J. and Roizman, B.,** Infection with herpes-simplex viruses 1 and 2, *N. Eng. J. Med.,* 289, 781, 1973.
5. **Morse, L. S., Buchman, T. G., Roizman, B., and Schaffer, P. A.,** Anatomy of herpes simplex virus DNA. IX. Apparent exclusion of some parental DNA arrangements in the generation of intertypic (HSV-1 × HSV-2) recombinants, *J. Virol.,* 24, 231, 1977.
6. **Morse, L. S., Pereira, L., Roizman, B., and Schaffer, P. A.,** Anatomy of herpes simplex virus (HSV) DNA. X. Mapping of viral genes by analysis of polypeptides and functions specified by HSV-1 × HSV-2 recombinants, *J. Virol.,* 26, 389, 1978.

7. **Courtney, R. J. and Powell, K. L.,** Immunological and biochemical characterization of polypeptides induced by herpes simplex virus types 1 and 2, *IARC Sci. Publ.*, 11, 63, 1975.
8. **Spear, P. G.,** Glycoproteins specific by herpes simplex virus type 1: their synthesis, processing and antigenic relatedness to HSV-2 glycoproteins, *IARC Sci. Publ.*, 11, 49, 1975.
9. **Pereira, L., Wolff, M. H., Fenwick, M., and Roizman, B.,** Regulation of herpesvirus macromolecular synthesis. V. Properties of α polypeptides made in HSV-1 and HSV-2 infected cells, *Virology*, 77, 733, 1977.
10. **Pereira, L., Klassen, R., and Baringer, J. R.,** Type-common and type-specific monoclonal antibody to herpes simplex virus 1, *Infect. Immun.*, 29, 724, 1980.
11. **Spear, P. G.,** Membrane proteins specified by herpes simplex viruses. I. Identification of four glycoprotein precursors and their products in type 1-infected cells, *J. Virol.*, 17, 991, 1976.
12. **Bauke, B. and Spear, P. G.,** Membrane proteins specified by herpes simplex viruses. V. Identification of an Fc-binding glycoprotein, *J. Virol.*, 32, 779, 1979.
13. **Norrild, B.,** Immunochemistry of herpes simplex virus glycoproteins, *Curr. Topics Microbiol. Immunol.*, 90, 67, 1980.
14. **Spear, P. G. and Roizman, B.,** Proteins specified by herpes simplex virus. V. Purification and structural proteins of the herpesvirion, *J. Virol.*, 9, 143, 1972.
15. **Heine, J. W., Spear, P. G., and Roizman, B.,** Proteins specific by herpes simplex virus. VI. Viral proteins in the plasma membrane, *J. Virol.*, 9, 431, 1972.
16. **Honess, R. W. and Roizman, B.,** Regulation of herpesvirus macromolecular synthesis. I. Cascade regulation of the synthesis of three groups of viral proteins, *J. Virol.*, 14, 8, 1974.
17. **Honess, R. W. and Roizman, B.,** Proteins specified by herpes simplex virus. XI. Identification and relative molar rates of synthesis of structural and nonstructural herpes virus polypeptides in the infected cell, *J. Virol.*, 12, 1347, 1973.
18. **Honess, R. W. and Roizman, B.,** Proteins specified by herpes simplex virus. XIII. Glycosylation of viral polypeptides, *J. Virol.*, 16, 1308, 1975.
19. **Cohen, G. H., Long, D., and Eisenberg, R. J.,** Synthesis and processing of glycoproteins gD and gC of herpes simplex virus type 1, *J. Virol.*, 36, 429, 1980.
20. **Eberle, R. and Courtney, R. J.,** gA and gB glycoproteins of herpes simplex virus type 1: two forms of a single polypeptide, *J. Virol.*, 36, 665, 1980.
21. **Courtney, R. J., Steiner, S. M., and Benyesh-Melnick, M.,** Effects of 2-deoxy D-glucose on herpes simplex virus replication, *Virology*, 52, 447, 1973.
22. **Knowles, R. W. and Person, S.,** Effects of 2-deoxyglucose, glucosamine, and mannose on cell fusion and the glycoproteins of herpes simplex virus, *J. Virol.*, 18, 644, 1976.
23. **Sarmiento, M. and Spear, P. G.,** Membrane proteins specified by HSV. IV. Conformation of the virion glycoprotein designated VP7(B_2), *J. Virol.*, 29, 1159, 1979.
24. **Savage, R., Roizman, B., and Heine, J. W.,** Immunologic specificity of the glycoproteins of herpes simplex virus subtypes 1 and 2, *J. Gen. Virol.*, 17, 31, 1972.
25. **Rawls, W. E. and Tompkins, W. A. F.,** Destruction of virus-infected cells by antibody and complement, in *Viral Immunology and Immunopathology*, Notkins, A. L., Ed., Academic Press, New York, 1975, 99.
26. **Rager-Zisman, B. and Bloom, B. R.,** Immunological destruction of herpes simplex virus infected cells, *Nature (London)*, 251, 542, 1974.
27. **Geder, L. and Skinner, G. R. B.,** Differentiation between type 1 and type 2 strains of herpes simplex virus by an indirect immunofluorescent technique, *J. Gen. Virol.*, 12, 179, 1971.
28. **Glorioso, J. C., Wilson, L. A., Fenger, T. W., and Smith, J. W.,** Complement-mediated cytolysis of HSV-1 and HSV-2 infected cells: plasma membrane antigens reactive with type-specific and cross-reactive antibody, *J. Gen. Virol.*, 40, 443, 1978.
29. **Norrild, B., Shore, S. L., and Nahmias, A. J.,** herpes simplex virus glycoproteins. Participation of individual herpes simplex virus type 1 glycoprotein antigens in immunocytolysis and their correlation with previously identified glycopolypeptides, *J. Virol.*, 32, 741, 1979.
30. **Norrild, B., Shore, S. L., Cromeans, T. L., and Nahmias, A. J.,** Participation of three major glycoprotein antigens of herpes simplex virus type 1 early in the infectious cycle as determined by antibody-dependent cell-mediated cytotoxicity, *Infect. Immun.*, 28, 38, 1980.
31. **Hoggan, M. D. and Roizman, B.,** The isolation and properties of a variant of herpes simplex producing multinucleated giant cells in monolayer cultures in the presence of antibody, *Am. J. Hyg.*, 70, 208, 1959.
32. **Ruyechan, W. T., Morse, L. S., Knipe, D. M., and Roizman, B.,** Molecular genetics of herpes simplex virus. II. Mapping of the major viral glycoproteins and of the genetic loci specifying the social behavior of infected cells, *J. Virol.*, 29, 1149, 1979.
33. **Sarmiento, M., Haffey, M., and Spear, P. G.,** Membrane proteins specified by HSV. III. Role of glycoprotein VP7(B_2) in virion infectivity, *J. Virol.*, 29, 1149, 1979.

34. **Manservigi, R., Spear, P. G., and Buchan, A.,** Cell fusion induced by herpes simplex virus is promoted and suppressed by different viral glycoproteins, *Proc. Natl. Acad. Sci. U.S.A.*, 74, 3913, 1977.
35. **McTaggart, S. P., Burns, W. H., White, D. O., and Jackson, D. C.,** Fc receptors induced by herpes simplex virus. I. Biologic and biochemical properties, *J. Immunol.*, 121, 726, 1978.
36. **Nakamura, Y., Costa, J., Tralka, T. S., Yee, C. L., and Rabson, A. S.,** Properties of the cell surface Fc-receptor induced by herpes simplex virus, *J. Immunol.*, 121, 1128, 1978.
37. **Eisenberg, R. J., Ponce de Leon, M., Pereira, L., and Cohen, G.,** Purification of glycoprotein gD of herpes simplex virus types 1 and 2 using monoclonal antibody, *J. Virol.*, March 1982.
38. **Powell, K. L., Buchan, A., Sim, C., and Watson, D. H.,** Type-specific protein in herpes simplex virus envelope reacts with neutralizing antibody, *Nature (London)*, 249, 360, 1974.
39. **Eberle, R. and Courtney, R.,** Preparation and characterization of specific antisera to individual glycoprotein antigens comprising the major glycoprotein region of herpes simplex virus type 1, *J. Virol.*, 35, 902, 1980.
40. **Vestergaard, B. F. and Norrild, B.,** Crossed immunoelectrophoretic analysis and viral neutralizing activity of five monospecific antisera against five different herpes simplex virus glycoproteins, *IARC Sci. Publ.*, 24, 225, 1979.
41. **Powell, K. L. and Watson, D. H.,** Some structural antigens of herpes simplex virus, *Intervirology*, 8, 18, 1975.
42. **Sim, C. and Watson, D. H.,** The role of type specific and crossreacting structural antigens in the neutralization of herpes simplex virus types 1 and 2, *J. Gen. Virol.*, 19, 197, 1973.
43. **Cohen, G. H., Katze, M., Hydrean-Stern, C., and Eisenberg, R. J.,** Type-common CP-1 antigen of herpes simplex virus is associated with a 59,000-molecular-weight envelope glycoprotein, *J. Virol.*, 27, 172, 1978.
44. **Para, M. F., Baucke, R. B., and Spear, P. G.,** Immunoglobulin G(Fc)-binding receptors on virions of herpes simplex virus type 1 and transfer of these receptors to the cell surface by infection, *J.Virol.*, 34, 512, 1980.
45. **Oi, V. and Herzenberg, L.,** Immunoglobulin producing hybrid cell lines, in *Selected Methods in Cellular Immunology*, Mishell, B. and Schiigi, S., Eds., W. H. Freeman, San Francisco, 1980.
46. **Pereira, L., Cassai, E., Honess, R. W., Roizman, B., Terni, M., and Nahmias, A.,** Variability in the structural polypeptides of herpes simplex virus 1 strains: potential application in molecular epidemiology, *Infect. Immun.*, 13, 211, 1976.
47. **Buchman, T. G., Roizman, B., Adams, G., and Stover, H.,** Restriction endonuclease fingerprinting of herpes simplex DNA: a novel epidemiology tool applied to a nosocomial outbreak, *J. Infect. Dis.*, 138, 488, 1978.
48. **Buchman, T. G., Roizman, B., and Nahmias, A. J.,** Exogeneous genital reinfection with herpes simplex 2 demonstrated by restriction endonuclease fingerprinting of viral DNA, *J. Infect. Dis.*, 140, 295, 1979.
49. **Wiktor, T. J. and Koprowski, H.,** Monoclonal antibodies against rabies virus produced by somatic cell hybridization: detection of antigenic variants, *Proc. Natl. Acad. Sci. U.S.A.*, 75, 3938, 1978.
50. **Yedwell, J. W., Webster, R. G., and Gerhard, W. U.,** Antigenic variation in three distinct determinants of an influenza type A haemagglutinin molecule, *Nature (London)*, 279, 246, 1979.
51. **Webster, R. G. and Laver, W. G.,** Determination of the number of nonoverlapping antigenic areas on Hong Kong (H3N2) influenza virus hemagglutinin with monoclonal antibodies and the selection of variants with potential epidemiological significance, *Virology*, 104, 139, 1980.
52. **Pereira, L., Dondero, D., Norrild, B., and Roizman, B.,** Differential immunologic reactivity and processing of glycoproteins gA and gB of herpes simplex viruses 1 and 2 made in Vero and HEp-2 cells, *Proc. Natl. Acad. Sci. U.S.A.*, 78, 5202, 1981.
53. **Zweig, M., Heilman, C. J., Rabin, H., and Hampar, B.,** Shared antigenic determinants between two distinct classes of proteins in cells infected with herpes simplex virus, *J. Virol.*, 35, 644, 1980.
54. **Dix, R. D., Pereira, L., and Baringer, J. R.,** Use of monoclonal antibody directed against herpes simplex virus glycoproteins to protect mice against acute virus-induced neurological disease, *Infect. Immun.*, 34, 192, 1981.
55. **Stevens, J. G. and Cook, M. L.,** Latent herpes simplex virus in spinal ganglia of mice, *Science*, 173, 843, 1971.
56. **Pereira, L., Dondero, D. V., Gallo, D., Devlin, V., and Woodie, J. D.,** Serological analysis of herpes simplex viruses 1 and 2 with monoclonal antibodies, *Infect. Immun.*, January 1982.
57. **Conley, A. J., Knipe, D. M., Jones, P. C., and Rolzman, B.,** Molecular genetics of herpes simplex virus, VIII, Characterization of a temperature sensitive mutant produced by *in vitro* mutagenisis and defective in DNA synthesis and accumulation of γ polypeptides, *J. Virol.*, 37, 191, 1981.

Chapter 7

HYBRIDOMAS IN IMMUNOPARASITOLOGY*

Graham F. Mitchell

TABLE OF CONTENTS

*The work referred to in this article from the Laboratory of Immunoparasitology of this Institute is currently supported by the Australian National Health and Medical Research Council, The Rockefeller Great Neglected Diseases of Mankind Network, the UNDP/World Bank/WHO Special Programme for Research and Training in Tropical Diseases, and the H. V. McKay Charitable Trust.

I. INTRODUCTION

Immunoparasitology, the study of the immunological aspects of host-parasite† relationships, is currently a major growth area in biomedical research and is dominated by the quest for antiparasite vaccines. The hybridoma technique is one of several ''newer biotechnologies'' which have added another dimension to this field and provided it with a potent shot-in-the-arm.[1-4] One activity in immunoparasitology which predates most others is the *serology* of parasitic infection and disease caused by various protozoan and helminth parasites in their hosts.[5] Clearly, the availability of single-specificity monoclonal antiparasite antibodies in milligram quantities will render some of the current armementarium of the parasite serologist reduntant. Already, hybridoma-derived antibodies have been used to demonstrate the power of this technique for the dissection of immune responses to parasite antigens, for the identification and isolation of parasite antigens, and for immunodiagnosis of parasitic infection.

The immunoparasitologist is faced with numerous difficulties in the objective of providing quantitative data on antiparasite antibody responses and in differentiating between ''relevant'' and ''irrelevant'' parasite antigens.[6,7] A lack of defined parasite starting material in many systems imposes restraints on strategies to be used for antigen identification, analyses, isolations, and characterization. Structural and life cycle complexities of most parasites add to the difficulties to be overcome by the molecular (immunochemical) immunoparasitologist. It is to be expected that defined parasite antigens, isolated by monoclonal antibody affinity chromatography, will enable precise analyses to be performed on the spectrum of antiparasite immune responses in infected, diseased, vaccinated, or naturally-resistant hosts. Possession of a ''functional'' hybridoma-derived antibody (that is one which mediates host protection or in vitro antiparasite effects) should automatically lead to the identification of ''relevant'' antigens (that is relevant to host protection).

In immunoparasitology, hybridoma-derived (monoclonal) antibodies are being used for three broad purposes:

1. As probes for antigenic determinants in the analysis of antigen location, organization, and ''availability''; exploration of antigenic heterogeneity (variability) in parasite populations; detection of expression of cloned DNA in various vectors; and parasite typing.
2. The development of immunodiagnostic reagents of high specificity.
3. The analysis of antibody-mediated, parasite-inhibitory effects, in vivo and in vitro.

Variations of the general theme are the uses of T cell hybridomas for analyses of T cell responses to parasite antigens and effects of T cell-derived mediators on parasites or parasitized cells (no publications are available as yet, however) and the fusion of modified myeloma cells with protozoa such as *Trypanosoma cruzi*[8] for antigen or mRNA production.

Considerable information is available on murine hybridoma-derived antiparasite antibodies and this article will be confined to a review of the use of such antibodies in the analysis of parasite antigens and host-vs.-parasite immune responses.

†Arbitrarily, the term parasite is generally confined to protozoa, metazoa, (helminths) such as nematodes, cestodes and trematodes, and arthropods (usually ectoparasites).

II. HYBRIDOMA-DERIVED ANTIBODIES AS PROBES FOR ANTIGENIC DETERMINANTS OF PARASITES

A. Location and Organization of Antigens in Parasites

Monoclonal antibodies are proving useful in the mapping of antigens to certain locations in parasites or parasitized cells using immunofluorescence, immunoperoxidase, and autoradiographic procedures. Monoclonal *myeloma*-derived antibodies have been used in the past to locate phosphorylcholine (PC) in the nematodes, *Ascaris suum* larvae[9] and *Nippostrongylus brasiliensis* worms.[10] For these studies, the anti-PC myeloma proteins were fluoresceinated (± affinity purified), reacted with intact or sections of parasites, and examined using fluorescence microscopy. Similar studies with various hybridoma antibodies and direct or indirect immunofluorescence are in progress using the trematode, *Fasciola hepatica*.[11]

Detailed structural analyses of the variant surface glycoprotein (VSG) antigens of the protozoan *T. brucei* are now possible using monoclonal antibodies and several laboratories are undertaking such work. In addition to using monoclonal antibodies in affinity chromatography for isolation of VSG antigens and their antigenic determinants,[12] information on the organization and "availability" (in the intact extracellular bloodstream trypanosome) of antigenic determinants and the extent of microheterogeneity in VSG can be anticipated in the near future.[13] Such hybridoma-derived antibodies will also be useful in the detection of expression of cloned trypanosome DNA.[14,15]

Analyses of labeled surface antigens with hybridoma-derived antibodies have been reported with extracellular *Toxoplasma gondii* tachyzoites.[16,17] In this study, hybridomas were prepared which produced antibodies against four major labeled proteins on the extracellular protozoan surface, and the antibodies used for immunoprecipitation of labeled solubilized antigens. Also, two antigens were coprecipitated with one of the hybridoma antibodies and it can thus be assumed that these two antigens share at least one determinant, or that one is a subunit of the other, or that they are associated in the solubilized products if not on the parasite surface itself. Other papers have reported on the production of anti *T. gondii* monoclonals.[18,19]

Using *Schistosoma mansoni* eggs in a circumoval precipitation (COP) reaction, the soluble antigen MSA_1 (which has immunodiagnostic potential for schistosomiasis mansoni) has been shown to be released from eggs as a "COP antigen". An anti-MSA_1 hybridoma-derived antibody was used for this study.[20]

B. Parasite Typing

One report has indicated the power of hybridoma-derived antibodies in identifying antigenic variability in protozoan parasite populations about which little information is currently available. Macroschizonts of two geographic isolates of the bovine intracellular protozoan *Theileria parva* were shown to differ in their reactivity using a monoclonal antibody raised against one of them.[21] Unpublished results of a study using American leishmania parasites has demonstrated very clearly that antigenic variability exists within and between the *Leishmania mexicana* and *L. brasiliensis* complexes. Hybridomas were prepared using cells from mice immunized with promastigote membrane preparations of *L. mexicana amazonensis* and *L. brasiliensis panamanensis*.[22]

No publications have yet appeared on the use of hybridoma-derived antibodies for the detection of expression of cloned parasite genomic DNA or cDNA in vectors for purposes of protein antigen production using recombinant DNA techniques. Of course this will be a major use for hybridoma-derived monoclonal antibodies in the immediate future particularly using those antibodies shown to have in vivo or in vitro parasite inhibitory effects (see below).

III. HYBRIDOMA-DERIVED ANTIBODIES IN IMMUNODIAGNOSIS OF PARASITIC INFECTION

The first indication that hybridoma-derived antibodies would be useful in the development of new immunodiagnostic tests (IDTs) of high specificity was provided in a model parasite system.[23] An IgG_1 monoclonal antibody (designated McH.105) was produced from the fusion of cells of mice infected with the proliferating larval cestode, *Mesocestoides corti,* and used in a competitive solid-phase radioimmunoassay (RIA) with the crudest of parasite homogenates. The binding of the labeled hybridoma to the antigen mixture on the RIA plate was inhibited by sera from all *M. corti*-infected mice (other than infected hypothymic nude mice) but not be sera from mice infected with 6 other parasites. With no false positive reactions, no false negatives using sera from immunocompetent mice, and positive reactions occurring as early as 7 days of infection, the test clearly had very high specificity and adequate sensitivity.

For the selection of the McH.105 hybridoma, living parasites from infected hypothymic nude mice (and which were depleted of surface Ig by mild in vitro acid treatment) were used together with culture supernatants and a labeled anti Ig reagent. *M. corti* larvae from infected intact mice are known to differ for parasites of nude mice in being coated with large amounts of IgG_1 including IgG_1 *antibodies.*[24,25] By using "denuded", yet intact, parasites for selection, the probability of obtaining a hybridoma secreting an antibody directed against a natural antigen (which was surface located and thus readily available to the mouse immune system) was presumably increased. Subsequently it was shown that the labeled hybridoma-derived antibody, selected for the model IDT, bound better to larvae from infected nude mice than to larvae from infected intact mice and, in vivo, ^{125}I-McH.105 was cleared more rapidly within the first 48 hr after injections to infected nude mice vs. infected intact mice.[23] Therefore the antigen to which the hybridoma-derived antibody McH.105 was directed was indeed a readily available antigen (and probably a strong immunogen) in intact mice.

It is noteworthy that a crude parasite antigen mixture was used in this design of the model IDT; no antigen purification was necessary. In many situations, even crude parasite antigens (such as whole worm homogenates) may be in short supply. For this reason, an attempt was made to substitute the crude parasite antigen mixture in the IDT with a large pool of antiidiotypic (anti Id) antibodies raised in SJL/J mice against the purified McH.105 IgG_1 antibody. When this anti-Id serum pool was used in a competitive RIA in lieu of the antigen, too many false negatives were obtained using sera from several strains of infected mice at various time points during infection. Presumably, the lack of sensitivity reflected the absence of appropriate idiotype-bearing antibodies in infected mice and directed against the antigen to which McH.105 was directed.[23]

Theoretically, single-specificity IDTs would be expected to suffer from sensitivity problems. In a test designed to detect antibodies directed against a single antigenic determinant, every infected individual will be required to produce antibody against that determinant. This difficulty can be expected to pertain in the immunodiagnosis of larval cestode infections (e.g., echinococcosis [hydatids] and cysticercosis) where, for reasons unknown, false negative reactions occur all too frequently with existing tests in man and livestock. With this in mind, an alternative approach to the use of monoclonal antibodies in the development of IDTs has been employed. Hybridoma-derived antibodies showing cross-reactions and directed against antigenic determinants shared between parasites have been used to deplete these shared antigens from crude mixtures.[26] In the work-up of the hybridoma antibodies, cross-reactions were demonstrated using a competitive RIA with sera from clinically-defined individuals believed to have monospecific infections with a particular parasite. We have found this approach to detection of shared antigens to be far more sensitive than direct binding studies of labeled hybridoma antibodies to various parasite antigen mixtures. Presumably the amplification provided by the host immune response uncovers the presence of minority antigens. In addition, the appropriate life cycle stage of the parasite which contains the shared antigen may simply not be available for the preparation of antigens to be used in direct binding RIAs. Using hybridoma-derived antibodies to process crude antigen mixtures and to deplete them of antigens shared with other parasites, an improved IDT for echinococcosis (*Echinococcus granulosis* infections) in sheep has been developed.[26] In this system, hybridoma antibodies were produced which showed cross-reactions with the parasites causing most confusion (false positives) in the available tests. This type of approach has been used previously with natural infection or heterologous antibody populations.[27,28]

Despite the theoretical difficulties with single-specificity IDTs, hybridoma-derived antibodies have been developed in two systems and which have high immunodiagnostic potential. In the case of *Taenia hydatigena* infections in sheep, a competitive hybridoma antibody-based RIA has been developed which has good sensitivity and specificity (in a limited series), although cross-reactions with the closely related *T. ovis* parasite were detected.[29] This system provides a good illustration of the point made previously: lack of binding to parasite antigens in a direct binding RIA is no reliable indication of parasite specificity of a hybridoma antibody. The anti-*T. hydatigena* antibody (ThH.23) had no binding to a *T. ovis* larval extract, yet two of six sheep with putative monospecific infections with *T. ovis* contained inhibitory serum activity in the RIA using ^{125}I-ThH.23 and *T. hydatigena* antigen.

Recently, a hybridoma-derived antibody with apparent high specificity for Philippine *Schistosoma japonicum* adult worms has been produced.[30,31] This antibody (designated IPH.134) does not bind to Philippine *S. japonicum* extracted egg antigens of adult worm extracts (AWEs) of *S. mansoni* and several other trematodes which can infect man, viz. *Fasciola hepatica, Paragonimus westermanii,* and *Clonorchis sinensis*. It also fails to bind to AWEs and other antigen preparations from several parasitic nematodes, cestodes, and protozoa. When ^{125}I-IPH.134 was used in a competitive RIA with 40 sera from known *S. japonicum*-infected individuals from the Philippines, a very low false negative reaction frequently was obtained. Moreover, most patients with high egg outputs or severe disease had high inhibitory activity in the serum. All evidence points to IgG anti-*S. japonicum* antibodies as being the inhibitors in serum rather than immune complexes, antiidiotypic antibodies, or circulating parasite-derived antigen.

Further studies[31] have demonstrated that infected mice and humans may have high inhibitory activity in their sera which, if it is all antibody (directed against the antigenic determinant to which IPH.134 is directed) computes out at up to 1 mg/mℓ. No false positive reactions have yet been obtained in this assay using sera from patients with various other parasitic infections.[30] However, sera from *S. mansoni* and *S. haematobium*-infected individuals have not yet been examined for inhibitory activity (neither of these two parasites is present in the Philippines) and carefully selected sera from patients in the areas in which *S. japonicum* is evident but which unequivocally do not have schistosomiasis japonica are also not yet available. In conclusion, the antigen to which the IPH.134 hybridoma antibody is directed has high immunodiagnostic potential in schistosomiasis japonica in the Philippines. It will be used in the field to determine whether a test based on detection of antibody will provide information not only on who is infected, but the level of infection and occurrence of disease in individual patients.

Solid-phase monoclonal antibodies against *Toxoplasma gondii* have been used in ELISA to detect antigens in the sera of patients with acute toxoplasmosis.[32] Chronically-infected individuals were negative in the test and a low false positive rate was demonstrated although no sera from patients infected with other systemic protozoa were used. A figure for false negatives is not available since only four individuals with acute toxoplasmosis were used for testing. The observation was made that the monoclonal antibodies offer no advantages over polyspecific rabbit anti-*T. gondii* antibodies in detection of circulating parasite antigens in this system.

IV. HYBRIDOMA-DERIVED ANTIBODIES AND PARASITE INHIBITION IN VIVO AND IN VITRO

In malaria immunoparasitology, there is a surprisingly large number of "functional" (i.e., with antiparasite effects in vivo or in vitro) monoclonal antibodies already generated. Mouse and rat-mouse hybridomas have been produced which secrete antibodies to *Plasmodium falciparum, P. knowlesi, P. gallinaceum, P. chabaudi, P. yoelii,* and *P. berghei* (either sporozoites, blood stages or gametes) and which were selected in simple parasite-binding assays as the primary screen. The major activity in the use of monoclonals in malaria is focussed on the identification and isolation of target antigens for host-protective or transmission-inhibiting immunity; this reflects the fact that the field of malaria immunology is dominated by the urgent need for vaccines against plasmodium infection, disease, or transmission. Other activities in several laboratories include the analysis of host cell recognition by merozoites (and sporozoites), the identification of cell surface molecular changes in infected cells, the development of immunodiagnostic reagents for the detection of circulating antigen, the search for antigenic variability within the various human plasmodium species, and the screening for expression of cloned DNA.

Host protection against the mouse parasite, *P. berghei,* has been demonstrated with an IgG_1 murine hybridoma antibody directed against a major surface protein (designated Pb 44) of the sporozoite.[33,34] All indications are that the 44,000 mol wt target antigen is a stage specific antigen and its species specificity is currently under investigation. Interestingly, a cross-reaction has been found with *P. yoelii nigeriensis,* a cross-reaction between the two species which was not detectable using polyspecific immune mouse sera.[35] Being a dominant surface antigen, it might be expected that antigenic variability in this molecule (or the equivalent molecules of other plasmodium species) may occur; however there is as yet no information on this point. Protection of recipient mice can be achieved with small quantities (10 μg) of the purified antibody and Fab fragments are effective when preincubated with sporozoites in vitro.[34] Nothing has been published as yet on the vaccination efficacy of Pb 44 isolated by antibody-affinity chromatography (± isoelectric focussing since Pb 44 has a low isoelectric point).

Freeman et al.[36] used two murine hybridoma antibodies (of IgG_1 and IgG_{2a} isotypes), with apparent binding specificity for merozoites, to reduce parasitemias in *P. yoelii*-infected mice. In this system, the hybridoma antibodies may operate to "give the host more time" to develop a protective response against the virulent *P. yoelii* parasite used. Efficacy of the hybridoma antibodies in infected nude mice would thus be of interest. Some evidence suggests that their mode of action is to inhibit red cell penetration particularly of mature red cells[37] but this has not been demonstrated directly. It is of some interest that the infected cells which remain after administration of the hybridoma antibodies to mice are reticulocytes; the possibility exists that effecting inhibition of invasion of such cells is more difficult than inhibition of invasion of more mature red cells or that different parasites invade the two host cell types. Analysis of this phenomenon may provide clues on mechanisms of invasion of reticulocytes vs. erythrocytes and population heterogeneity in murine plasmodia. It was further reported in this system[36] that hybridoma antibodies directed against several other blood stage antigens (by immunofluorescence) were not protective on passive transfer. No information has been provided on the stage or species specificity of the two "functional" hybridoma antibodies and the minimal amount of antibody required for parasitemia reduction in infected mice is not known. In another series,[38] no protective hybridoma antibodies were produced from fusion of spleen cells from *P. berghei*-resistant mice.[39]

Various hybridoma cell lines secreting antibodies to surface antigens of *P. knowlesi* merozoites have been produced.[40] Some correlation has been found between merozoite agglutinability of the antibodies and the efficiency of rhesus red cell invasion inhibition; the "functional" hybridoma antibodies had specificity for a high molecular weight biosynthetically-labeled protein. Several other groups are producing hybridoma antibodies to *P. knowlesi* merozoites, this system being amenable to experimentation since merozoites of this plasmodium species can be obtained in large quantities from rhesus monkeys with synchronized infections.

Large amounts of a combination of two murine monoclonal antibodies (of IgM and IgG_1 isotypes) directed against *P. gallinaceum* gametes mediate transmission-blocking immunity.[41] Although these antibodies bind to both male and female gametes, their mode of action in mediating transmission inhibition appears to be by agglutination of male gametes and prevention of detachment from the residual body of the gametocyte. Infectivity of *P. gallinaceum*-infected chicken blood for the mosquito vector *Aedes aegypti* is suppressed in the presence of the two hybridoma antibodies (but not as well as the inhibition following incubation with gamete-immune chicken serum).

Numerous groups are involved in the production of murine monoclonal antibodies to blood stages of *P. falciparum*[42] and there are already reports of in vitro inhibitory antibodies being obtained.[43] A strategy being used in this laboratory is to select hybridomas which secrete antibodies binding to biosynthetically-labeled Papua New Guinea *P. falciparum* antigens and which are differentially immunoprecipitated by sera from older individuals in an endemic area (and which inhibit in vitro *P. falciparum* growth) vs. sera from infected children in the same endemic area (and which do not inhibit in vitro growth).[44,45] In this way, it is hoped that hybridoma antibodies will be produced against candidate host-protective "natural" antigens of *P. falciparum*. Recent studies by Perrin and colleagues[43] have identified 96,000 and 41,000 mol wt biosynthetically labeled proteins as being targets for inhibitory anti-*P. falciparum* hybridomas.

Antierythrocyte hybridoma antibodies (including hybridoma autoantibodies) which inhibit plasmodium or babesia penetration of erythrocytes would be of enormous value in the dissection of red cell recognition, attachment, and penetration by merozoites. No reports on this are available to date and attempts in this laboratory to produce in vitro inhibitory antihuman and antibovine erythrocyte hybridoma antibodies (in *P. falciparum* and *Babesia bovis* systems, respectively) have been unsuccessful. Considerable progress would be made in hemoprotozoal and other parasite systems if it was possible to seed infected cells or parasites into wells in which hybridomas were growing and to select, early in the procedure, those in which parasite growth or persistence was inhibited.

Antibody-dependent effects (± cellular involvement) are well known in *Schistosoma mansoni*/rat and mouse systems. No systematic study on the effects of monoclonal antibodies of various isotype (± cells of various types such as eosinophils, neutrophils, mast cells, and macrophages) has been published but a preliminary report using concentrated hybridoma culture supernatants indicates that this approach will be highly instructive.[46] It is clear that analyses of plasmodium systems using hybridoma-derived antibodies are well advanced but a flurry of activity can be expected in the next 2 to 5 years in other parasite systems in which antibodies have proven antiparasite effects.

V. CONCLUDING COMMENTS AND SPECULATION

The movement of the hybridoma technology into immunoparasitology is accelerating, there being greatest activity at the present time in systems involving human, monkey, and mouse malarial protozoa (*Plasmodium* spp.) and those where improved immunodiagnostic or parasite typing reagents are required (e.g., *Schistosoma* spp., *Toxoplasma gondii, Leishmania* spp., *Trypanosoma* spp., veterinary larval cestodes, etc.). This chapter has documented some of this activity.

Attempts to use antiparasite hybridoma-derived antibodies for the focussing of conjugated drugs and toxic moieties to parasites are in progress and will proceed along in parallel with similar studies in tumor systems.

Much activity can be expected in the next few years in the use of immunogenic monoclonal anti-Id antibodies directed against host-protective monoclonal antibodies to sensitize hosts for accelerated response to parasite antigens following natural exposure to parasites. (Little promise for the approach of using hybridoma antibodies plus anti-Id antibodies in immunodiagnosis was found in one host-parasite system[23] although this will in no way dampen enthusiasm for the approach in other systems.) It is predicted that "presensitization" with immunogenic monoclonal anti-Id may prejudice the establishment of a particular parasite especially in those systems where there is evidence that the invasive form of the parasite is vulnerable to pre-existing or inducible immune responses (antibody and/or cell-mediated) early in the course of the infection.[47–49] Although the approach needs careful testing in various systems, it should not be assumed that this is a proven, well-established method of inducing "functional" immune responses in hosts. One expects that the heterogeneity of the immune response induced, or the state of sensitization established, by anti-Id injection will be highly restricted in terms of clonality.

Methods for in vitro induction of antiparasite antibody-secreting cells for fusion with modified mouse or human myeloma cells must be developed as a matter of urgency. Conceivably, the spectrum of antibody production in vitro may exceed that induced in vivo if immune regulation operates to limit certain antibody responses to certain antigenic determinants. Such influences may be inoperative in vitro and cell cultures may provide the investigator with a wider range of antibody specificities from which to select those appropriate for the particular investigation. This requirement for in vitro induction of antibody-secreting cells is particularly important in the case of human cells to be used for fusion with the various modified human myeloma cells being developed at the present time.

The demonstration of functional activity with a monoclonal antibody in vivo or in vitro does not automatically mean that antibody-affinity purification and effective active immunization with the isolated antigen is simply a couple of weeks work. A heavily-labeled band on an autoradiograph of an SDS-polyacrylamide gel, and a functional hybridoma antibody obtained by reacting with labeled parasite antigens, may give a false impression of the representation of the antigen in the mixture from which the immunoprecipitate was made. Difficulties can be expected in eluting antigens from columns containing high-affinity monoclonal antibodies. Moreover, achieving the levels of antibody possible with passive immunization, or in vitro incubation, may be difficult in vivo following stimulation of the regulated intact immune system with the isolated antigen. The powerful adjuvants which are often required to induce high-titered responses may not be suitable for use in man or livestock. In heterologous systems, a molecule which is highly antigenic in the immunized mouse (from which cells were obtained for hybridoma production) may be weakly immunogenic in the natural host species and in fact may resemble an autoantigen. Great care is therefore required in testing the safety, long before testing for efficacy, of human parasite antigens isolated by murine hybridoma-derived antibodies in human subjects. Perhaps these cautionary words are appropriate at the end of a chapter which, I hope, has illustrated the analytical power and the revolutionary impact the hybridoma technique will have in the discipline of immunoparasitology.

REFERENCES

1. **Cox, F. E. G.,** Monoclonal antibodies and immunity to malaria, *Nature (London)*, 284, 304, 1980.
2. **Rowe, D. S.,** The role of monoclonal antibody technology in immunoparasitology, *Immunol. Today*, 1, 30, 1980.
3. **Mitchell, G. F. and Cruise, K. M.,** Monoclonal antiparasite antibodies: a shot-in-the-arm for immunoparasitology, in *Monoclonal Antibodies and T Cell Hybridomas*, Hämmerling, G. J., Hämmerling, U., and Kearney, J. F., Eds., Elsevier, Amsterdam, 1981, 303.
4. **McMichael, A. J. and Bastin, J. M.,** Clinical applications of monoclonal antibodies, *Immunol. Today*, 1, 56, 1980.
5. **Cohen, S. and Sadun, E. H.,** Eds., *Immunology of Parasitic Infection*, Blackwell Scientific, Oxford, 1976.
6. **Mitchell, G. F. and Anders, R. F.,** Parasite antigens and their immunogenicity in infected hosts, in *The Antigens*, Vol. 6, Sela, M., Ed., Academic Press, New York, 1981, 70.
7. **Anders, R. F., Howard, R. J., and Mitchell, G. F.,** Parasite antigens, in *The Immunology of Parasitic Diseases*, Vol. 2, Cohen, S. and Warren, K. S., Eds., Blackwell Scientific , Oxford, in press.
8. **Crane, M. St. J. and Dvorak, J. A.,** Vertebrate cells express protozoan antigen after hybridization, *Science*, 208, 194, 1980.
9. **Gutman, G. A. and Mitchell, G. F.,** *Ascaris suum:* location of phosphorylcholine in lung larvae, *Exp. Parasitol.*, 43, 161, 1977.
10. **Péry, P., Luffau, G., Charley, J., Petit, A., Rouze, P., and Bernard, S.,** Phosphorylcholine antigens from *Nippostrongylus brasiliensis*. I. Anti-phosphorylcholine antibodies in infected rats and location of phosphorylcholine antigens, *Ann. Immunol. (Inst. Pasteur)*, 130C, 879, 1979.
11. **Gorrell, M. D. and Howell, M. J.,** personal communication.
12. **Pearson, T. and Anderson, L.,** Analytical techniques for cell fractions. Dissection of complex antigen mixtures using monoclonal antibodies and two-dimensional gel electrophoresis, *Anal. Biochem.*, 101, 377, 1980.
13. **Pearson, T. W., Pinder, M., Roelants, G. E., Kar, S. K., Lunden, L. B., Mayor-Withey, K. S., and Hewett, R. S.,** Methods for derivation and detection of anti-parasite monoclonal antibodies, *J. Immunol. Methods*, 34, 141, 1980.
14. **Hoeijmakers, J. H. J., Frasch, A. C., Bernards, A., Borst, P., and Cross, G. A. M.,** Novel expression-linked copies of the genes for variant surface antigens in trypanosomes, *Nature (London)*, 284, 78, 1980.
15. **Williams, R. O., Young, J. R., and Majiwa, P. A. O.,** Genomic rearrangements correlated with antigenic variation in *Trypanosoma brucei*, *Nature (London)*,282, 847, 1979.
16. **Handman, E. and Remington, J. S.,** Serological and immunochemical characterization of monoclonal antibodies to *Toxoplasma gondii*, *Immunology*, 40, 579, 1980.
17. **Handman, E., Goding, J. W., and Remington, J. S.,** Detection and characterization of membrane antigens of *Toxoplasma gondii*, *J. Immunol.*, 124, 2578, 1980.
18. **Sethi, K. K., Endo, T., and Brandis, H.,** Hybridoma secreting monoclonal antibody with specificity for *Toxoplasma gondii*, *J. Parasitol.*, 66, 192, 1980.
19. **Johnson, A. M., McNamara, P. J., Neoh, S. H., McDonald, P. J., and Zola, H.,** Hybridomas secreting monoclonal antibody to *Toxoplasma gondii*, *Aust. J. Exp. Biol. Med. Sci.*, 59, 303, 1981.
20. **Hillyer, G. V. and Pelley, R. P.,** The major serological antigen (MSA_1) from *Schistosoma mansoni* eggs is a "circumoval" precipitinogen, *Amer. J. Trop. Med. Hyg.*, 29, 582, 1980.

21. **Pinder, M. and Hewett, R. S.,** Monoclonal antibodies detect antigenic diversity in *Theileria parva* parasites, *J. Immunol.*, 124, 1000, 1980.
22. **Pratt, D. M. and David, J. R.,** personal communication.
23. **Mitchell, G. F., Cruise, K. M., Chapman, C. B., Anders, R. F., and Howard, M. C.,** Hybridoma antibody immunoassays for the detection of parasitic infection: development of a model system using a larval cestode infection in mice, *Aust. J. Exp. Biol. Med. Sci.*, 57, 287, 1979.
24. **Mitchell, G. F., Marchalonis, J. J., Smith, P. M., Nicholas, W. L., and Warner, N. L.,** Studies on immune responses to larval cestodes. Immunoglobulins associated with the larvae of *Mesocestoides corti, Aust. J. Exp. Biol. Med. Sci.*, 55, 187, 1977.
25. **Chapman, C. B., Knopf, P. M., Anders, R. F., and Mitchell, G. F.,** IgG_1 hypergammaglobulinaemia in chronic parasitic infections in mice: evidence that the response reflects chronicity of antigen exposure, *Aust. J. Exp. Biol. Med. Sci.*, 57, 389, 1979.
26. **Craig, P. S., Hocking, R. E., Mitchell, G. F., and Rickard, M. D.,** Murine hybridoma-derived antibodies in the processing of antigens for the immunodiagnosis of hydatid (*Echinococcus granulosus*) infection in sheep, *Parasitology*, in press.
27. **Suzuki, T., Sato, Y., Yamashita, T., Sekikawa, H., and Otsuru, M.,** *Angiostrongylus cantonensis:* preparation of a specific antigen using immunoadsorbent columns, *Exp. Parasitol.*, 38, 191, 1975.
28. **Welch, J. W. and Dobson, C.,** Immunodiagnosis of parasitic zoonoses: comparative efficacy of three immunofluorescence tests using antigens purified by affinity chromatography, *Trans. R. Soc. Trop. Med. Hyg.*, 72, 282, 1978.
29. **Craig, P. S., Mitchell, G. F., Cruise, K. M., and Rickard, M. D.,** Hydridoma antibody immunoassays for the detection of parasitic infection: attempts to produce an immunodiagnostic reagent for a larval taeniid cestode infection, *Aust. J. Exp. Biol. Med. Sci.*, 58, 339, 1980.
30. **Mitchell, G. F., Cruise, K. M., Garcia, E. G., and Anders, R. F.,** A hydridoma-derived antibody with immunodiagnostic potential for schistosomiasis japonica, *Proc. Natl. Acad. Sci. U.S.A.*, 78, 3165, 1981.
31. **Cruise, K. M., Mitchell, G. F., Garcia, E. G., and Anders, R. F.,** Hybridoma antibody immunoassays for the detection of parasitic infections: further studies on a monoclonal antibody with immunodiagnostic potential for schistosomiasis japonica *Acta Trop.*, in press.
32. **Araujo, F., Handman, E., and Remington, J. S.,** Use of monoclonal antibodies to detect antigens of *Toxoplasma gondii* in serum and other body fluids, *Infect. Immun.*, 30, 12, 1980.
33. **Yoshida, N., Nussenzweig, R. S., Potocnjak, P., Nussenzweig, V., and Aikawa, M.,** Hybridoma produces protective antibodies directed against the sporozoite stage of malaria parasite, *Science*, 207, 71, 1980.
34. **Potocnjak, P., Yoshida, N., Nussenzweig, R. S., and Nussenzweig, V.,** Monovalent fragments (Fab) of monoclonal antibodies to a sporozoite surface antigen (Pb 44) protect mice against malarial infection, *J. Exp. Med.*, 151, 1504, 1980.
35. **Nussenzweig, R. S.,** personal communication.
36. **Freeman, R. R., Trejdosiewicz, A. J., and Cross, G. A. M.,** Protective monoclonal antibodies recognize stage-specific merozoite antigens of a rodent malaria parasite, *Nature (London)*, 284, 366, 1980.
37. **Freeman, R. R., Trejdosiewicz, A. J., Bushby, L. E., and Cross, G. A. M.,** Passive protection against lethal *Plasmodium yoelii* infection with monoclonal antibodies, Abstract 12.8.9 of the 4th Int. Cong. Immunology, Paris, July 1980.
38. **Howard, M. C., Howard, R. J., Cruise, K. M., and Mitchell, G. F.,** Identification of malaria antigens using hybridoma antibodies. Proc. WHO Conf. Immunodiagnostic Aspects Malaria, June 1979, 43.
39. **Mitchell, G. F., Handman, E., and Howard, R. J.,** Protection of mice against plasmodium and babesia infection: attempts to raise host-protective sera, *Aust. J. Exp. Biol. Med. Sci.*, 56, 553, 1978.
40. **Epstein, N.,** personal communication.
41. **Rener, J., Carter, R., Rosenberg, Y., and Miller, L. H.,** Anti-gamete monoclonal antibodies synergistically block transmission of malaria by preventing fertilization in the mosquito, *Proc. Natl. Acad. Sci. U.S.A.*, 77, 6797, 1981.
42. **Perrin, L. H., Raminez, R., Er-Hsiang, L., and Lambert, P. H.,** *Plasmodium falciparum:* characterization of defined antigens by monoclonal antibodies, *Clin. Exp. Immunol.*, 41, 91, 1980.
43. **Perrin, L. H.,** personal communication.
44. **Brown, G. V., Anders, R. F., Stace, J. F., Alpers, M. P., and Mitchell, G. F.,** Immunoprecipitation of biosynthetically-labelled proteins from different Papua New Guinea *Plasmodium falciparum* isolates by sera from individuals in the endemic area, *Parasite Immunol.*, in press.

45. **Knopf, P. M., Brown, G. V., Howard, R. J., and Mitchell, G. F.,** Immunoprecipitation of biosynthetically-labeled products in the identification of antigens of murine red cells infected with the protozoan parasite, *Plasmodium berghei, Aust. J. Exp. Biol. Med. Sci.*, 57, 603, 1979.
46. **Verwaerde, C., Grzych, J-M., Bazen, H., Capron, M., and Capron, A.,** Production of monoclonal antibodies to *Schistosoma mansoni*. Preliminary studies on their biological activities, *C. R. Acad. Sci. Ser. D.*, 289, 725, 1979.
47. **Mitchell, G. F., Rajasekarish, G. R., and Rickard, M. D.,** A mechanism to account for mouse strain variation in resistance to the larval cestode, *Taenia taeniaeformis, Immunology*, 39, 481, 1980.
48. **Mitchell, G. F.,** Effector cells, molecules and mechanisms in host-protective immunity to parasites, *Immunology*, 38, 209, 1979.
49. **Mitchell, G. F.,** Responses to metazoan and protozoan parasites in mice, *Adv. Immunol.*, 28, 451, 1979.

Chapter 8

HYBRIDOMA ANTIBODIES SPECIFIC FOR HUMAN TUMOR ANTIGENS

Kenneth F. Mitchell, Zenon Steplewski, and Hilary Koprowski

TABLE OF CONTENTS

I. TUMOR IMMUNOLOGY

The search for chemical or biochemical characteristics which are unique to tumor cells has been pursued with some vigor in recent years. The reasons for this undertaking fall into two main areas. First, the distinct behavioral characteristics of tumors with respect to their growth rate and invasive properties suggest that these cells are different from the normal cells from which, presumably, they derive. The apparently "unregulated" behavior of tumor cells suggests that they are unable to perceive the modulating influences by which the body controls the behavior of normal cells. Second, the belief that tumors may be susceptible to suppression or control by the action of the autologous immune system encourages the search for structural (antigenic) differences between tumor cells and other kinds of cells present in the host either of the same lineage or of different types. The fact that tumors do, on occasion, spontaneously regress and disappear[1] encourages the speculation that the immune system is responsible for these events. Similarly, the presence of infiltrating lymphocytes in the bed of primary tumors[2] and the ability of some investigators to elicit hypersensitivity responses with tumor extracts[3] also supports the notion that patients can mount immune responses directed to their own tumors. Serological tests have often shown the presence of antibodies which bind to autologous tumors[4–6] and, frequently, to other tumors of similar histologic types.[7] Sera from many patients, however, do not show this effect, presumably because these individuals are unable to recognize or to respond immunologically to their tumors. The failure of some patients to recognize their tumors raises questions about the tumor-specific nature of the antigens in question since three possible interpretations may be applied: (1) the patient may be unable to recognize the antigen because it is, in fact, a normal constituent of their tissues and they are, therefore, naturally tolerent to it; (2) conversely, the recognition of tumors by some patients may be because of an autoimmune response to a normal antigen rather than a response to a neoantigen; and (3) the patient may be either immunosuppressed or tolerized to the antigen in question, as a result of the growth of the tumor.

Despite the problems, claims have been made and continue to be made that tumor-specific or tumor-associated antigens are detectable by the use of autologous, allogeneic, or xenogeneic antisera. These three kinds of reagents each have their problems which will be described in order to establish the rationale behind the use of monoclonal antibodies.

II. AUTOLOGOUS ANTITUMOR IMMUNE RESPONSES

The autologous immune responses of patients to their own tumors should, in theory, lead to the highest degree of tumor specificity because of the innate self-tolerance exhibited by the immune system. In practice there are good reasons for thinking that the normal self-tolerance may well be partially abrogated in tumor-bearing patients and that the serological responses may be of an autoimmune type directed to normal antigens which occur on tumor cells. Responses of this type can occur because B cells with specificity for self-antigens probably exist at low frequency in all individuals but fail to respond to their target antigens because of either the lack of T cell help or because of the presence of T suppressor cells. The recognition of minor antigenic differences, however, seems to be most readily perceived by T cells in many systems. The primary result of a change in antigenic expression, therefore, may well be a facilitation of the recognition of tumor cells by T helpers which then initiate the proliferation of B cells reactive with normal surface antigens. Concomitant to this serological reactivity a T cell-mediated sensitivity may be expected to occur and, indeed, this is the case,

The ability of patients to respond immunologically to their own and to allogeneic tumors seems to be well established.[8–13] What is lacking is a clear demonstration of the tumor specificity of the responses and a clear identification of the antigens detected. Attempts to isolate antigens by the use of autologous or allogeneic sera have generally failed, the problem appearing to be the low titer and/or low affinity of the antibodies in question. This result is, however, predictable if the responses are due to autoimmunity to a normal antigenic species. A final difficulty in the use of autoantisera lies in the complexity of these reagents. This complexity problem is common to all antisera and occurs because a variety of different B cells may respond to each antigenic determinant. The autologous response gives rise to a mixture of antibodies with varied specificities and affinities. The presence of these heterogeneous elicited antibodies, in addition to the other immunoglobulin of the serum, hampers the analysis of the specificity of the autologous immune response.

III. IMMUNE RESPONSES TO ALLOGENEIC TUMORS

The opportunity to study the immune responses of patients to allogeneic tumors is available mainly because of the attempts that have been made to treat patients with extracts of tumors, or irradiated- or virus-disrupted tumor or tissue culture cells. The problems associated with interpreting the results of binding assays performed with such sera are similar to those which afflict autoantisera but, in addition, the presence of alloantibodies further complicates the issues. The general preamble to the use of such sera involves absorption on a variety of nontumor target cell types to remove nonspecifically binding antibodies and antibodies directed to alloantigens of common occurrence. The presence of tumor-specific antibodies, and from this the occurrence of tumor-specific antigens, is inferred from the results of binding assays which may be radioimmunoassays, various kinds of adherence, or complement fixation assays.

Difficulties in interpretation arise from the fact that absorption may be either quantitatively or qualitatively incomplete. Reduction of binding to an undetectable level on the absorbing cell does not necessarily preclude binding of residual antibody to a tumor cell with a much higher surface density of the antigenic epitope in question. Another fundamental problem with this approach is that antibodies may be raised to normal antigens which occur only on the population of patients but which are not specific for the tumor. A specific instance may be suggested. Particular variants of the HLA-D locus are believed to be associated with the occurrence of certain tumors such as melanoma. D-related antigens occur on melanoma cells[14,15] and antisera recognizing such antigens may well react only with melanoma cells and not be absorbed by tissues from other sources.

In general, sera from patients who have been immunized even multiple times with allogeneic tumor material, exhibit low titers of antibody. Obviously, such phenomena may result from the presence of low affinity antibody or low amounts of antibody and may reflect the general nonimmunogenic nature of tumor cells.[16] In either case, the phenomenon contributes to the difficulties experienced by most investigators who have attempted to identify the antigenic targets of the alloantisera.

IV. TUMOR ANTIGENS IDENTIFIED BY XENOGENEIC ANTISERA

The identification of tumor antigens by xenoantisera[14,17–20] is complicated by the vastly greater number of normal antigens which can be expected to be immunogenic in this situation. To accommodate this complexity, extensive absorption on normal human tissues and on serum are often performed to remove antibodies reactive with normal cells.

Attempts to minimize the range of specificity exhibited by antisera have been made by the use of primates for immunization. This strategem is based on the belief that fewer antigenic differences exist between the normal antigens of these species and those of human beings and the likelihood of recognition of tumor-specific antigens is thus increased. However, *Cercopithecus aethiops* antisera raised against human tissue culture melanoma cells were found to require absorption on red cells, leukocytes, and liver before specificity for melanoma cells could be revealed.[18]

Numerous other publications have described binding studies, fluorescence antibody detection, mixed hemagglutination assays, and a variety of other experimental techniques to show the presence in various human and xenoantisera of antibodies which bind to tumor cells. The use of monoclonal antibodies has, however, revolutionized the analysis of cell surface antigens because of the ability of each of these reagents to react specifically to a particular antigenic epitope. Binding of a monoclonal antibody to a target cell is an unequivocal demonstration that the antigen is present and quantitative distinctions between different types of cells can be readily made.

V. PRODUCTION OF HYBRIDOMAS

Various procedures for the production of hybrid cells have been described[21] but the most useful method appears to be that in which the two types of lymphoid cells are induced to fuse by the addition of polyethylene glycol.[22] After fusion hybrid cells are selected by virtue of their ability to grow in an appropriate medium.[23] In much work the hypoxanthine, aminopterin, thymidine (HAT) medium of Szybalski[24] has been used to suppress the growth of mutant parental myeloma cells which lack the enzyme hypoxanthine guanine phosphoribosyl transferase necessary for growth under these selective conditions. The other parent of the hybrid cell, the spleen cell, lacks the immortal trait of the myeloma but does contribute the missing enzyme along with its own particular antibody. Surviving cells under these conditions are, of necessity, hybrids and the growth and multiplication of these cells gives rise to microscopic colonies which can be detected in hybrid cultures usually by about 7 to 10 days after fusion. These colonies are removed into fresh culture vessels and their progeny are subsequently cloned to ensure that the antibody produced is truly monoclonal in origin.

HAT-sensitive myeloma cells were originally derived from the BALB/c myeloma MOPC-21 and were designated P3.[25] A variant of this line P3 × 63Ag8 was described by Köhler and Milstein[26] and is frequently used for fusion. A disadvantage of this cell line is that it continues to produce the IgG1 of the myeloma parent. More recently, derivatives of this line that have lost the ability to produce IgG1 but retain the HAT sensitivity and efficiency in fusion have been isolated. P3 × 63Ag8.653 was isolated by use of a cell sorter, selection being made for cells which did not bind fluorescent antimouse immunoglobulin.[27] These cells neither secrete nor contain the γ1 and kappa chain of the parental myeloma. A second line which has come into common use is also derived from MOPC-21 and is called P3-NS1/1Ag4.1 and is known by the abbreviation 'NS1'.[28] This line produces intracellular kappa chains but does not secrete them. Hybrids formed from this cell line do, however, incorporate the parental myeloma light chain into the secreted immunoglobulin.

The production of hybrid cells leaves three problems to be solved: (1) the identification of those cells that produce immunoglobulin; (2) the determination of which of these clones makes antibody with an appropriate specificity; and, (3) the characterization of the target antigen to ensure that distinct specificities are being recognized. This last task can be undertaken in one of two ways, by isolation of the antigen and an unequivocal demonstration that reactivity is directed to distinct structural entities, or, by demonstration that different antibodies have distinct patterns of reactivity on different targets thus precluding that the reaction is occurring with the same determinant.

To determine the binding specificity of the antibodies, the usual strategy is to utilize an indirect radioimmunoassay on a variety of targets. Hybridoma culture supernatants which show binding to the target cells are tested on larger panels of cells to examine whether the antigen occurs on many other types of human cells or has an expression only on the target of interest. At this point decisions are made based on the level of binding detected, and many antibodies with a broad specificity for many types of human cells are usually discovered which, for reasons of expediency, are often eliminated from further study. Antibodies with the desired specificities, in contrast, are subjected to further study. Biochemical studies are undertaken to isolate and characterize the target antigens and the principal technique used for characterization of tumor antigens is immune precipitation of antigens from radiolabeled cells followed by sodium dodecyl sulfate polyacrylamide gel electrophoresis to determine the molecular weight of the isolated radioactive antigens.

VI. MONOCLONAL ANTIBODIES TO LYMPHOID CELLS AND LYMPHOID TUMORS

The lymphoid cell pool can be divided into two functional subsets of cells, thymus-derived "T" cells and immunoglobulin-producing "B" cells. These two kinds of cells act in concert to bring about the full range of immunological phenomena seen in normal animals and each kind has a distinct range of biological activities. Intuitively, one would expect that these distinct functions occur because of the presence of different surface structures which initiate and control the biological activities of the cells. This expectation has been well borne out in the mouse by use of antisera raised by immunization of congenic strains. In the human, antisera with such restricted activities cannot be obtained, but several monoclonal antibodies have been reported which show the presence of distinct structures. Intuitively, again, it seems reasonable that tumors are initially clonal in origin and, therefore, despite subsequent differentiation, these cells might bear markers characteristic of normal lymphoid cells. Again, this expectation is borne out by studies with monoclonal antibodies.

VII. MONOCLONAL ANTIBODY-DEFINED T LYMPHOID CELL ANTIGENS

A hybridoma secreting a monoclonal antibody reactive with cortical thymocytes was established from the spleen of a BALB/c mouse immunized with human thymus cells.[29] Spleen cells were fused with myeloma line NS1[28] and selected in the usual way in HAT medium.[24] The antibody (NAI/34-HLK) reacted with cortical thymocytes and with the leukemia cells of 9 of 11 patients with thymic acute lymphoblastic leukemia (ALL).[30] This antibody, which recognizes an antigen designated HTA-1, did not react with medullary thymus lymphocytes or with peripheral blood T cells or B cells. The antigen HTA-1 has a molecular weight of 45,000 daltons and appears to be a marker for one of the earlier stages of the T cell differentiation pathway occurring on 2 to 5% of normal cortical thymus cells and on the ALL cells believed to arise from this population. A second antibody isolated by the same group[30] reacted with cortical and medullary thymocytes and also with peripheral T and B cells. This antibody (2D1) detects a common lymphoid antigen (HLe1) which was also expressed weakly on tumor cells of three thymic ALL cases, but not on three other cases of this disease. The antigen was strongly expressed on 18 B lymphomas, four B-type chronic lymphocytic leukemias (CLL), and one case of T-type CLL, but not on cells of four cases of non-T, non-B ALL. Physicochemical characterization of this antigen has not been reported but the different distribution precludes its identity with HTA-1.

Antibody to a distinct antigen with a similar distribution to HTA-1 has been reported.[31] These authors also fused spleen cells from immunized BALB/c mice with NS-1 and screened 1877 clones to find 2 with this reactivity. The two antibodies, designated 12E7 and 21D2 reacted with cortical thymocytes but did not react with medullary thymocytes, with peripheral lymphoid cells, B lymphomas, or leukemias. The antibodies did react with T ALL cells, but immunochemical characterization showed that the target antigen had a molecular weight of 28,000 daltons and thus is distinct from HTA-1.

A third antigen which occurs on T cells has been detected with a monoclonal antibody prepared from C57Bl/6 × BALB/c F_1 hybrid mice immunized with human peripheral blood mononuclear cells.[32] The fusion, made with NS-1, yielded a clone producing an antibody (9-3) which bound to 50 to 60% of peripheral T cells and to 20 to 30% of thymocytes. The antigen has been tentatively designated HuLyt-1 and despite a similar molecular weight (44,000 daltons), has a distribution different from HTA-1. This antigen was expressed by four of six T leukemia lines tested.

A fourth T-cell antigen which appears to be distinct from those described above has been detected by a monclonal antibody designated OKT-1.[33] This antigen appears to be a marker for mature T cells and occurs on 5 to 10% of thymus cells and on all peripheral blood T cells. This antibody was produced from a BALB/c mouse immunized with peripheral blood T cells and spleen cells from this mouse were fused with the myeloma cell line P3 × 63AgU1. The detected antigen is not expressed on B cells, null cells, or macrophages. T-type ALL cells (which are believed to represent a proliferation of a T precursor) are antigen-negative, but T-type chronic lymphocytic leukemia (CLL) which represent a more mature cell type are antigen-positive. Of three established T cell tissue culture lines, two were positive (HJD-1 and CEM), but a third was negative (HSB-2). The molecular weight of this antigen has not been reported.

A fifth antigen, which is expressed by mature and immature cells of the T cell lineage, has been detected by a monoclonal antibody T-101.[34] This antibody also binds to neoplastic cells which have characteristics of the B cell lineage, namely, immunoglobulin-bearing CLL cells (12 patients). In contrast, surface immunoglobulin-negative CLL cells were also negative for the antigen (3 patients) as were lymphosarcoma cell leukemias (4 patients) and hairy cell leukemias (3 patients). The antigen is distinct from those previously described and has a molecular weight of 65,000 daltons. This antigen, designated the T65 antigen, has been extracted from normal T cells and from surface IgG-positive CLL cells.

VIII. MONOCLONAL ANTIBODY-DEFINED B LYMPHOID CELL ANTIGENS

An antigen (DR) which is known from conventional serology to be a marker for B cells has also been identified by a variety of monoclonal antibodies, as will be discussed further in the section on melanoma. In the context of lymphoid cells, an antibody designated 7-2, produced from a C57Bl/6 × BALB/c spleen fused with the cell line NS-1, has been shown to precipitate the characteristic antigen with two components of 34,000 and 29,000 daltons.[32] The antibody reacted strongly with normal B cells, with six cultured B cell lines, two pre-B lines, a Burkitt lymphoma line, and three CLL lines. Another monoclonal antibody with a similar pattern of reactivity, but whose antigen has not been characterized, was produced from a C57Bl/6 mouse immunized with phytohemagglutin (PHA)-stimulated human peripheral blood lymphocytes.[35] The fusion was performed with the cell line P3-NS/1-A4-1 (2/K-M) and the antibody designated FMC4. This antibody was shown to react with B lymphocytes, blood monocytes, null lymphocytes, B-type CLL, null-type ALL, and some myeloid leukemias, but did not react with T lymphocytes, T-type CLL cells, T-type ALL and certain other myeloid lines.

An antigen which defines a subset of B lymphomas was identified with a monoclonal antibody (Ab 89) which was produced from a BALB/c mouse immunized with cryopreserved poorly differentiated lymphocytic lymphoma cells (D-PDL).[36] Spleen cells from the mouse were fused with NS1 cells and the isolated monoclonal antibody was shown to react only with cells from 2 of 18 D-PDL and 2 of 17 CLL patients. No other leukemia or lymphoma (66 in all) or any normal lymphoid cell tested (65 in all) bound this antibody. Preliminary evidence suggested that an antigen was present in serum of antigen-positive patients with a bimolecular structure of 20,000 and 75,000 daltons. Of particular interest is the observation that antigen 89-positive D-PDL patients had a survival rate of almost twice that of antigen 89-negative P-PDL individuals and in this respect, resembled CLL patients.

An antigen which seems to be a characteristic of certain myeloid cells has been described. A number of different monoclonal antibodies were isolated from a BALB/c spleen/NS1 fusion, with similar reactivities and one (J-5), was studied in some detail.[37] This antibody precipitates an antigen with a molecular weight of 95,000 daltons which is expressed on 21 of 34 non-T ALL cell lines and on three of five chronic myelocytic leukemia patients in blast crisis, and which has been referred to as the common ALL antigen, CALLA. The antibody did not react with peripheral blood lymphocytes, mononuclear cells or concanavalin-A T cell blasts.

Each of the antigens described above, with the exception of antigen 89, has been shown to occur on both normal cells and on neoplastic cells. These lymphoid markers do not have the characteristics of tumor-specific or tumor-associated antigens. In contrast, the markers have a distribution which would be predicted if the tumor cells do, in fact, represent a particular developmental stage of a particular type of normal cells. The availability of the normal cells has permitted this observation and, as will be seen, the problem with establishing the tumor-specific or tumor-associated nature of antigens on other cell types is frequently the unavailability of normal cells with which to compare the tumor cells.

IX. MONOCLONAL ANTIBODY-DEFINED ANTIGENS OF HUMAN MELANOMAS

The earliest report of monoclonal antibodies with specificity for human melanoma cells appeared in 1978.[38] In this study hybridoma cultures were established from a fusion between melanoma immunized BALB/c spleen cells and P3 × 63Ag8 myeloma cells. Hybridoma antibodies were tested for binding to a panel of six melanoma cell lines, five colorectal carcinoma cell lines, and three fibroblast lines by radioimmunoassay. The pattern of reactivities observed is a perfect example of the kinds of results obtained in this type of work. The majority of the antibodies bound to most of the test panel without respect to the target cell type. Negative results were obtained in specific instances presumably because the particular cell line did not express the antigen in question. There were three antibodies which did show melanoma specificity in that they did not bind to nonmelanoma cell lines in the test panel; clones derived from these cultures were subjected to further study and form the subject of subsequent papers from this group.

An antibody of particular interest is designated 691I5Nu-4-B. This immunoglobulin was elicited by immunization with a hybrid cell line formed from a human melanoma, SW 691, and a mouse fibroblast IT 22. This cell line lost human chromosomes until only three could be detected, numbers 14, 17, and 21. Despite this loss the cell line retained the tumorigenicity of the human parent in nude mice and, as was shown, also retained expression of a characteristic melanoma surface antigen. The antigen occurs on all melanoma lines tested to date and also on some, but not all, astrocytoma lines, low levels of binding to human embryonal fibroblasts could also be observed, but these cells were unable to absorb measurable quantities of the antibody. Tests on fresh tumor specimens showed that the antigen was present on melanoma cells from patients but not on fibroblasts from the same patients.[39] The antigen was not present on nonmalignant pigmented cells from giant hairy nevi,[39] nor could it be detected on normal melanocytes in skin adjacent to primary melanomas.[40] Structural studies on the target antigen revealed a tetramolecular structure composed of three disulphide-linked polypeptide chains with molecular weights of 116,000, 29,000, and 26,000 daltons noncovalently associated with a fourth polypeptide chain of 95,000 daltons.[41,42]

Another antibody, 691-13-17, originally described in 1978[38] was subsequently shown to react with all normal human lymphocytes and Epstein-Barr transformed lymphocyte lines[43] and to precipitate DR antigens.[41] This antibody has been used in conjunction with a second DR-specific monoclonal antibody, 37-7, to study the expression of DR on melanoma cells. These studies showed that 37-7 and 691-13-17 recognize different common determinants expressed on the 31,000 dalton β chain of the DR dimer. The studies also indicate that melanoma cells express free chains on their surfaces in addition to $\alpha:\beta$ complexes.[44] This result contrasts with the situation on cells of the lymphoid lineage and the biological significance of the phenomenon remains to be established.

Antibody from hybridoma clone 691-19-19[38] also appears to react with melanoma cells and some astrocytoma cells.[41] This antibody, however, detects an antigen on surface iodinated melanoma cells distinct from that of 691I5Nu-4-B with a major component with a molecular weight of 260,000 daltons, and two less well-labeled entities with molecular weights of 240,000 and 220,000 daltons appear to be associated with the 260,000 molecule in immune precipitates.

A report in 1979 described three clones of an antibody which reacted with an antigenic determinant found to be strongly expressed only on the immunizing line.[45] These clones, designated 3.1, 3.2, and 3.3, were formed by fusion of BALB/c spleen cells and the myeloma line NS1. The antibody bound strongly to M1804, the immunizing line, weakly to two allogeneic melanoma lines and one breast carcinoma line, but did not bind to 5 carcinomas, 1 sarcoma, 17 fibroblasts, or 10 lymphoblastoid lines. Peripheral blood lymphocytes from 68 normal individuals and from 12 chronic lymphocytic leukemia patients did not bind this antibody. Molecular characterization of the target antigen has not been reported.

Two distinct melanoma-associated antigens have been detected by both monoclonal antibodies and xenoantisera.[46,47] These molecules are antigenically distinct and are shed by cells into tissue culture medium. One antigen is a glycoprotein designated MGP-1 and has a subunit molecular weight of 240,000 daltons, appears to be unique to melanoma cells, and is bound by lentil lectin. The second antigen is designated MGP-2, is also a glycoprotein, exists as a monomer with a molecular weight of 94,000 daltons, is bound by ricin lectin and is also found on carcinoma cells and fetal melanocytes.

Three melanoma-specific hybridomas were identified by selection from a large panel[48] formed by fusing the spleen from a BALB/c mouse immunized with membranes from ME-43 cells to myeloma NS1. There were 26 hybrid lines generated of which 7 were shown to secrete an antibody that reacted with melanoma cells; 3 of these reacted specifically with melanomas and were designated anti-MEL 5, anti-MEL 14, and anti-MEL 7. Both anti-MEL 5 and anti-MEL 14 reacted with 15 out of 16 melanoma lines tested, but the pattern of reactivity precluded that they reacted with the same antigen. Anti-MEL 7 reacted with 5 of 16 melanoma lines tested, however, in none of these three cases has characterization of the antigen been reported.

The identification of eight distinct monoclonal antibody-defined antigenic systems recognized by BALB/c × NS1 hybridomas have been described.[49] Of these antigens, one is detected by an antibody named 96.5, has a molecular weight of 97,000 daltons, and is not present on autologous fibroblasts. The relationship of this antigen to a 97,000 dalton molecule detected on melanoma cells by the same group[50] with a monoclonal antibody named 4.1 has not been reported. This latter antibody reacted with 90% of melanoma lines tested (23 of 25) and with 23 of 35 nonmelanoma lines. The antibody showed minimal reactivity with 15 fibroblast lines and 3 lymphoid lines. Another publication from this group described five antigenic systems shared by melanoma cells and autologous fibroblasts which were shown to exist[49] with a panel of antibodies produced from a mouse immunized with a melanoma cell line (G.D.). Antibody 96.1 detects an antigen with two components whose molecular weights are 33,000 and 50,000 daltons; antibody 96.2 reacts with an antigen of 23,000 daltons; 96.3 precipitates an antigen of 27,000 daltons; 96.4 a molecule of 200,000 daltons; and 96.10 a molecule of 40,000 daltons. Antibody 96.6 precipitated a structure which contained three components with molecular weights of 27,000, 80,000, and 110,000 daltons; however, whether these are antigenically cross-reacting distinct entities or, alternatively, whether they are covalently or noncovalently bonded together at the cell surface has not been reported. A final melanoma-specific antigen, which did not occur on fibroblasts, was described in this publication[49] which differed from the others in that it was not expressed at the cell surface. This antigen is recognized by antibody 96.7 and has a molecular weight of 60,000 daltons.

Another group of investigators[51] has used C57Bl/6 × BALB/c mice immunized with SK-MEL 28 and fused the immune spleen cells with NS1 myeloma cells to produce about 17 monoclonal antibodies which define five distinct antigenic groups. Six antibodies were identified in a gp95 group which recognized a glycoprotein with a molecular weight of 95,000 daltons. Antibodies of this group reacted with 11 of 16 melanoma lines, with 3 of 5 astrocytomas, 2 of 4 renal cancers, 1 bladder carcinoma and with normal kidney epithelium. Many melanomas, astrocytomas, and carcinomas of breast, lung, and cervical origin, and a variety of normal tissues did not expess the antigen. Antibodies of the gp150 group, defined by reaction with a glycoprotein of 150,000 daltons, bound to 13 of 15 melanoma lines, 3 of 5 astrocytomas, a renal, a bladder, and a colon carcinoma line. The antibody also bound strongly to normal kidney epithelium and fetal brain but weakly to normal melanocytes and fibroblasts. Antibodies of this group did not bind to tumors of a variety of different kinds including some melanomas and various carcinomas. In this respect, the range of reactivity of the gp95 and gp150 antibody types is similar.

An antigenic system defined by two antibodies has a molecular weight in the range of 50,000 to 70,000 daltons and is thus distinct from those described above. These antibodies also bind to some, but not all, cell lines of a variety of different types including melanomas, astrocytomas, renal, and ovarian carcinomas and also bind to normal melanocytes, kidney epithelium, and fibroblasts.

Antibodies of the R_{24} group define an antigen which is heat-stable in contrast to the target antigen of the three groups described above. This antigen has the characteristics of a glycolipid and was found on 16 melanoma lines and on 2 of 5 astrocytomas but not on a variety of carcinomas or on normal cells. The final type of reactivity described by these authors is shown by a single antibody designated O_5 which reacts with all human cells tested.

Monoclonal antibodies reactive with products of the HLA complex on melanoma cells have been produced by fusion of mouse spleen cells and myeloma cells.[52] Antibody 28 reacted with products of the HLA-A and B loci without regard to the numbered specificities expressed by these molecules. Similarly, antibody 70 reacted with products of the HLA-DR locus and showed the expected pattern of reactivity with melanoma cells, and lymphoid cells of the β lineage.

A number of new antigenic structures have been recently described on melanoma cells some of which also occur on other cell types.[53] Antibody 9-11-24 precipitates an antigen of about 60,000 daltons from iodinated melanoma cells and bound in a radioimmunoassay to 9 of 11 melanoma lines, 2 astrocytomas, and 2 of 3 lung carcinomas, but did not bind to colon carcinomas or normal fibroblasts or lymphocytes.[54] Antibody 56-1 precipitated an antigen which migrates as a 60,000 dalton species when unreduced but which exhibits a molecular weight of 28,000 daltons after reduction. This antigen can be detected on 7 of 11 melanomas but does not occur on any other type of cell tested. An antigen with a molecular weight of 196,000 daltons is precipitated from melanoma cells by antibody 51-52. This antigen can be detected by radioimmunoassay on five of eight melanomas, on two astrocytomas, on one lung carcinoma, and on the Burkitt lymphoma cell line Raji. An antibody generated by immunization with melanoma cells but which exhibits reactivity with a variety of cell tyes is 691-6-37.[41,54] This antibody reacts strongly with 13 melanoma lines and less strongly with three others. Only one melanoma line was unreactive, however five out of seven colorectal carcinoma lines were negative as were normal fibroblasts and lymphocytes. Three lung carcinomas, two astrocytomas, one laryngeal carcinoma, two lymphomas, and two EBV-transformed lines were positive.

X. MONOCLONAL ANTIBODY-DEFINED ANTIGENS OF NONMELANOMA TUMORS

Antibodies with specificity for colorectal carcinoma cells were described in 1979.[55] These authors prepared 104 hybridomas by immunization of mice with five different colorectal carcinoma cell lines and screened them against nine colorectal carcinoma lines, five melanoma lines, two astrocytomas, and a variety of other lines and normal cells. There were 25 hybridomas identified which bound to human cells of one kind or another, but only two were discovered which bound only to colorectal cells. The two specific antibodies, 1083-17-1A and 1116-56-2, showed distinct patterns of reactivity on a panel of target cells indicating reaction with different antigens but the antigenic targets were not identified. In the same paper, antibodies reactive with all human cells were described and designated 480-1-4 and 480-4-12. Again, however, the nature of the antigen was not reported.

Later in 1979, a further group of antibodies with specificity for colorectal carcinoma cells was prepared.[56] These antibodies were isolated from a single immunization of a BALB/c mouse with colorectal carcinoma cell line SW 1116 and fusion of the immune splenocytes with the nonsecreting variant of P3, P3 × 63Ag8.653.[27] The isolated antibodies showed a range of reactivities which suggested that they recognized various different antigens but immunoprecipitation did not permit identification of a proteinaceous target except in one case in which the antigen was identified as carcinoembryonic antigen (CEA). This antibody, 1116NS-3d, was subsequently studied in some detail and shown to be specific for the 180,000 dalton form of CEA and not to crossreact with the normal colon antigen (NCA) which is recognized by many xenoantisera.[57] Studies carried out on the antibodies which did not recognize protein antigens subsequently showed that four of these were directed against neutral glycolipids and two others against gangliosides.[58] One of this group of antibodies, 1116NS-10, is reactive with the Le^b blood group substance.[67] One antibody, 1116NS-52a, has been shown to bind to a previously unknown monosialoganglioside which migrates on thin-layer chromatography between GM1 and GD1a.[59] Other antibodies, 1116NS-3a, 1116NS-33a, and 1116NS-38a, react with colorectal carcinoma and with a glycolipid substance present in the serum of some individuals but not others.

Several monoclonal antibodies reactive with lung carcinomas have been prepared[60] which precipitate surface protein antigens from iodinated cells. Antibodies 9812-16A6 and 9812-16B13 precipitate an antigen consisting of two components with molecular weights of 37,000 and 19,000 daltons. This antigen occurs on all tumor cells tested and on normal red blood cells and lymphocytes. The antigen does not, however, occur on normal fibroblasts. Another monoclonal antibody, elicited by immunization with a lung carcinoma A427 and fused with P3 secretes an antibody, 427-2, which precipitates from iodinated cells a heavily labeled antigen with a molecular weight of 127,000 daltons together with two additional polypeptide chains which are more lightly iodinated of 145,000 and 113,000 daltons. This antibody binds to four of six lung carcinomas, all five colon carcinomas tested, three of six melanomas, one of three breast carcinomas, two of five fibroblast cell lines, but did not bind to normal lymphocytes or red blood cells. Antibody 900-1 bound strongly to the immunizing cell line SW 900 but not to five other lung carcinomas or to five colon carcinomas. The antibody does bind to five of six melanomas, to four of five normal lymphocytes, and one of three breast carcinomas. Normal lymphocytes and red blood cells were antigen-negative. The antibody precipitates a polypeptide antigen with a molecular weight of 126,000 daltons from iodinated SW 900 but did not precipitate an antigen from iodinated WM 9 cells, despite the fact that this cell line binds the antibody strongly. An antibody which seems to be largely specific for the immunizing cell line has been raised by immunization with the lung carcinoma WL 1680. The antibody 1680-25 binds strongly to the carcinoma line and less strongly to a fibroblast line grown from the same tumor specimen. This antibody binds weakly to a few other lung carcinoma lines and to no other tested line except one melanoma, WM 9. The antibody precipitates an iodinated dimeric antigen with components that have molecular weights of 149,000 and 119,000 daltons from the two parental cell lines and from WM 9.

XI. THE NATURE AND PROPERTIES OF TUMOR ANTIGENS

The ideal situation would be to find an antigen that would be characteristic of the tumor under study. Such a molecule would be found only on the cells of one type of tumor; however, proof of such a situation may be difficult to obtain for several reasons: (1) we can only ever show that we cannot detect an antigen on normal cells, we can never prove that the antigen is not there, (2) the important event may not be the appearance of a new antigen, but the presence of an abnormal amount of an antigen. Indeed, the relationship between the amounts of the various antigens on the cell surface may distinguish a tumor cell from a normal cell.

With these considerations in mind, we should survey tumor cells and normal cells for the relative amounts of various molecules and attempt to relate the presence of changed concentrations of surface molecules to the phenomenon of tumorigenicity. At the same time, we should continue our search for tumor-specific antigens (TSA).

We can, from the first principles, however, do a thought experiment as to what form TSA might take. For the present purpose, we should assume that TSA are molecules found in or on tumor cells and not elsewhere. In common with all other biological macromolecules, TSA must be either protein, carbohydrate, or lipid, although lipids are poor antigens in general. For a proteinaceous antigen we may ask the question: what is the origin of the genetic information which encodes the substance? For carbohydrate and lipid antigens the question is a great deal more complex since the assembly of these structures requires the integrated action of a number of enzymes.

The origin of the information for a protein antigen can be endogenous or exogenous. Let us consider the endogenous case first in which the antigen could be the product of a normal gene abnormally expressed.

1. Oncofetal antigens fall into this category since these molecules presumably have some function in the fetus and thus are normal proteins but are expressed in tumor cells as the result of a relaxation (or imposition) of an inappropriate regulatory control.
2. Molecules expressed preferentially during the rapid growth of cells could appear to be TSAs since their expression would not be observed on normal cells.
3. Many proteins are synthesized with a "leader" sequence which is selectively cleaved before the protein becomes functional or after the protein is inserted in the cell membrane; if such sequences were left attached to the finished molecules they could appear as TSA.
4. The antigen could be the expression of a gene with a point mutation which would be observed as an essentially normal product but with unique antigenic determinants. (Care should be taken to distinguish such molecules from allelic variants!)
5. Frameshift mutants may occur but are unlikely to be found for several reasons. First, membrane proteins are inserted in the membrane by virtue of a leader sequence at the N terminal end. Second, retention of the protein in the membrane requires that the protein have a suitable hydrophobic region at the C terminus, therefore, to get a viable protein both the C and N termini must be read in correct frame and the occurrence of a small frameshifted region in the interior of a protein is an unlikely event.
6. Deletion mutants should have certain characteristics in common with normal proteins and could be identified by peptide mapping.

A brief consideration of the structure of carbohydrates leads to the conclusion that the appearance of an entirely new sugar residue is unlikely because this would require the presence of a battery of enzymes for the synthesis of the sugar and another enzyme to place it on the oligosaccharide. Similarly, the occurrence of a new pattern (new arrangement) of sugars in the oligosaccharides of glycoproteins or glycolipids would require the operation of a new set of synthetic enzymes with different substrate specificities. Additional copies of normal oligosaccharides or the presence of incompletely synthesized oligosaccharides on a protein would, however, be more likely since a "minor" deregulation of the enzymes involved would yield this type of effect.

In the case of exogenous genetic material by which, of course, we mean viruses, information coding for membrane proteins could be normal virus constituents. Alternatively, viruses could carry with them some nonessential material which could be expressed in the host cell as a TSA.

Let us turn now to the consideration of the process by which antigens come to be expressed. Again, we may restrict ourselves to an internal or external cause. First, internal causes: (1) random occurrence of genetic rearrangement during somatic division could lead to the removal of (or insertion of inappropriate) control elements and thus to abnormal expression of antigens; (2) loss by deletion of processing enzymes could lead to the retention of peptides usually not present in the final proteins; (3) excessive production of glycosylating enzymes could lead to over glycosylation of proteins, and, thus, to incorrect processing and changed antigenicity. Second, external causes are probably viral and these entities could bring about their effect in various ways: (1) the presence of a viral enzyme could lead to an abnormal scission of a protein and thus to the expression of a new antigen; (2) the integration of a virus in the host genome could lead to the separation of a control element from its structural target; (3) genetic rearrangements could be caused by the presence of virus or by the insertion of virus material into the genome.

Consideration of the structure of antigens discussed above allows a variety of predictions to be made. Examples of over expression of normal components should be identifiable by use of a more sensitive technique by which the antigen may be detectable on the nonmalignant cellular counterpart of the tumor cell and may be seen on many different types of cells from different individuals.

In contrast, point mutations or deletion mutants would give rise to antigens that would be unique to the cell line that bore them. These antigens would have normal counterparts that could be identified. The opposite extreme would be antigens encoded by a viral genome which would be common to all tumors of a given type and also perhaps to tumors of other types if they were elicited either directly or indirectly by the action of a virus. Antigens of this type would have no counterpart on normal cells.

A more complex situation would arise if TSA arose from abnormal processing of normal molecules. The "leader" sequences present on many different proteins are thought to be similar since they all function in the same way (to facilitate the insertion of the protein into the cell membrane). If TSA of this type exist then an antigenic determinant might be found to be associated with different proteins on different cells or within the same cell. Antigenic determinants of this type would be characteristically on molecules larger than normal molecules but which would be otherwise similar to normal molecules in many of their antigenic determinants.

XII. PROBLEMS IN SCREENING FOR SPECIFICITY

In order to establish that the antigen recognized by a monoclonal antibody is found on tumor cells but not on other kinds of cells a binding assay is frequently undertaken. The occurrence of binding can be assessed by radioactive means (radioimmunoassay), by use of an enzyme to permit detection of binding (ELISA) or by visual inspection, often a hemagglutination assay (mixed hemagglutination).

Binding assays, however, have a dependence on the intrinsic association constant of the antibodies involved. This feature is of critical importance for monoclonal antibodies but of less significance for an antiserum which contains a variety of different antibodies with different affinities and specificities. In the case of a monoclonal antibody the functional affinity "Kf" may be enhanced by bivalent binding (the monogamous bivalency of Karush[61]) by a factor of 10^2 to 10^3 over the intrinsic equilibrium association constant "Ko". Bivalent interaction can only occur when the number and spacing of determinants is appropriate. Demonstration of binding at high level on tumor cells may depend on Kf and thus may encourage the belief that an antibody is "tumor-specific". Binding which occurs to a cell which has a much lower level of antigen expression may, however, depend on Ko if the spacing of determinants is too great to be spanned by individual antibody molecules.

Monovalent interactions will differ from bivalent interactions in several respects: (1)

the dissociation rate constant ''k_d'' will be much greater for antibody molecules bound by a single site and this will permit antibody molecules to dissociate and be removed during the washing procedures, (2) the proportion of antigen sites occupied ''r'' at a given antibody concentration will be lower in a manner related to the enhancement factor contributed by bivalent binding. Thus, by use of the relationship $K \times C = r/n - r$ it can be readily calculated that at certain antibody concentrations the proportion of sites occupied will be 90 times greater if the antibody can bind bivalently than if only a monovalent interaction is possible. The net effect of these considerations is that below a certain critical surface antigen concentration the ease with which binding may be detected suddenly decreases by several orders of magnitude. Antigens expressed on normal cells may, thus, remain undetected if present at low levels because the apparent inability of certain antibodies to bind to normal cells may result not from the absence of the antigen but, rather, from antigen expression below a certain critical level.

XIII. BIOLOGICAL FUNCTIONS OF MONOCONAL ANTIBODIES

It is to be expected that monoclonal antibodies will behave like normal immunoglobulins in terms of their ability to fix complement; mediate antibody-dependent, cell-mediated cytotoxicity (ADCC); and other functions. The in vivo distribution of antibodies, with a restriction of IgM to the intravascular space and the penetration of IgG, in addition, to the interstitial space, should also be normal. The specific ability of monoclonal antibodies to affect their tumor cell targets has been tested in a number of cases. Three antibodies with specificity for melanoma antigens and one with specificity for colorectal cacinoma cells were shown to specifically mediate ADCC against their respective targets.[62] The IgG2a colorectal carcinoma-specific antibody, 1083-17-1A, was subsequently shown to inhibit the growth of human colorectal carcinomas implanted in nude mice.[63] Of interest, and in line with the in vivo distribution expected for IgM antibodies, a group of monoclonal antibodies of this class with specificity for human colorectal cells were unable to inhibit the growth of these tumors in nude mice despite an efficient killing of cells by complement-mediated cytolysis in vitro.

Efforts to use the specificity of monoclonal antibodies to target toxic moieties onto tumor cells in vitro have proved successful. Ricin or diphtheria toxin A chains which by themselves are nontoxic because of an inability to bind to cell surfaces were rendered specifically toxic towards colorectal carcinoma cells by conjugating them to antibodies via a disulfide bridge.[64] In these experiments cytotoxicity was measured by the cessation of protein synthesis and while complete inhibition of colorectal carcinoma cells was achieved, melanoma cells were virtually unaffected.

XIV. FUTURE PROSPECTS FOR MONOCLONAL ANTIBODIES

From studies reported to date it seems clear that a tremendous range of different antigenic moieties have been, and will be, discovered on the surfaces of tumor cells. The origin, structure, and occurrence of these antigens remains, in most cases, to be fully elucidated but already in the case of lymphoid tumor markers, which may be taken as a model system, it seems clear that the identified antigens mark both tumor cells and subsets of the normal population. Particularly, it appears that the tumors themselves may consist of cells in a differentiated state which may mimic or be identical with that of a normal precursor stage. These molecules are most probably onco-developmental antigens. With tumor cells of other lineages the establishment of an antigen as an onco-developmental product is much more difficult simply because one cannot identify the precursor population in question. This may be because such cells occur in the adult organism at very low frequencies or may even not occur at all and only be found in the fetus. Some inferences may be drawn from studies such as those perfomed on the antigen defined by the antibody 691I5Nu-4-B.[41,42] This antigen occurs on all melanoma cells tested and has an apparently identical structure in each case. The molecule is complex, as described, and presumably has some function at the cell surface. The most consistent interpretation is that the molecule appears on the surface of these cells as a result of the expression (perhaps reexpression) of a carefully orchestrated set of genes and, thus, is likely to be the product of a normal component of the human genome. The determination of "tumor specificity" is bound to be a difficult task.

Tumor specificity, in the strictest sense, is not necessary for purposes of utility. Antibodies may bind to tumor cells with an "operational specificity" if the antigen density is much higher on tumor cells than it is on other cells of the body. Alternatively, binding may be tumor-specific if the antigen is an onco-fetal structure not present in the adult. The detection of tumor products in the serum or urine of patients may well be possible by use of appropriate monoclonal antibodies[65] and may provide early indication of the occurrence of a malignant growth or of the recurrence of tumor growth. Finally, monoclonal antibodies with tumor specificity may provide the long sought "magic bullets" of Paul Ehrlich when used in conjunction with an appropriate toxic agent.[66]

ACKNOWLEDGMENTS

This work was supported by Grants CA 25874, CA 10815, and CA 21124 from the National Cancer Institute, by RR 05540 from the Division of Research Resources, and by funds from the Pew Memorial Trust.

REFERENCES

1. **Bodurtha, A., Berkelhammer, J., Kim, Y. H., Laucius, J. F., and Mastrangelo, M. J.,** A clinical and immunologic study of a case of metastatic malignant melanoma undergoing spontaneous remission, *Cancer,* 37, 735, 1967.
2. **Edelson, R. L., Hearing, V. J., Dellon, A. L., Frank, M., Edelson, K. K., and Green, I.,** Differentiation between B cells, T cells and histiocytes in melanocytic lesions: primary and metastatic melanoma and halo and giant pigmented Nevi, *Cancer Immunol. Immunopathol.,* 4, 557, 1975.
3. **Bluming, A. Z., Vogel, O. L., Ziegler, J. L., and Kiryabwire, J. M. W.,** Delayed cutaneous sensitivity reactions to extracts of autologous malignant melanoma: a second look, *J. Natl. Cancer Inst.,* 48, 17, 1972.
4. **Irie, R. F., Giuliano, A. E., and Morton, D. L.,** Oncofetal antigen: tumor-associated fetal antigen immunogenic in man, *J. Natl. Cancer Inst.,* 63, 367, 1979.
5. **Sidell, N., Irie, R. F., Nathanson, S. D., and Morton, D. L.,** Immune cytolysis of human malignant melanoma by antibody to oncofetal antigen-1 (OFA-1), *Cancer Immunol. Immunother.,* 9, 49, 1980.
6. **Gupta, R. K., Silver, H. K. B., Reisfeld, R. A., and Morton, D. L.,** Isolation and immunochemical characterization of antibodies from the sera of cancer patients which are reactive against human melanoma cell membranes by affinity chromatography, *Cancer Res.,* 39, 1683, 1974.
7. **Embleton, M. J., Price, M. R., and Baldwin, R. W.,** Demonstration and partial purification of common melanoma-associated antigen(s), *Eur. J. Cancer,* 16, 575, 1980.
8. **Lewis, M. G., Ikonopisov, R. L., and Nairn, R. C.,** Tumor-specific antibodies in human malignant melanoma and their relationship to the extent of the disease, *Br. Med. J.,* 3, 547, 1969.
9. **Morton, D. L., Malmgren, A. L., and Holmes, E. C.,** Demonstration of antibodies against human malignant melanoma by immunofluorescence, *Surgery,* 64, 233, 1968.
10. **Garrett, T. J., Takahashi, T., Clarkson, B. D., and Old, L. J.,** Detection of antibody to autologous human leukemia cells by immune adherence assays, *Proc. Natl. Acad. Sci. U.S.A.,* 74, 4587, 1977.

11. **Cornain, S., deVries, J. E., Collard, J., Vennegoor, C., van Wingerden, I., and Rumke, P.,** Antibodies and antigen expression in human melanoma detected by the immune adherence test, *Int. J. Cancer,* 16, 981, 1975.
12. **Carey, T. E., Takahashi, T., Resnick, L. A., Oettgen, H. F., and Old, L. J.,** Cell surface antigen of human malignant melanoma: mixed hemadsorption assays for humoral immunity to cultured autologous melanoma cells, *Proc. Natl. Acad. Sci. U.S.A.,* 73, 3278, 1976.
13. **Bell, C. E., Jr., Seetharam, S., and McDaniel, R. C.,** Endodermally-derived and neural crest-derived differentiation antigens expressed by a human lung lesion, *J. Immunol.,* 116, 1236, 1976.
14. **Wilson, B. S., Indiveri, F., Pellegrino, M. A., and Ferrone, S.,** DR (Ia-like) antigens on human melanoma cells, *J. Exp. Med.,* 149, 658, 1979.
15. **Winchester, R. J., Wang, C.-Y., Gibofski, A., Kunkel, H. G., Lloyd, K. O., and Old, L. J.,** Expression of Ia-like antigens on cultured human malignant melanoma cell lines, *Proc. Natl. Acad. Sci. U.S.A.,* 75, 6235, 1978.
16. **Bray, A. E.,** The immunology in cancer, *Surg. Gyn. Obst.,* 147, 103, 1978.
17. **Galloway, D. R., McCabe, R. P., Pellegrino, M. A., Ferrone, S., and Reisfeld, R. A.,** Tumor-associated antigens in spent medium of human melanoma cells: immunochemical characterization with xenoantisera, *J. Immunol.,* 126, 62, 1981.
18. **Liao, S. K., Kwong, P. C., Thompson, J. C., and Dent, P. B.,** Spectrum of melanoma antigens on cultured human malignant melanoma cells as detected by monkey antibodies, *Cancer Res.,* 39, 183, 1979.
19. **Mutzner, P. A., Stuhlmiller, G. M., and Seigler, H. F.,** Characterization of melanoma cell membrane tumor-associated antigens using xenoantiserum, alloserum and autoserum 1. Immunofluorescence, *J. Surg. Oncol.,* 14, 367, 1980.
20. **Suter, L., Bruggen, J., Vakilzadeh, F., Kovary, P. M., and Macher, E.,** Human malignant melanoma: assay of tumor-associated antigens by use of rabbit antisera, *J. Invest. Dermatol.,* 75, 235, 1980.
21. **Pontecorvo, G., Croce, C. M., and Sisskin, E.,** Cell fusion, *Adv. Pathobiol.,* 6, 258, 1977.
22. **Pontecorvo, G.,** Production of mammalian somatic cell hybrids by means of polyethylene glycol treatment, *Somat. Cell Genet.,* 1, 397, 1975.
23. **Littlefield, J. W.,** Selection of hybrids from mating of fibroblasts *in vitro* and their presumed recombinants, *Science,* 145, 709, 1964.
24. **Szybalski, W., Szybalka, E. H., and Regnie, G.,** Genetic studies with human cell lines, *Cancer Inst. Monogr.,* 7, 75, 1962.
25. **Horibata, K. and Harris, A. W.,** Mouse myelomas and lymphomas in culture, *Exp. Cell Res.,* 60, 61, 1970.
26. **Köhler, G. and Milstein, C.,** Continuous cultures of fused cells secreting antibody of predefined specificity, *Nature (London),* 257, 495, 1975.
27. **Kearney, J. F., Radbruch, A., Liesegang, B., and Rajewski, K.,** A new mouse myeloma cell line that has lost immunoglobulin expression but permits the construction of antibody-secreting hybrid cell lines, *J. Immunol.,* 123, 1548, 1979.
28. **Köhler, G., Howe, S. C., and Milstein, C.,** Fusion between immunoglobulin-secreting and nonsecreting myeloma cell lines, *Eur. J. Immunol.,* 6, 292, 1976.
29. **McMichael, A. J., Pilch, J. R., Galfre, G., Mason, D. Y., Fabre, J. W., and Milstein, C.,** A human thymocyte antigen-defined by a hybrid myeloma monoclonal antibody, *Eur. J. Immunol.,* 9, 205, 1979.
30. **Bradstock, K. F., Janossy, G., Pizzolo, G., Hoffbrand, A. V., McMichael, A., Pilch, J. R., Milstein, C., Beverly, P., and Bollum, F. J.,** Subpopulations of normal and leukemic human thymocytes: an analysis with the use of monoclonal antibodies, *J. Natl. Cancer Inst.,* 65, 33, 1980.
31. **Levy, R., Dilley, J., Fox, R. I., and Warnke, R.,** A human thymus-leukemia antigen defined by hybridoma monoclonal antibodies, *Proc. Natl. Acad. Sci. U.S.A.,* 12, 6552, 1979.
32. **Hansen, J. A., Martin, P. J., and Nowinski, R. C.,** Monoclonal antibodies identifying a novel T cell antigen and Ia antigens of human lymphocytes, *Immunogenetics,* 10, 247, 1980.
33. **Reinherz, E. L., Kung, P. C., Goldstein, G., and Schlossman, S. F.,** Monoclonal antibody with selective reactivity with functionally mature human thymocytes and all peripheral human T cells, *J. Immunol.,* 123, 1312, 1979.
34. **Royston, I., Majda, J. A., Baird, S. M., Meserve, B. A., and Griffiths, J. C.,** Human T cell antigens defined by monoclonal antibodies: the 65,000-dalton antigen of T cells (T65) is also found on chronic lymphocytic leukemia cells bearing immunoglobulin, *J. Immunol.,* 125, 725, 1980.
35. **Beckman, I. G. R., Bradley, J., Brooks, D. A., Kupa, A., McNamara, P. J., Thomas, M. E., and Zola, H.,** Human lymphocyte markers defined by antibodies derived from somatic cell hybrids, *Clin. Exp. Immunol.,* 40, 593, 1980.

36. **Nadler, L. M., Stashenko, P., Hardy, R., and Schlossman, S. F.,** A monoclonal antibody defining a lymphoma-associated antigen in man, *J. Immunol.*, 125, 570, 1980.
37. **Ritz, J., Pesando, J. M., Notis-McConanty, J., Lazarus, H., and Schlossman, S. F.,** A monoclonal antibody to human acute lymphoblastic leukemia antigen, *Nature (London)*, 283, 583, 1980.
38. **Koprowski, H., Steplewski, Z., Herlyn, D., and Herlyn, M.,** Study of antibodies against human melanomas produced by somatic cell hybrids, *Proc. Natl. Acad. Sci. U.S.A.*, 75, 3403, 1978.
39. **Steplewski, Z., Herlyn, M., Herlyn, D., Clark, W. H., and Koprowski, H.,** Reactivity of monoclonal anti-melanoma antibodies with melanoma cells freshly isolated from primary and metastatic melanoma, *Eur. J. Immunol.*, 9, 94, 1979.
40. **Thompson, J., Herlyn, M. J., Elder, D. E., Clark, W. H., Steplewski, Z., and Koprowski, H.,** Use of monoclonal antibodies in detection of melanoma associated antigens in intact human tumors, *Hybridoma*, 2, 1982, in press.
41. **Mitchell, K. F., Fuhrer, J. P., Steplewski, Z., and Koprowski, H.,** Biochemical characterization of human melanoma cell surfaces: dissection with monoclonal antibodies, *Proc. Natl. Acad. Sci. U.S.A.*, 77, 7287, 1980.
42. **Mitchell, K. F., Fuhrer, J. P., Steplewski, Z., and Koprowski, H.,** Structural characterization of the "melanoma-specific" antigen detected by monoclonal antibody 691I5Nu-4-B, *Mol. Immunol.*, 18, 207, 1981.
43. **Herlyn, M., Clark, W. H., Jr., Mastrangelo, M. J., Guerry, D. P., IV, Elder, D. E., LaRossa, D., Hamilton, R., Bondi, E., Tuthill, R., Steplewski, Z., and Koprowski, H.,** Specific immunoreactivity of hybridoma-secreted monoclonal anti-melanoma antibodies to cultured cells on freshly derived human cells, *Cancer Res.*, 40, 3602, 1980.
44. **Mitchell, K. F., Ward, F. E., and Koprowski, H.,** Analysis of DR antigens on melanoma cells with monoclonal antibodies, *Human Immunol.*, in press.
45. **Yeh, M.-Y., Hellstrom, I., Brown, J. P., Warner, G. A., Hansen, J. A., and Hellstrom, K. E.,** Cell surface antigens of human melanoma identified by monoclonal antibody, *Proc. Natl. Acad. Sci. U.S.A.*, 76, 2927, 1979.
46. **Reisfeld, R. A., Galloway, D., Imai, K., Ferrone, S., and Morgan, A. C.,** Molecular profiles of human melanoma-associated antigens, *Fed. Proc.*, 39, 351, 1980.
47. **Imai, K., Molinaro, G. A., and Ferrone, S.,** Monoclonal antibodies to human melanoma-associated antigens, *Trans. Proc.*, 12, 380, 1980.
48. **Carrel, S., Accolla, R. S., Carmagnola, A. L., and Mach, J. P.,** Common human melanoma-associated antigen(s) detected by monoclonal antibodies, *Cancer Res.*, 40, 2523, 1980.
49. **Brown, J. P., Wright, P. W., Hart, C. E., Woodbury, R. G., Hellstrom, K. E., and Hellstrom, I.,** Protein antigens of normal and malignant human cells identified by immunoprecipitation with monoclonal antibodies, *J. Biol. Chem.*, 255, 4980, 1980.
50. **Woodbury, R. G., Brown, J. P., Yeh, M.-Y., Hellstrom, I., and Hellstrom, K. E.,** Identification of a cell surface protein, p97, in human melanomas and certain other neoplasms, *Proc. Natl. Acad. Sci. U.S.A.*, 77, 2183, 1980.
51. **Dippold, W. G., Lloyd, K. O., Li, L. T. C., Ikeda, H., Oettgen, H. F., and Old, L. J.,** Cell surface antigens of human malignant melanoma: definition of six antigenic systems with mouse monoclonal antibodies, *Proc. Natl. Acad. Sci. U.S.A.*, 77, 6114, 1980.
52. **Wilson, B. S., Indiveri, F., Molinaro, G. A., Quaranta, V., and Ferrone, S.,** Characterization of DR antigens on cultured melanoma cells by using monoclonal antibodies, *Trans. Proc.*, 12, 125, 1980.
53. **Mitchell, K. F., Steplewski, Z., and Koprowski, H.,** Human malignant melanoma cell surface antigens identified by monoclonal antibodies, *Br. J. Med.*, submitted.
54. **Steplewski, Z., Mitchell, K. F., and Koprowski, H.,** Biologic studies of antimelanoma monoclonal antibodies, in *Melanoma Antigens and Antibodies*, Reisfeld, R., Ed., Plenum Press, in press.
55. **Herlyn, M., Steplewski, Z., Herlyn, D., and Koprowski, H.,** Colorectal carcinoma-specific antigen: detection by means of monoclonal antibodies, *Proc. Natl. Acad. Sci. U.S.A.*, 76, 1438, 1979.
56. **Koprowski, H., Steplewski, Z., Mitchell, K. F., Herlyn, M., Herlyn, D., and Fuhrer, J. P.,** Colorectal carcinoma antigens detected by hybridoma antibodies, *Somat. Cell Genet.*, 5, 597, 1979.
57. **Mitchell, K. F.,** A carcinoembryonic antigen (CEA)-specific monoclonal antibody that reacts only with high molecular weight CEA, *Cancer Immunol. Immunother.*, 10, 1, 1980.
58. **Magnani, J. L., Brockhaus, M., Smith, D. F., and Ginsburg, V.,** Detection of glycolipid antigens by direct binding of monoclonal antibodies to thin-layer chromatograms of total lipid extracts of tissues, *Fed. Proc.*, (Abstr. 1613), 65th Annu. Meet., Atlanta, 1981.
59. **Magnani, J. L., Brockhaus, M., Smith, D. F., Ginsburg, V., Blasczyzyk, M., Mitchell, K. F., Steplewski, Z., and Koprowski, H.,** A monosialoganglioside is a monoclonal antibody defined antigen of colorectal carcinoma, *Science*, 212, 55, 1981.

60. **Mazauric, T., Mitchell, K. F., Letchworth, G. J., III, Koprowski, H., and Steplewski, Z.**, Monoclonal antibody-defined human lung cell surface protein antigens, *Cancer Res.*, 42, in press.
61. **Hornick, C. L. and Karush, F.**, The interaction of hapten-coupled bacteriophage $\phi \times 174$ with anti-hapten antibody, *Israel J. Med. Sci.*, 5, 163, 1969.
62. **Herlyn, D., Herlyn, M., Steplewski, Z., and Koprowski, H.**, Monoclonal antibodies in cell-mediated cytotoxicity against human melanoma on colorectal carcinoma, *Eur. J. Immunol.*, 9, 657, 1979.
63. **Herlyn, D., Steplewski, Z., Herlyn, M., and Koprowski, H.**, Inhibition of growth of colorectal carcinomas in nude mice by monoclonal antibody, *Cancer Res.*, 40, 717, 1980.
64. **Gilliland, D. G., Steplewski, Z., Collier, R. J., Mitchell, K. F., Chang, T. H., and Koprowski, H.**, Antibody directed cytotoxic agents: use of monoclonal antibody to direct the action of toxin A chains to colorectal carcinoma cells, *Proc. Natl. Acad. Sci. U.S.A.*, 77, 4539, 1980.
65. **Koprowski, H., Sears, H. F., Herlyn, M., and Steplewski, Z.**, Specific antigen in serum of patients with colon carcinoma, *Science*, 212, 53, 1981.
66. **Davies, T.**, Magic bullets, *Nature (London)*, 289, 12, 1981.
67. **Brockhaus, M.**, personal communication.

Chapter 9

MURINE MACROPHAGE DIFFERENTIATION ANTIGENS DEFINED BY MONOCLONAL ANTIBODIES

Timothy A. Springer

TABLE OF CONTENTS

I. INTRODUCTION

Recently, the Köhler-Milstein myeloma-hybrid technique has given great impetus to the analysis of cell surface complexity.[1] Its most revolutionary feature is the ability to use highly complex antigens such as whole cells in xenogeneic immunization. The resultant multispecific response may then be resolved by cloning into a set of hybrid lines each secreting a monoclonal antibody (MAb) recognizing a single antigenic determinant on a single cell surface molecule. This paper will review some previously published as well as new work from this laboratory on the use of this technology for the identification and study of macrophage antigens.

II. MAC-1 ANTIGEN

M1/70 antibody, identifying the Mac-1 antigen, was obtained by a serendipitous route. Rats were immunized with mouse spleen cells and 10 cloned hybridoma lines were obtained.[2] The M1/70 line gave barely significant, twofold over background binding to spleen cells in the indirect ^{125}I-anti-rat IgG sandwich assay. Screening on a tumor cell panel revealed that the P388D1 macrophage-like cell line bound 100-fold more M1/70 antibody than spleen cells, but a series of B and T lymphoid lines gave no significant binding. This led to further studies on the cell distribution and molecular properties of this antigen.[3] In normal tissues M1/70 gave binding to the adherent and nonadherent fraction of peritoneal exudate cells that was proportional to the number of macrophages in each. Fluorescence activated cell sorter analysis showed that Mac-1 is expressed on thioglycollate-induced peritoneal exudate macrophages, 50% of bone marrow cells (Figure 1), and on granulocytes and blood monocytes but is found on only a small proportion of spleen cells and is absent from thymocytes (Table 1). Mac-1 is also expressed on peritoneal resident macrophages and those induced by peptone, *Corynebacterium parvum, Listeria monocytogenes,* lipopolysaccharide, and concanavalin A. In splenic thin sections, M1/70 stains macrophages in the marginal zone and red pulp and also granulocytes in the red pulp.[4]

Mac-1 contains two polypeptide chains of 190,000 and 105,000 mol wt (Figure 3b) and much greater quantities are precipitated from peritoneal exudate cells (PEC) than spleen. Peritoneal exudate macrophages express about tenfold greater amounts of M1/70 than positive cells in bone marrow (Figure 1g, h), about eightfold more than M1/70$^+$ spleen cells, and much more than granulocytes or blood monocytes.[3] The increase in M1/70 expression during maturation of monocytes to exudate macrophages is paralleled by a decrease in another antigen, the M1/69 heat stable antigen (HSA).[3] Because of its phagocyte-specificity and strong expression on macrophages, the M1/70 antigen has been designated Mac-1.

M1/70 also cross-reacts with an antigen on human monocytes, granulocytes, and natural killer and antibody-dependent cytotoxic cells.[5] Presence on the latter cells was determined by FACS sorting of monocyte-depleted blood mononuclear cells using F(ab')$_2$ M1/70 and FITC second antibody followed by testing for functional activity. M1/70$^+$ cells were enriched for NK and ADCC activity, while M1/70$^-$ cells were depleted compared to stained but unsorted cells.

III. IMMUNOADSORBENT-CELL HYBRIDIZATION CASCADES

To obtain lineage-specific MAb, animals are usually immunized with whole cells of one lineage and MAb recognizing widely shared antigens are screened out by testing on other types of cells. A major problem with this approach is that widely shared an-

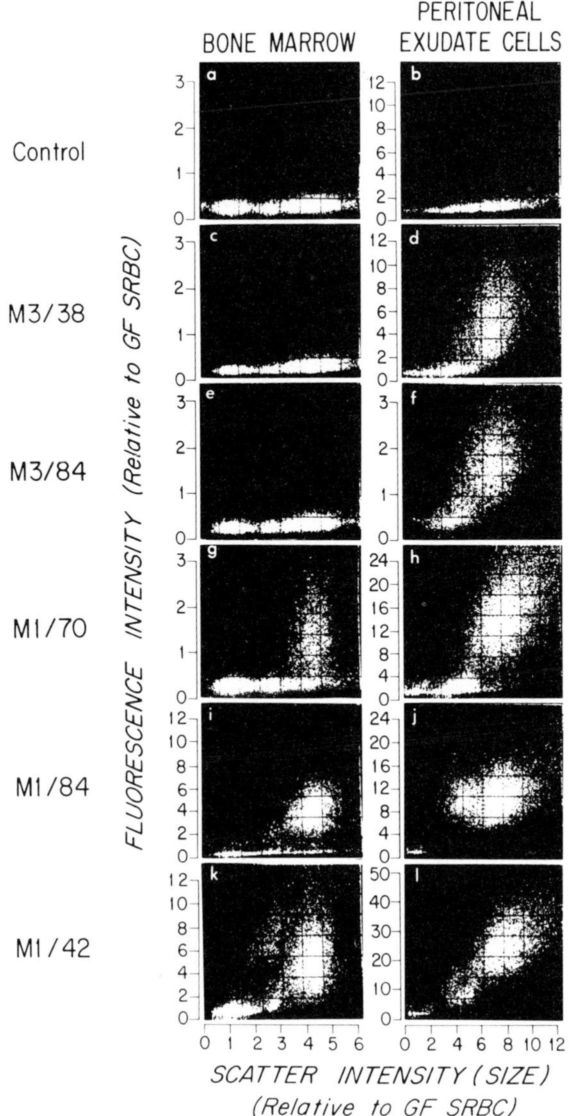

FIGURE 1. FACS dot plot analysis of staining of Mac-2 (M3/38), Mac-3 (M3/84), Mac-1 (M1/70), M1/84, and H-2 (M1/42) on B6/J bone marrow and thioglycollate-induced 4 day PEC. Cells were labeled with rat MAb, then FITC-rabbit $F(ab')_2$ antirat IgG absorbed with mouse IgG as described previously.[3] Mouse RBC, polymorphs, and macrophages appear at scatter intensities of 1, 4 to 5, and 7 to 10, respectively. GF SRBC = glutaraldehyde-fixed sheep red blood cells.

tigens as well as the more readily identified macrophage-specific antigens may be immunodominant and thus may nonspecifically suppress the response to other antigens.[6] In the M1 experiment, for example, the widely shared HSA and common leukocyte antigen (CLA) appeared immunodominant, since they accounted for 7/10 of the MAb obtained.[2] These two antigens are also on peritoneal exudate cells. Immunization with whole PEC resulted in comparable titers of antibodies to Mac-1, HSA, and CLA as

Table 1
MONOCLONAL RAT ANTIMOUSE MACROPHAGE ANTIBODIES

Antibody	Subclass	Antigen	Polypeptide chains	Distribution[a] Positive	Negative	Ref.
M1/70	IgG2b	Mac—1	190,000 105,000	(PP, LM, LPS, Con A, TG)—PEM, SM, M, G, PM, 50% BM	T, PLN	3 9
M3/31	IgM			TG—PEM	>97% (LM, LPS, Con A)—PEM, PM, SM, G, T,	7
M3/38	IgG2a	Mac—2	32,000	20% PP—PEM[b]	PLN, >99% BM	9
M3/84	IgGl	Mac—3	110,000	TG—PEM	T, PLN, >99% BM	7, 13
M3/37[c]	?	Mac—4	180,000	TG—PEM	T, >99% BM	7, 13

[a]Abbreviations used: PEM: peritoneal exudate macrophages, PM: unelicited peritoneal macrophages, SM: splenic macrophages, M: monocytes, G: granulocytes, BM: bone marrow cells, T: thymus cells; PLN: peripheral lymph node cells, TG: thioglycollate, PP: protease peptone, LM: L. monocytogenes, LPS: lipopolysaccharide, Con A: concanavalin A.
[b]Weakly positive.
[c]Not cloned.

determined by competitive inhibition of the binding of ^{3}H-labeled MAb to target cells;[7] therefore, in order to increase the chance of obtaining macrophage-specific MAb, these two antigens were removed by an immunoadsorbent procedure shown in Figure 2. As illustrated, one of the attractive features of this method is that it may be indefinitely extended in a cascade so that the immunogenic stimulus is always limited to those antigens not yet identified by MAb.

IV. MAC-2, 3, AND 4 ANTIGENS

To obtain further antimacrophage MAb, rats were immunized with immunoadsorbent-depleted purified macrophage glycoproteins and their spleen cells fused with NSI as described in the legend of Figure 2. Hybrid culture supernatants were screened for binding to macrophages, and all binders were screened for immunoprecipitation of ^{125}I-labeled cell surface antigens.[7] Then five supernatants precipitated polypeptides of 190,000 and 105,000 mol wt which resemble those of Mac-1, 11 cultures precipitated a 32,000 mol wt polypeptide, 1 a 110,000 mol wt, and another a 180,000 mol wt polypeptide; however, none of the cloned lines precipitated the 200,000 mol wt CLA polypeptide.[1] Analysis of the sera from animals immunized with cascade-purified antigen also showed absence of CLA competing or precipitating antibodies, although these antibodies were elicited by whole macrophages.[7]

There were three stable subcloned lines obtained by the cascade procedure. (For brevity, subclone designations will be omitted.) A 32,000 mol wt polypeptide (Mac-2), is precipitated by M3/31 and M3/38, while a 110,000 mol wt polypeptide (Mac-3) is precipitated by M3/84 (Figure 3a). A 180,000 mol wt polypeptide (Mac-4) is precipitated by an uncloned line, M3/37 (Figure 3b). (A cloned line, 54-1 has been independently obtained which appears to recognize the same antigen as determined by comigration in SDS-PAGE.)[8]

The cell distributions of all three antigens are very similar (Table 1). They are present on essentially all thioglycollate-induced peritoneal exudate macrophages (Figure 1) but

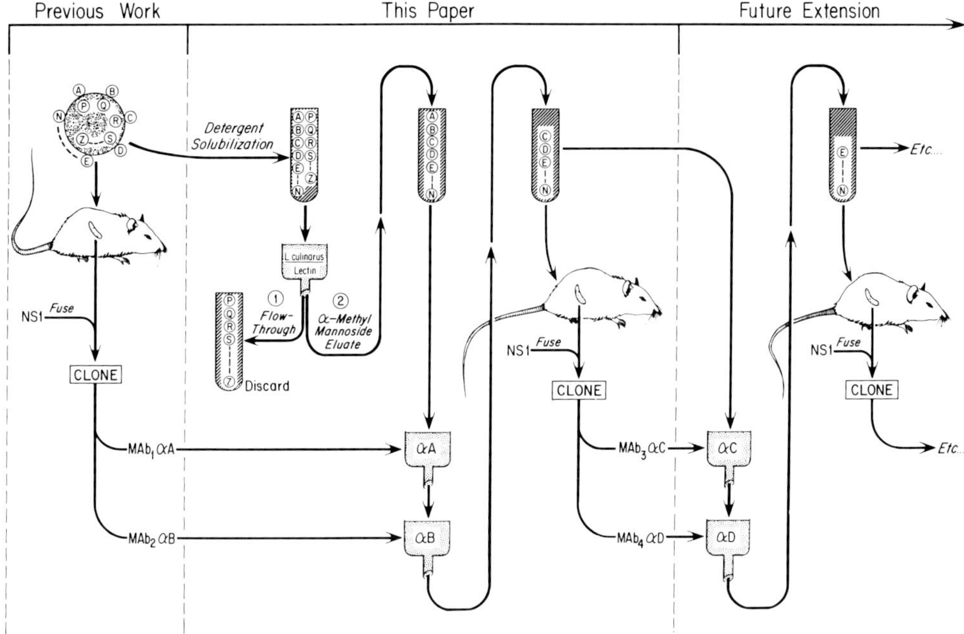

FIGURE 2. Cascade immunoadsorbent procedure for focusing hybridoma production on unrecognized antigens. B6/J PEC (8×10^8 4 days thioglycollate-induced, 84% macrophages, 2.5% neutrophils, 7.5% eosinophils, 4.5% lymphocytes, 1.5% RBC) in 20 mℓ PBS + 0.5 m*M* phenylmethylsulfonyl fluoride were N_2 cavitated after 10 min at 600 psi. Membranes were prepared, solubilized with sodium deoxycholate (NaDC), and glycoproteins purified on *Lens culinaris* lectin columns. Samples were then passed through columns containing approximately 1 mℓ of Sepharose CL-4B coupled with 1 mg of purified MAb M1/69.16 (to remove HSA) and M1/89.23 (to remove CLA). The sample was dialyzed 7 days vs. 2 changes daily of 0.01 *M* tris HCℓ, pH 8.2, to remove NaDC. Rats were injected twice with 40 μg protein of antigen in Complete Freund's Adjuvant and 4 months later with 100 μg in saline, and spleen cells fused 3 days later with NSI and grown in 5 × 96 well 0.2 mℓ culture trays. Full details have been described elsewhere.[7]

on 0% of thymocytes and <10% of spleen cells. Recent studies show that Mac-2 defines a macrophage subpopulation. It is present on >90% of thioglycollate-induced macrophages but on only 10 to 20% of peptone induced cells and <2% of peritoneal resident and *L. monocytogenes,* lipopolysaccharide, or concanavalin A induced macrophages.[9] Mac-2, 3, and 4, in contrast to Mac-1, are not expressed on bone marrow cells (0 to 1% positive, Figure 1). These results rule out expression on granulocytic precursors, but not on promonocytes, which constitute only 0.3% of bone marrow cells;[10] thus, Mac-2, 3, and 4 appear to be expressed on the monocytic line of differentiation at some stage after divergence from the granulocytic line, while Mac-1 is found on both branches. Mac-1, 2, and 3 all appear to be expressed in lower amounts on macrophages than H-2 antigen (Figure 1, note the changes in fluorescence scale).

The antigens described here all appear to be on the macrophage cell surface on the basis of fluorescent and ^{125}I-labeling. ^{35}S-methionine incorporation into the polypeptides by the adherent fraction of thioglycollate-induced PEC also suggests these antigens are synthesized by macrophages (Figure 3a, data not shown for Mac-1). Many preparations of Mac-2 antigen show in addition to the 32,000 mol wt chain fourfold less of a 30,000 mol wt chain. Much smaller amounts of slightly lower molecular weight polypeptides precipitated by M3/38 but not M3/31 have also been seen (Figure 3a). The working hypothesis is that the smaller polypeptides are degradation products bearing the M3/38 but not the M3/31 determinant. The M3/84 (Mac-3) 110,000 mol wt band is char-

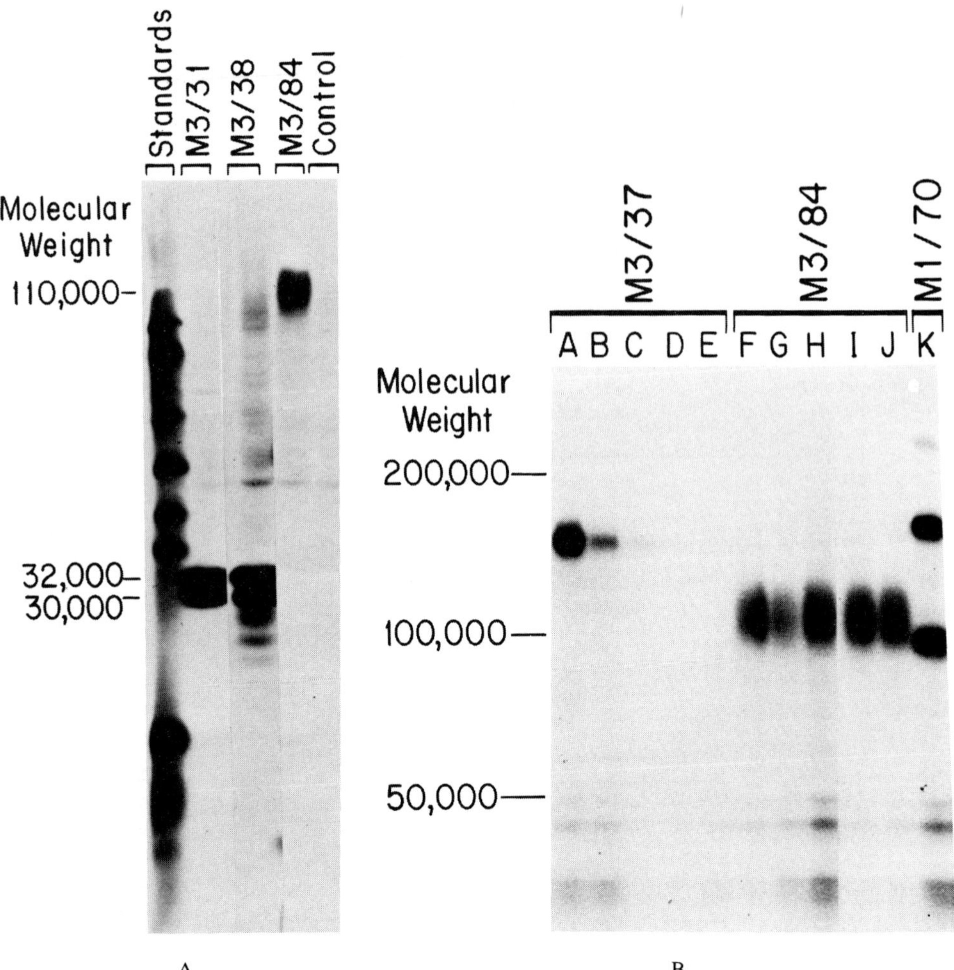

FIGURE 3. SDS-PAGE of Mac-1, 2, 3, and 4 antigens immunoprecipitated from 4 day thioglycollate-induced macrophages. Triton® X-100 lysates of labeled cells were incubated with MAb, then with rabbit antirat IgG second antibody and precipitates analyzed after 2-mercaptoethanol reduction.[3] (A) Cells adherent to tissue culture flasks were internally labeled with {^{35}S}- methionine; (B) Cells were vectorially labeled with ^{125}I using lactoperoxidase. A-E: M3/37, uncloned supernatants at weekly intervals; F-H: M3/84 uncloned supernatants at weekly intervals; I, M3/84.6 clone; J, M3/84.6.34 subclone; K, M1/70.15.1 subclone.

acteristically "fuzzy" after both ^{35}S-met and ^{125}I-labeling (Figures 3a, b). Side-by-side comparison of the high molecular weight Mac-4 (M3/37), Mac-3 (M3/84), and Mac-1 (M1/70) chains shows them all to have different molecular weights and thus, they are all clearly unique antigens (Figure 3b). The molecular weight and tissue distributions of these antigens differ from the macrophage Fc receptor II.[11] Their relationship to the genetically defined Mph-1 antigen[12] is unknown.

V. SUMMARY

These studies have defined four different antigens which are present on macrophages but not lymphocytes, demonstrating the distinctiveness of macrophage cell surface architecture (Table 1). This also suggests that classical antimacrophage sera, even after extensive absorption, recognize a complex of cell surface antigens. Classical antimacrophage sera have been reported to block a number of macrophage functional activities such as phagocytosis. The MAb described here are being used as probes to inhibit a panel of macrophage functions. In this way, it should be possible to link the molecular structures described here with specific macrophage cell surface activities.

ACKNOWLEDGMENTS

This work was supported by USPHS Grants CA 31798 and CA 31799 and the Council for Tobacco Research Grant 1307.

REFERENCES

1. **Springer, T. A.,** Cell-surface differentiation in the mouse. Characterization of ''jumping'' and ''lineage'' antigens using xenogeneic rat monoclonal antibodies, in *Monoclonal Antibodies,* Kennett, R. H., McKearn, T. J., and Bechtol, K. B., Eds., Plenum Press, New York, 1980, 185.
2. **Springer, T. A., Galfre, G., Secher, D. S., and Milstein, C.,** Monoclonal xenogeneic antibodies to murine cell surface antigens: identification of novel leukocyte differentiation antigens, *Eur. J. Immunol.,* 8, 539, 1978.
3. **Springer, T. A., Galfre, G., Secher, D. S., and Milstein, C.,** Mac-1: a macrophage differentiation antigen identified by monoclonal antibody, *Eur. J. Immunol.,* 9, 301, 1979.
4. **Ho, M. K. and Springer, T. A.,** Rat anti-mouse macrophage monoclonal antibodies and their use in immunofluorescent studies of macrophages in tissue sections, in *Monoclonal Antibodies and T Cell Hybridomas,* Hämmerling, U., Hämmerling, G., and Kearney, J., Eds., Elsevier, Amsterdam, in press.
5. **Ault, K. A. and Springer, T. A.,** Cross reaction of a rat-anti-mouse phagocyte-specific monoclonal antibody (anti-Mac-1) with human monocytes and natural killer cells, *J. Immunol.,* 126, 359, 1980.
6. **Pross, H. F. and Eidinger, D.,** Antigenic competition. A review of nonspecific antigen-induced suppression, *Adv. Immunol.,* 18, 133, 1974.
7. **Springer, T.,** Monoclonal antibody analysis of complex biological systems: combination of cell hybridization and immunoadsorbents in a novel cascade procedure and its application to the macrophage cell surface, *J. Biol. Chem.,* 256, 3833, 1981.
8. **Leblanc, P. A., Katz, H. R., and Russell, S. W.,** A discrete population of mononuclear phagocytes detected by monoclonal antibody, *Infect. Immun.,* 8, 520, 1981.
9. **Ho, M. K. and Springer, T.,** Mac-2, a novel 32,000 Mr macrophage subpopulation-specific antigen defined by monoclonal antibody, *J. Immunol.,* in press.
10. **Van Furth, R.,** Modulation of monocyte production, in *Mononuclear Phagocytes in Immunity Infection and Pathology,* Van Furth, R., Ed., Blackwell Scientific, Oxford, 1975, 161.
11. **Unkeless, J.,** Characterization of a monoclonal antibody directed against mouse macrophage and lymphocyte Fc receptors, *J. Exp. Med.,* 150, 580, 1979.
12. **Archer, J. R. and Davies, D. A. L.,** Demonstration of an alloantigen on the peritoneal exudate cells of inbred strains of mice and its association with chromosome 7 (linkage group I), *J. Immunogen.,* 1, 113, 1974.
13. **Springer, T. A.,** Mac-1,2,3, and 4; murine macrophage differentiation antigens identified by monoclonal antibodies, in *Heterogeneity of Mononuclear Phagocytes,* Förster, O. and Landy, M., Eds., Academic Press, New York, 1981, 37.

Chapter 10

APPLICATION OF MONOCLONAL ANTIBODIES TO THE STUDY OF HUMAN LYMPHOCYTE SURFACE ANTIGENS

C. S. Hosking and G. M. Georgiou

TABLE OF CONTENTS

I. INTRODUCTION

The lymphocyte surface membrane consists of a number of protein, glycoprotein, lipoprotein, and carbohydrate moieties floating in a lipid bilayer.[1] These molecules are mobile within the cell wall and evidence suggests that they can move independently of each other. Each molecule represents at least one antigenic determinant and in most cases more than one. As the number of distinct structural and other molecules that can be displayed antigenically can probably be numbered in the hundreds, the potential number of antibodies that can be directed against one of these cells can probably be numbered in the thousands.

The picture painted above describes lymphocytes as though they were a homogeneous class of cells; however, further variability is added by there being functional and probably antigenically distinct subclasses within one individual. Complicating the picture still further are the allotypic differences between individuals and a further degree of complexity is provided by the lymphocytes in any of the above compartments having to pass through developmental stages during which they may gain or lose antigenic determinants.

One can thus picture the lymphocyte surface as being a mass of antigenic sites. Some of these sites may share antigenic structures with most human cell types, some with other hemopoietic cells, some with all lymphocytes and still others may be distinct for the subclass of lymphocyte to which the index cell belongs (Figure 1).

The types and proportions of antibodies produced will be dependent on the amount and antigenicity of each of these epitopes on the surface membrane. Thus if one was to have 50% of the surface occupied with antigens that were common to all injected cells, then one might expect to have 50% of antibody positive primary monoclonal cultures producing antibodies to these structures. Of course, if the antigenic structure is present on only a small portion of the cell membrane of a minor population, then few splenic lymphocytes will be producing antibody to that particular structure. Thus many cultures will need to be screened before a monoclonal antibody to that particular antigen is found.

Let us consider the example of producing antibodies to surface membrane immunoglobulin of B cells. If B cells represent 20% of the population of the injected cells and the proportion of total antigenic determinants on the surface of a B cell represented by immunoglobulin was say 2%, then one would need to screen 500 cultures before finding one that had antibody to the particular antigen sought.

The above example presupposes a simple and sensitive test for the desired antibody. Thus if the aim of the project was to gain some knowledge about the density of antigenic determinants, then one would probably test for antibodies using a radioimmunoassay for serum immunoglobulin (Ig). This would have the benefit of simplicity as well as being relatively inexpensive. On the other hand, if the experiments were being done to seek unique determinants of the immunoglobulin chains on lymphocytes compared to serum immunoglobulins then one would need to test by enriching for those cells having immunoglobulin chains on their surface because of their relatively low frequency. This would be particularly so because of the subgroups of those cells with surface membrane immunoglobulin of the various heavy and light chain classes.

One could, of course, increase the statistical chances of finding the right antibody(s) by purifying either the lymphocytes containing surface membrane Ig chains or by going a further step and purifying the Ig from the surface membrane. In both these steps, particularly the latter, one would run the risk of altering the antigenic structure; thus while antibodies might be produced to the purified antigen they may not react with the antigen on the surface of the lymphocyte.

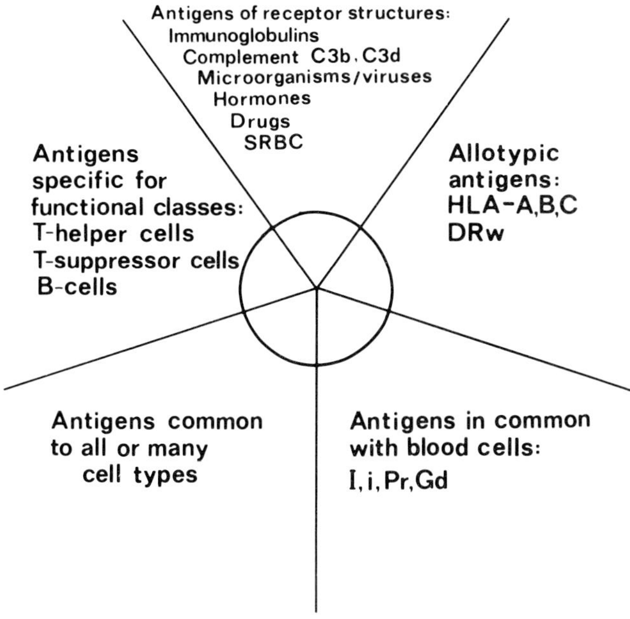

FIGURE 1. An illustration of some of the types of antigens to be found on the lymphocyte surface.

With normal heteroantisera, antibodies can be raised to many of the determinants described above. Many of the undesired antibodies can be absorbed out by using cells that are related to the cells in question but do not have the features being sought in the antisera. Perhaps the best example of this is the use of thymocytes and lymphoid cell lines from the same patient for producing and absorbing complementary heteroantisera. Thus to raise antibodies to structures unique to thymocytes, one injects thymocytes into a rabbit then absorbs the antiserum with a cell line produced by Epstein-Barr virus transformation of that same patient's lymphocytes. The cell line will be derived from B lymphocytes and have many of the characteristics of B cells but will have the same allotype (HLA) as the thymus cells. Thus one removes from the antiserum the antiallotypic element as well as many of the antibodies to antigens common to all lymphocytes or all human cells.

This approach, however, cannot be used with hybridoma antisera as these are directed to only one antigenic determinant which either is, or is not, the one sought.

II. LYMPHOCYTE POPULATIONS

Studies of the cells inolved in the immune response led to the discovery of two populations of lymphocytes, namely T and B lymphocytes.

The T lymphocyte is responsible for cell-mediated immunity which involves defense against fungi, facultative intracellular bacteria, viruses, delayed cutaneous hypersensitivity, graft-vs.-host reaction, allograft rejection, and some forms of tumor immunity.

B lymphocytes are responsible for humoral- or antibody-mediated immunity which involves synthesis of antibodies which may be of several immunoglobulin classes. Cells of both T and B cell lineage develop from a common lymphoid precursor (Figure 2).

Immature T cells termed prothymocytes migrate from the bone marrow to the thymus, where, under the inductive influence of thymic hormones in this microenvironment,

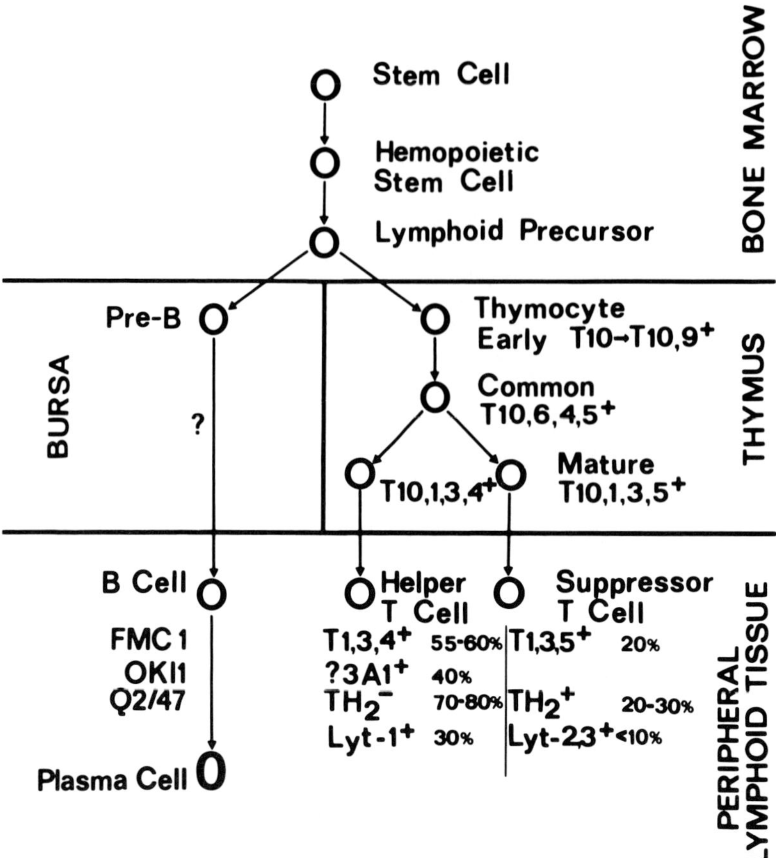

FIGURE 2. Antigens detected with monoclonal antibodies present on human T and B cells. The monoclonal antisera with the T label are of the OKT series and describe a developmental pathway of human T cells. Anti-TH_2 is a heteroantiserum. The Lyt antigens are murine and appear to be equivalent to the human helper and suppressor T cell subsets. Proportions of cells identified by the antisera are indicated by the number percent.

they differentiate into functional mature T cells. They are then exported into the peripheral lymphoid compartment which includes blood, spleen, and lymph nodes. These stages of T cell ontogeny are associated with changes in cell surface antigens.[2] The lymphoid precursors destined to become B cells come under the influence of the Bursa of Fabricius in chickens and its equivalent in mammals where they mature and gain surface membrane immunoglobulin. The cells then migrate to the peripheral lymphoid tissues to await further differentiation and maturation following antigenic challenge. The end cell of this series is the antibody-producing plasma cell.

III. SURFACE MEMBRANE MARKERS OF LYMPHOCYTES

A. Murine Lymphocyte Classes

The early studies in lymphocyte population identification were carried out in the murine system. The availability of different genetic strains allowed ontogenic and functional subpopulations to be identified

This involved production of antisera from mice immunized with allogeneic thymocytes. These antisera contained antibodies that reacted with the mouse T-cell-specific antigen Thy-1 (formerly called theta, antigen). The antibody did not react with mouse B cells.

Antisera were also produced against mouse immunoglobulin (Ig) which was used to detect surface membrane immunoglobulin (sIg) on B cells.

In a typical experiment to study functional properties, isolated mouse lymphocytes were treated with anti-Thy-1 serum plus complement, thus lysing cells with Thy-1 antigen. It was found that the ability of treated cell populations to transfer cellular immunity to irradiated mice was abolished, thus illustrating T cell function.

Similarly, treatment of lymphocytes with anti-immunoglubulin antisera inhibited humoral antigen recognition without affecting cellular immunity. This type of experiment has continued with the finding of other murine lymphocyte membrane antigens.

The differentiation of murine stem cells follows a path of antigenic change. Initially, the stem cells acquire TL (thymus-leukemia), Thy-1, and Lyt-1, 2, 3 antigens. The vast majority of lymphocytes within the thymus gland are Lyt-1, 2, 3, TL, and Thy-1. As maturation continues, a subset of thymic lymphocytes becomes TL^-, i.e., loses the TL antigen. At the same time there is a diminution of Thy-1 antigen and an increase in H2 antigens which are the products of the major histocompatibility region in the mouse. This latter phenotype is characteristic of the vast majority of peripheral T cells. In addition, some cells that are Lyt-1, 2, 3^+ diverge into two subsets of T cells having lost either Lyt-1 or Lyt-2, 3 markers, thus becoming Lyt-2, 3^+ and Lyt-1^+ cells, respectively. These cells have different functional properties.

When T cells are released from the thymus to localize in peripheral tissues, they contain roughly 50% cells with Lyt-1, 2, 3, about 30% Lyt-1, and less than 10% Lyt-2, 3 populations.

Antibody and complement lysis showed that the Lyt-1 cells function as helper cells in the T-B cell interaction necessary to produce antibody against thymus-dependent antigens and in the T-T cell interactions which generate suppressor or cytolytic cells.

Allogeneic cells which differ at the Ir (immune-response) gene region activate the Lyt-1 subpopulation of T cells in the mixed lymphocyte reaction (MLR).

The Lyt-2, 3 are responsible for the inhibition of humoral- and cell-mediated immune responses and are thus termed suppressor cells. They are also responsible for cytotoxicity of allogeneic lymphocytes or tumor cells by directing their activity against histocompatibility antigens.[3–5]

B. Human Lymphocyte Classes

1. Lymphocyte Populations Not Defined by Antilymphocyte Antibodies

In 1969 it was reported that sheep red blood cells (SRBC) attach spontaneously to about 60% or more of human peripheral blood lymphocytes, thus forming "erythrocyte rosettes".[6] The population of lymphocytes that rosette with SRBC have characteristics of T cells' absence of surface membrane immunoglobulin, as well almost all thymocytes form rosettes. This provides a relatively simple method to quantitate numbers of T cells and allows separation of the cells for functional studies. Technical variations in the formation of E-rosettes, particularly the time and temperature of incubation, have divided the rosette-forming cell into two categories termed active and late rosettes. This may relate to different subpopulations of T cells.

Although reproducibility in determining T cell rosette numbers is usually obtained within a laboratory, differences exist between laboratories. Therefore, attempts to evaluate small changes in the T cell population in certain diseases, other than immunodeficiencies or leukemias, are difficult.

Attempts to demonstrate subpopulations of T cells led to the discovery of Fc receptors on T lymphocytes.[7] These subpopulations were identified by a rosetting technique using oxRBC IgM, oxRBC IgG, oxRBC TNP IgA, and oxRBC IgE coated cells. The populations detected have been named Tμ, Tγ, Tα, and Tϵ cells, respectively. Further experiments as to functional properties of the Tμ (helper) and Tγ (suppressor) cells has led to contradictory data from different laboratories.[8–11] According to a study by Reinherz et al.[12] there appears to be little functional correlation between Tμ and Tγ cells and those populations identified by monoclonal antibodies. They suggest these cells may be of monomyeloid rather than T cell lineage.

The results of these experiments illustrate only too well the difficulties encountered in trying to identify subpopulations of T cells. Reproducible results between different laboratories have not been achieved mainly due to the limitations and nature of the techniques. Thus, efforts have continued to develop antibodies that will identify antigenic markers on T cells. The monoclonal method has overcome many of the limitations of the earlier techniques.

2. Naturally Occurring Antilymphocyte Antibodies in Disease

In 1973, Huang and Hong[13] showed that during certain viral infections a transient lymphopenia was observed in patients. Infections with influenza A and B, adenovirus, varicella, herpes simplex, measles, and rubella could produce a severe lymphopenia. The patients' sera contained an IgM antilymphocyte antibody.

Systemic lupus erythematosus (SLE) is a multisystem disease in which there are various autoantibodies suggesting overactive B cells. Previous investigations have attempted to show that the pathological defect reflects inactive or absent suppressor T lymphocyte control of B cells. Using a concanavalin A (Con A) stimulation system to generate suppressor cells, a decreased suppressor response has been demonstrated.[14] More recently it has been suggested that an autoantibody to suppressor T cells shown to be present in the serum of SLE patients is responsible for their dysfunction. Although the mechanism(s) causing the production of such an antibody are unknown, it is postulated that genetic factors combined with viral infection may alter receptors on the suppressor cell subpopulation to permit the formation of antisuppressor antibody.[15]

Another group of antibodies termed cold agglutinins and directed against I and i antigens react in a cytotoxity test with red blood cells at temperatures below 37° C. Using enzymatically treated erythrocytes, new antigenic determinants have been found and now designated Pr_1, Pr_2, Pr_3, and Gd. These antigens have been shown to be present on human peripheral blood, tonsil, and thymus lymphocytes, polymorphonuclear leukocytes, and monocytes.[16]

The search for functional populations of lymphocytes has also made use of a "naturally occurring" antibody present in the serum of patients with active juvenile rheumatoid arthritis (JRA).[17,18] This antibody reacted with 30% of peripheral human T cells (JRA^+) but not with B cells. The JRA^+ T cells reacted poorly in response to allogeneic cells, responded to Con A but not to phytohemagglutinin (PHA) and also did not help in the synthesis and secretion of immunoglobulin by B cells. In contrast, the JRA^- T cells respond to allogeneic cells, proliferate in response to PHA but not Con A and also greatly enhance the secretion of immunoglobulins by B cells. In a comparative study to determine similarities between the serum from JRA patients and heteroantibody TH_2, approximately 40 to 45% of the TH_2^- subset was shown to be JRA^+, whereas less than 5% of the TH_2^+ subset was JRA^+. It was concluded that the TH_2^+ and JRA^+ T cell subsets define different T cell populations.[19]

3. *Nonmonoclonal Heteroantibodies to Lymphocytes*

Many different antigenic sources and preparations have been used for raising heteroantibodies. Some of these have included normal human peripheral blood lymphocytes, T enriched lymphocytes, B enriched lymphocytes, null cells, thymocytes, tonsil cells, and splenocytes. Owing to the difficulty in obtaining specific heteroantibodies, conventional biochemical methods have been used to purify antigens before injection. Although enrichment of antigens has occurred, there is little evidence that surface membrane constituents have been purified to homogeneity.

Abnormal cells have also been used which have included leukemias of both B and T cells, and nonleukemic diseases such as SLE.

Roberts and Greaves[20] produced an antibody to human thymocytes that detected an antigen(s) shared by thymocytes, T cell acute lymphatic leukemia (T-ALL), activated peripheral T cells, and a subset of peripheral T cells. With this reaction pattern against different cell populations, this antibody appears to detcct antigen expressed at different maturational stages. Another antibody produced, by Andersson et al.[21], again to thymocytes, identified membrane glycoproteins which carry T cell specific antigens on human T lymphocytes and thymocytes. After polyacrylamide gel electrophoresis (PAGE) of T lymphocytes, or thymocytes, precipitation with the antibodies identified four proteins with molecular weights (mol wt) of 200,000, 180,000, 165,000, and 160,000. The 200,000 and 180,000 proteins were not present on high-density cortical thymocytes. Antibody to mouse Thy-1 antigen was also tested on the PAGE preparations of cells and it was found that a human equivalent of the Thy-1 antigen with the same molecular weight was precipitated by the anti-Thy-1. Another antiserum to human thymocytes recently developed by Foon et al.[22] was evaluated as an anti-T cell specific antibody with cytotoxic properties. The antibody was not cytotoxic to myeloid progenitor cells and therefore has potential for in vitro treatment of allogeneic bone marrow to prevent human graft-vs.-host disease (GvHD) following bone marrow transplantation.

One of the first antibodies identifying a functional population of human lymphocytes was produced against human lymphocytes.[23] The antiserum identified a subpopulation of human T cells termed TH_2^+. This subset of cells was shown to contain the cytotoxic effectors in cell-mediated lympholysis, as well as the immunoregulatory suppressor cell of T and B cell function.

The findings mentioned above illustrate important aspects of the differentiation and function of lymphocytes in various diseases and the complex structure and composition of lymphocytes. Molecular antigens expressed on lymphocytes appear to be closely related to disease processes. There are subpopulations of lymphocytes identified by distinct antigens or quantitative differences in the amount of certain antigens. Although a number of hetero- and naturally occurring antibodies have helped in identifying these cells, complexity of both the lymphocyte membrane and of the humoral immune responses to it has limited progress.

C. Human Lymphocyte Classes Defined by Monoclonal Antibodies

As shown in Table 1, many monoclonal antibodies identifying lymphocyte antigens have already been produced. Most of these are useful in identifying population marker antigens, and will eventually help in classifying populations of cells. Some have potential as therapeutic agents. As with the heteroantibodies many different lymphoid preparations have been used as antigens. The monoclonal antibodies produced, identify three broad but overlapping classes of cells. These are cells with T cell ontogeny and functional markers, B cell markers, and leukemic antigen markers. Antibodies to the

Table 1
A summary of the reactivity against a variety of cell types of many of the monoclonal antisera described in the text

	Monoclonal antibody											
Target cells	**Ta**	**3A1**	**T1**	**T3**	**T4**	**T5**	**T6**	**T8**	**T9**	**T10**	**OKI1**	**Q5/13**
Peripheral blood mononuclear cells	24*	41	100	100							5	
Peripheral T cells	33	68	100	>95	57	30	—	30	—	5		—
Thymocytes			10	10	80	80	70	80	<10	95		
Peripheral B cells	—		—	±	±	—					+	+
Monocytes	—	—	—			—					+	
T leukemias		+										
Null ALL												
CLL												
T cell lines	+	+	+	±, —	—	+, —	+		+	+		—
B cell lines	+	—	+, —	—	—							+

Key: * = % reactivity, + = reacts with (up to 100%), — = not reactive with, ± = low or background levels reacting, +, — = reacts with some but not all of this type, and blank = no data available.

histocompatibility HLA molecules will only be mentioned briefly as this topic is discussed elsewhere in this volume.

1. Antibodies to T Cells

Monoclonal antibodies defining lymphocyte maturation antigens as well as functional subpopulations have been developed by various research groups. The antibody anti-Ta discriminated between B and T lymphocytes and even between peripheral T lymphocyte subpopulations.[24] This specificity did not extend to cultured lymphoid cell lines where both B and T cells reacted. Enrichment for Ta^{+}T cells accounted for 30 to 35% of peripheral blood (PB) T cells. These cells responded well to Con A, PHA, pokeweed mitogen (PWM), and allogeneic stimulation. Although the Ta^{-} population is responsive to allogeneic, PHA and PWM stimulation, it is refractory to Con A stimulation.

The antibody 3A1 indentifies a trypsin-sensitive antigen on PB T cells which did not block sheep E-rosette formation, and did not block the detection of IgG or IgM Fc receptors or complement receptors.[26–28] $3A1^{+}$ cells were Con A and PHA responsive as well as helping B cell response to PWM and of intracytoplasmic production of Ig. $3A1^{-}$ cells suppressed B cell Ig synthesis in vitro. It is possible that Ta cells are a subset of the $3A1^{+}$T cells, but comparisons are difficult because parallel experiments have not been performed.

Reinherz et al.[12] have developed a panel of antibodies which have identified functional subpopulations of T cells and a possible T cell differentiation pathway.

Antibodies recognizing cells with functional properties are the OKT (i.e., T) series of antibodies. Antibodies anti-T4 and anti-T5 recognize subpopulations of human T lymphocytes now classed as helper and suppressor/cytotoxic cells, respectively. The two populations are distinct with no overlap.

The $T4^{+}$T cell population provides help for B cell Ig production and is also required for generation of $T5^{+}$ cytotoxic effector cells. The $T4^{+}$ population responds in mixed lymphocyte culture (MLC), and to Con A, PHA, and soluble antigens.[29–32]

$T5^{+}$T cells are responsible for cytotoxic effector functions as well as suppression of

Table 1 (continued)
A summary of the reactivity against a vareity of cell types of many of the monoclonal antisera described in the text

Monoclonal antibody														
FMC1	FMC3	FMC4	W6/32	N16, N24a, N26	TA-1	F10-89-4	F10-44-2	12E7	NA1/34	J5	A50	T101	Leu-1	Ab89
14	66	18	+	+	75	99	95	±	±	—		77		
	80	±		+	100	+		+	±	—	80	100	90	—
			+		67	100	29		85		47	+	>95	
+	50	+			10	+				—		—	—	—
—	100	100	+		100	100				—		—		—
—	+	±, —			+, —					—	—	+		—
±	+	+			—					+				—
	+	+			—	+				—	+, —	+, —	+, —	+, —
—	+, —	—	+	+	+, ±				+			+		
+	+, —	+	+	+					±			—	—	

both T and B cell function.[33] This subpopulation is equivalent to the heteroantibody TH_2^+ cells discussed earlier. The $T5^+$ population also responds well in MLC reaction and to Con A while response to PHA is lower than for $T4^+$. The $T4^+$ population may be a subset of the $3A1^+$ cells discussed previously.

Other antibodies developed by this group which include anti-T10, anti-T9, anti-T8 (equivalent to anti-T5), anti-T6, anti-T3, and anti-T1 have allowed for apparent definition of distinct intrathymic stages of T cell differentiation.[34–36]

Anti-T9 and anti-T10 antibodies define the earliest lymphoid cells because these cells share some antigens with bone-marrow cells, but are absent on mature T cells. In the first stage there is apparent loss of antigen T9, but detection of new antigens by antibodies T3, T4, T5, and T6 is possible. It was shown in a previous study that antibody T1 defines a mature T cell differentiation antigen. The $T1^+$ cells are MLC responsive, however, neither $T1^+$ or $T1^-$ are responsive to Con A or PHA.[37] Antibody T3 has a similar staining pattern to anti-T1 but varies when testing against T cell lines.

The next stage involves differentiation of this thymocyte population into two functionally distinct populations identified by the antibodies T4 and T5.

The $T4^+$ population is identified by antibodies T10, T1, T3, and T4, thus losing antigens T5 and T6 while gaining antigen T1 and T3. The $T5^+$ population is identified by antibodies T10, T1, T3, and T5, thus losing antigens T4 and T6 while gaining antigens T1 and T3. These differentiation stages take place within the thymus. The two major ''functional'' populations of thymocytes are exported to the peripheral lymphoid compartment, and antigen T10 is lost. These cells now represent the mature circulating helper and cytotoxic/suppressor populations, respectively. (Figure 2).

Studies on the lymphocyte membrane antigens recognized by antibodies T4 and T5 have attempted to define these molecules biochemically. The antigen on human thymocytes or peripheral T cells identified by T4 was shown after immunoprecipitation and sodium dodecyl sulfate polyacrylamide gel electrophoresis (SDS-PAGE), to be a single glycoprotein of 62,000 mol wt. The antigen identified by anti-T5 is a glycoprotein complex of apparently 76,000 mol wt, under reducing conditions, subunits of 30,000 and 32,000 mol wt are detected.

The murine thymocyte antigen Lyt-1.1 has a molecular weight of between 67,000 and 87,000 depending on the assay used; thus, both human and murine helper cells have an antigen of comparable molecular weight. Lyt-2 and Lyt-3 antigens present on murine suppressor cells have a molecular weight of 35,000 as detected by an alloantiserum. A monoclonal rat antibody precipitated a complex of two proteins of 30,000 and 35,000 mol wt under reducing conditions. Under nonreducing conditions a single glycoprotein of 65,000 was detected. These molecular sizes are in the range of those recognized by anti-T5 antibody; thus, the Lyt-1 and Lyt-2, 3 cells in the mouse not only have an analogous function to the human $T4^+$ and $T5^+$ populations but also have similar molecular and biochemical properties.[38]

2. *Antibodies to B Cells*

The data at present indicate that a major antigenic marker present on B cells is the human equivalent of the mouse Ia antigen; however, it is also present on monocytes, a subset of null cells and on activated T cells.[39] This set of histocompatibility antigens has a two chain structure composed of noncovalently associated glycoproteins. The smaller chain, which displays extensive structural polymorphism and carries the serologically defined allospecificities, has an apparent molecular weight of 28,000 to 32,000, whereas the larger chain has a molecular weight of 34,000. In the human these antigens are designated HLA-DRw.

Monoclonal antibodies have been produced against these human Ia-like molecules and include antibody OKI1 which defines the invariant region of the Ia-like molecule in man.[40] The antibodies Q2/47, Q2/61, Q2/70, Q2/80 recognize framework determinants of the Ia-like antigens. Q1/28 reacts with determinants expressed on the heavy chain of HLA-A and B antigens.[41] Another antibody Q5/13 reacts with a subset of human Ia-like antigens which is probably an HLA-DR allospecificity.[42] The antibody FMC4 also identifies the Ia molecule.[43]

In the authors' laboratory, a number of monoclonal antibodies have been raised against malignant cells from a patient with CLL and another patient with null ALL. Of these antibodies, 2G12 and 1G5 derived from each cell type, respectively, two have demonstrated a similar staining pattern by indirect immunofluorescence on the target cells tested. There was no reactivity with normal peripheral mononuclear cells, thymocytes, tonsil cells, neutrophils, or the T cell line CEM. There was reactivity with the non T, non B cell line NALM-1, and the DAUDI lymphoblastoid cell line which lacks HLA antigens and β_2-microglobulin; however three of five lymphoblastoid cell lines reacted with these antisera though the reaction of individual lines to each was identical. This suggests that an identical antigen was present on both CLL and ALL cells and an antigen commonly, but not invariably present on B lymphoblastoid cell lines.

An antibody which appears specific for B cells is FMC1. This B cell marker is distinct from sIg^+, Fc receptor, C3b receptor, mouse E-rosette receptor, and Ia antigens.[44] Such an antibody may overcome problems in enumerating B cells because of poor anti-immunoglobulin reagents, technical problems encountered in rosetting assays, and the presence of Fc, C3 receptors, and Ia antigens on cells other than B cells.

3. *Other Monoclonal Antilymphocyte Antibodies Against Normal Tissues*

β_2-microglobulin—Many antibodies reacting with HLA and β_2-m have been produced. Antibody W6/32 is against a determinant common to most, if not all of the 43,000 mol wt chain of the HLA-A, B, and C antigens.[45] This was determined using somatic cell genetics and immunoprecipitation techniques. Antibodies N16, N24a, and N26 identify the β_2-m chain which is associated with HLA antigens.[46]

Cross population antibodies—Two monoclonal antibodies have shown an unusual reaction pattern. FMC3 detects an antigenic determinant present on most T cells, B cells, and myeloid leukemias. While T cells and myeloid leukemias are distantly related, this antibody identifies 80% of T cells.[47] Antibody TA-1 detects an antigen present at some stage of intrathymic differentiation which is still present on peripheral T lymphocytes and cells of monocyte-macrophage lineage. It could distinguish acute myelomonocytic leukemia (AMML) cells from acute myelocytic leukemia cells (AML).[48] Although not identical, the staining pattern of these antibodies is similar.

Antibodies to antigenic sites in common with other tissues—The monoclonal antibody F10-89-4 identifies a human leukocyte-specific membrane glycoprotein of 190,000 to 215,000 mol wt which is probably homologous to the leukocyte-common (L-C) antigen of the rat, which is present on all T lymphocytes, B lymphocytes, thymocytes, granulocytes, and monocytes, but absent from other tissues.[49] Another antibody F10-44-2 identifying a glycoprotein of 105,000 mol wt on human brain, granulocytes, and T lymphocytes is probably homologous to the W3/13 antigen of the rat.[50]

4. Leukemic Cell Markers Identified by Monoclonal Antibody

Monoclonal antibody 12E7 detects a 28,000 mol wt antigen present on ALL cells and on a population of normal cells found in the cortex of the thymus. The tissue distribution is reminiscent of the mouse 45,000 dalton TL antigen associated on the cell surface with β_2-m. By contrast the antigen defined by 12E7 is not associated with β_2-m.[51]

The antibody NA1/34-HLK recognizes a 45,000 mol wt antigen expressed on thymocytes and the T-ALL cell line MOLT-4.[52] In the thymus, 85% of the cells were stained, and these cells expressed little or no HLA-A, B, or C antigens as recognized by the monoclonal antibody W6/32. The antibody did not precipitate β_2-m. A comparative study may show a similarity between these antibodies.

A monoclonal J5 specific for common (non T-non B) ALL has been developed by Ritz et al.[53,54] This antibody does not bind to T ALL or other leukemias with the exception of chronic myeloid leukemia in blast crisis.

Antibody A50 recognizes PB T cells as well as B-CLL and other T cell leukemias.[55] Antibody T101, precipitates a 65,000 mol wt protein found on immature and mature normal T cells, T cell lines, and T cells from acute leukemia and lymphomas.[56] Although this antibody did not react with B cell lines, B cell lymphomas, or B cells with surface immunoglobulin, it precipitated an antigen present on sIg^+ CLL cells; thus, there are apparently two major subtypes of chronic lymphocytic leukemia CLL (sIg^+, $T101^+$, and sIg^-, $T101^-$). This study supports the hypothesis that the leukemic cells in sIg^+ CLL, despite their mature appearance, are functionally immature and appear to be arrested at a very early stage of lymphocyte differentiation sharing an antigen common to both B and T cells.

The antibody Leu-1 recognizes an antigen complex of 69,000 and 71,000 mol wt shared by T cells and cells from patients with CLL but not detectable on normal B cells and B cell lines.[57] In the mouse, such an antigen is exemplified by the G_{IX} system because its distribution on normal lymphoid cells is restricted to thymus dependent lymphocytes of certain strains, but it is found on both thymic and nonthymic leukemias of G_{IX}^+ and G_{IX}^- strains. It is also notable that G_{IX} is associated with a membrane complex of 69,000 and 71,000 mol wt and that this complex shares biochemical and antigenic properties with the major glycoprotein component of the murine leukemia virus envelope. Investigations of a relationship between the human p69, 71 complex and the murine G_{IX} system are continuing.

It is also possible that antibodies Leu-1 and T101 recognize the same antigen, based on the data that both T cells, B CLL but not B cells or B cell lines are recognized. Also, T101 recognizes a 65,000 mol wt protein in the range of the p69, 71 complex.

Antibody Ab89 supports the notion that there is a greater heterogeneity of B cell lymphomas than was previously believed.[58] Groups of patients with lymphomas reactive with Ab89 did not coincide with histopathologic classification systems. The antibody raised against a poorly differentiated B cell lymphocytic lymphoma was specific for these cells. It did not show any activity with normal leukocytes but only with B cell lymphomas and B CLL. Therefore, Ab89 probably recognizes an antigen unique to B cell lymphomas.

IV. CLINICAL APPLICATION OF MONOCLONAL ANTIBODIES

A. Lymphocyte Populations in Disease

The many different monoclonal antibodies already produced have proved extremely useful in the study of lymphocyte ontogeny and function in both health and disease. The diagnostic and therapeutic potential of monoclonals is exciting, particularly as heteroantibodies have proved disappointing.

Many studies are now proceeding to evaluate methods and techniques for using these antibodies. These include ascertaining lymphocyte populations present in different diseases, treatment of bone marrow to remove abnormal cells, or T cells responsible for causing graft-vs.-host reaction, the location of tumors, and the delivery of ''hot'' isotopes or other cytotoxins to malignancies for therapeutic purposes. It may also prove possible to manipulate the immune system in immunodeficient or hyperreactive states.

The OKT series of antibodies has been used to determine functional lymphocyte subpopulations in SLE and multiple sclerosis (MS). Reinherz et al.[59] found that anti-T-cell antibodies from patients with active SLE reacted with 80% of an enriched suppressor cell population ($T4^-$) from controls. This indicates the presence of antisuppressor cell antibodies in SLE. A similar study with patients with active MS demonstrated a selective decrease in the $T5^+$ (suppressor cell) population, although a smaller decrease was observed with the $T4^+$ (helper) population.[60] Thus, immunoregulatory T cells seem important in these diseases.

The potential clinical application of monoclonals to treat hematologic malignancies and the prevention of GvHD is being evaluated as new monoclonal antibodies are developed. The pan-T-cell-specific monoclonal antibody (T101) has complement dependent cytotoxic activity. This activity did not effect blood and bone marrow granulocyte, macrophage, and erythroid progenitors but was cytotoxic to T-colony-forming cells from blood and bone marrow. This antibody therefore may be used in the treatment of T cell malignancies and prevention of GvHD.

B. Diagnosis and Therapy of Malignancy

Following experiments in the mouse, monoclonal antibodies are now expected to open a new era in the diagnosis and treatment of malignancies in man. The tumor seeking radiopharmaceuticals currently available lack specifity. The tumor imaging occurs because of nonspecific secondary changes in neoplasms, i.e., altered microvascularity and blood flow and nonspecific trapping of labeled substances. In this and previous studies, the authors have used a I-heteroantibody to locate primary and/or metastatic tumors by radionuclide imaging. The trapping of this heteroantibody by reticuloendothetial cells in the liver, spleen, and lungs as well as impurity (<1% specific antibody) and the circulating antibody-antigen complexes limits its usefulness.[62]

More recent experiments using monoclonal antibody indicate that this problem will be overcome. A monoclonal antibody raised to murine teratocarcinomas, was labeled with ^{131}I. Another ^{125}I-labeled indifferent antibody of the same immunoglobulin class as the tumor-specific antibody was also injected into the mouse with a teratocarcinoma induced after subcutaneous injection of these cells. This allows for a similar metabolism of the antibodies except for the binding to the tumor. Following γ-ray scintigraphy, this double-isotope method allowed for subtraction of the nontumor specific antibody activity, although this was not required using the monoclonal antibody. Localization was accomplished with great accuracy.[63]

Bernstein et al.[64] produced a monoclonal antibody to Thy-1.1 antigen which was used in the therapy of a transplanted mouse leukemia. The leukemia (SL2) was an AKR mouse lymphoma which was derived from a spontaneous thymoma. Passive immunization with the monoclonal antibody resulted in high titer of cytotoxic antibody in the serum of treated mice and the suppression of metastatic tumor cells. Antibody with exogenous complement therapy resulted in the cure of the induced leukemia in a significant proporation of the treated animals.

V. CONCLUSION

The introduction of the hybridoma monoclonal antibody technique by Köhler and Milstein in 1975, has resulted in dramatic changes in immunology. Within immunology, the study of the lymphocyte surface membrane antigens has been revolutionized. Previous reliance on production of heteroantisera to identify lymphocyte populations has been virtually replaced by the hybridoma method.

Distinct functional populations of lymphocytes in the mouse identified by alloantisera have also been detected by monoclonal antibodies. Similar T cell populations in humans, have also been identified using monoclonal antibodies. A maturation pathway for T cells in the human thymus has been proposed.

The specificity of the different antibodies already produced have assisted in the classification of lymphoid subpopulations in several diseases. The future will almost certainly expand their diagnostic possibilities. Experiments in mice suggest that the use of monoclonal antibody may allow nonspecific diagnosis and therapy of malignancies.

Technology now available has also greatly facilitated the characterization of the lymphocyte populations to which the monoclonal antibody is directed. The cytofluorograph and the fluorescence activated cell sorter (FACS) have been invaluable in this regard.

The rapid advances made in producing monoclonal antibodies to lymphocyte antigens have also resulted in a number of problems. Nomenclature and cross characterization of antibodies produced by different laboratories are among such difficulties. To allow better cross characterization between laboratories, an identical series of cells and cell extracts need to be tested with a broad spectrum of antibodies. Thus the monoclonal antibody should be tested against a series of normal lymphocytes, normal lymphocyte subpopulations, lymphoid cell lines of various types, lymphoid malignancies, and extracts of some or all of these cells to characterize the antigen involved physicochemically.

What is required is the equivalent of the HLA workshops designed to evaluate new antilymphocyte antibodies and their reaction patterns. This will allow the direct comparison of one antibody with another. Useful antibodies to the various cell types can then be made available for experimental, diagnostic, and therapeutic use.

REFERENCES

1. **Singer, S. J. and Nicolson, G. L.,** The fluid mosaic model of the structure of cell membranes, *Science,* 175, 720, 1972.
2. **Raff, M. C.,** Surface antigenic markers for distinguishing T and B lymphocytes in mice, *Transplant. Rev.,* 6, 52, 1971.
3. **Cantor, H. and Boyse, E. A.,** Functional subclasses of T lymphocytes bearing different Ly antigens. I. The generation of functionally distinct T cell subclasses as a differentiative process independent of antigen, *J. Exp. Med.,* 141, 1376, 1975.
4. **Cantor, H. and Boyse, E. A.,** Functional subclasses of T lymphocytes bearing different Ly antigens. II. Cooperation between subclasses of Ly cells in the generation of killer activity, *J. Exp. Med.,* 141, 1390, 1975.
5. **Cantor, H., Shen, F. W., and Boyse, E. A.,** Separation of helper T cells from suppressor T cells expressing different Ly components. II. Activation by antigen: after immunization, specific suppressor and helper activities are mediated by distinct T cell subclasses, *J. Exp. Med.,* 143, 1391, 1976.
6. **Coombs, R. R. A., Gurner, B. W., Wilson, A. B., Holm, G., and Lindgren, B.,** Rosette formation between human lymphocytes and sheep red blood cells not involving Ig receptors, *Int. Arch. Allergy Appl. Immunol.,* 39, 658, 1970.
7. **Gupta, S. and Good, R. A.,** Markers of human lymphocyte subpopulations in primary immunodeficiency and lymphoproliferative disorders, *Semin. Hematol.,* 17, 1, 1980.
8. **Moretta, L., Mingari, M. C., Moretta, A., and Cooper, M. D.,** Human T lymphocyte subpopulations: studies of the mechanism by which T cells bearing Fc receptors for IgG suppress T-dependent B cell differentiation induced by pokeweed mitogen, *J. Immunol.,* 122, 984, 1979.
9. **Williams, R. C. and Strand-Montano, J. D.,** Subpopulations of T cells (Tγ and Tμ) in patients with chronic liver disease, *Clin. Immunol. Immunopathol.,* 15, 616, 1980.
10. **Durandy, A., Fischer, A., and Griscelli, C.,** Active suppression of B lymphocyte maturation by two different newborn T lymphocyte subsets, *J. Immunol.,* 123, 2644, 1979.
11. **Matsumoto, K., Osakabe, K., Ohi, H., Yoshizawa, N., Harada, M., and Hatano, M.,** Alteration of T-lymphocyte subpopulations in patients with primary renal diseases and systemic lupus erythematosus, *Scan. J. Immunol.,* 11, 187, 1980.
12. **Reinherz, E. L., Moretta, L., Roper, M., Breard, J. M., Mingari, M. C., Copper, M. D., and Schlossman, S. F.,** Human T lymphocyte subpopulations defined by Fc receptors and monoclonal antibodies, *J. Exp. Med.,* 151, 969, 1980.
13. **Huang, S. W. and Hong, R.,** Lymphopenia and multiple virus infections *JAMA,* 225, 1120, 1973.
14. **Bresnihan, B., and Jasin, H. E.,** Suppressor function of peripheral blood mononuclear cells in normal individuals and in patients with systemic lupus erythematosus, *J. Clin. Inves.,* 59, 106, 1977.
15. **Sagawa, A. and Abdou, N. I.,** Suppressor-cell antibody in systemic lupus erythematosus: possible mechanism for suppressor-cell dysfunction, *J. Clin. Invest.,* 63, 536, 1979.
16. **Pruzanski, W., Roelcke, D., Armstrong, M., and Manly, M. S.,** Pr and Gd antigens on human B and T lymphocytes and phagocytes, *Clin. Immunol. Immunopathol.,* 15, 631, 1980.
17. **Evans, R. L., Breard, J. M., Lazarus, H., Schlossman, S. F., and Chess, L.,** Detection, isolation, and functional characterization of two human T cell subclasses bearing unique differentiation antigens, *J. Exp. Med.,* 145, 221, 1977.
18. **Strelkauskas, A. J., Schauf, V., Wilson, B. S., Chess, L., and Schlossman, S. F.,** Isolation and characterization of naturally occurring subclasses of human peripheral blood T cells with regulatory functions, *J. Immunol.,* 120, 1278, 1978.
19. **Reinherz, E. L., Strelkauskas, A. J., O'Brien, C., and Schlossman, S. F.,** Phenotypic and functional distinctions between the TH_2^+ and JRA^+ T cell subsets in man, *J. Immunol,* 123, 83, 1979.
20. **Roberts, M. M. and Greaves, M. F.,** Restricted expression of a human T cell lineage membrane antigen, *Eur. J. Immunol.,* 10, 46, 1980.
21. **Andersson, L. C., Karhi, K. K., Gahmberg, C. G., and Radt, H.,** Molecular identification of T cell-specific antigens on human T lymphocytes and thymocytes, *Eur. J. Immunol.,* 10, 359, 1980.
22. **Foon, K. A., Fitchen, J. H., Billing, R. J., Belzer, M. B., Terasaki, P. I., and Cline, M. J.,** An antithymocyte serum noncytotoxic to myeloid progenitor cells. Candidate serum for prevention of graft-versus-host diseases in bone marrow transplantation, *Clin. Immunol. Immunopathol.,* 16, 416, 1980.
23. **Evans, R. L., Lazarus, A. C., Penta, S. F., and Schlossman, S. F.,** Two functionally distinct populations of human T cells that collaborate in the generation of cytotoxic cells responsible for cell mediated lympholysis, *J. Immunol.,* 120, 1423, 1978.
24. **Goldsby, R. A., Osborne, B. A., and Engleman, E. G.,** Identification isolation and characterization of a human T cell population by a monoclonal antibody, *Curr. Microbiol.,* 3, 141, 1979.

25. **Engleman, E. G., Benike, C., Osborne, B., and Goldsby, R.,** Functional characteristics of human T-cell subpopulations distinguished by a monoclonal antibody, *Proc. Natl. Acad. Sci. U.S.A.*, 77, 1607, 1980.
26. **Eisenbarth, G. S., Haynes, B. F., Schroer, J. A., and Fauci, A. S.,** Production of monoclonal antibodies reacting with peripheral blood mononuclear cell surface differentiation antigens, *J. Immunol.*, 124, 1237, 1980.
27. **Haynes, B. F., Eisenbarth, G. S., and Fauci, A. S.,** Human lymphocyte antigens: production of a monoclonal antibody that defines functional thymus-derived lymphocyte subsets, *Proc. Natl. Acad. Sci. U.S.A.*, 76, 5829, 1979.
28. **Haynes, B. F., Mann, D. L., Hemler, M. E., Schroer, J. A., Shelhamer, J. H., Eisenbarth, G. S., Strominger, J. L., Thomas, C. A., Mostowski, H. S., and Fauci, A. S.,** Characterization of a monoclonal antibody that defines an immunoregulatory T cell subset for immunoglobulin synthesis in humans, *Proc. Natl. Acad. Sci. U.S.A.*, 77, 2914, 1980.
29. **Kung, P. C., Goldstein, G., Reinherz, E. L., and Schlossman, S. F.,** Monoclonal antibodies defining distinctive human T cell surface antigens, *Science*, 206, 347, 1979.
30. **Reinherz, E. L., Kung, P. C., Goldstein, G., and Schlossman, S. F.,** Further characterization of the human inducer T cell subset defined by monoclonal antibody, *J. Immunol.*, 123, 2894, 1979.
31. **Reinherz, E. L., Kung, P. C., Breard, J. M., Goldstein, G., and Schlossman, S. F.,** T cell requirements for generation of helper factor(s) in man: analysis of the subsets involved, *J. Immunol.*, 124, 1883, 1980.
32. **Reinherz, E. L., Chikao, M., Penta, A. C., and Schlossman, S. F.,** Regulation of B cell immunoglobulin secretion by functional subsets of T lymphocytes in man, *Eur. J. Immunol.*, 10, 570, 1980.
33. **Reinherz, E. L., Kung, P. C., Goldstein, G., and Schlossman, S. F.,** A monoclonal antibody reactive with the human cytotoxic/suppressor T cell subset previously defined by a heteroantiserum termed TH_2 *J. Immunol.*, 124, 1301, 1980.
34. **Reinherz, E. L., Kung, P. C., Goldstein, G., Levy, R., and Schlossman, S. F.,** Discrete stages of human intrathymic differentiation; analysis of normal thymocytes and leukemic lymphoblasts of T-cell lineage, *Proc. Natl. Acad. Sci. U.S.A.*, 77, 1588, 1980.
35. **Reinherz, E. L. and Schlossman, S. F.,** The differentiation and function of human T lymphocytes, *Cell*, 19, 821, 1980.
36. **Reinherz, E. L. and Schlossman, S. F.,** Regulation of the immune response-inducer and suppressor T-lymphocyte subsets in human beings, *N. Engl. J. Med.*, 303, 370, 1980.
37. **Reinherz, E. L., Kung, P. C., Goldstein, G., and Schlossman, S. F.,** A monoclonal antibody with selective reactivity with functionally mature human thymocytes and all peripheral human T cells, *J. Immunol.*, 123, 1312, 1979.
38. **Terhost, C., Agthoven, A. van., Reinherz, E. L., and Schlossman, S. F.,** Biochemical analysis of human T lymphocyte differentiation antigens T4 and T5, *Science*, 209, 520, 1980.
39. **Fu, S. M., Chiorazzi, N., Wang, Y., Montazeri, G., Kunkel, H. G., Ko, H. S., and Gottlieb, A. B.,** Ia bearing T lymphocytes in man. Their identification and role in the generation of allogeneic helper activity, *J. Exp. Med.*, 148, 1423, 1978.
40. **Reinherz, E. L., Kung, P. C., Pesando, J. M., Ritz, J., Goldstein, G., and Schlossman, S. F.,** Ia determinants on human T-cell subsets defined by monoclonal antibody: activation stimuli required for expression, *J. Exp. Med.*, 150, 1472, 1979.
41. **Fitchen, J. H., Ferrone, S., Quaranta, V., Molinaro, G. A., and Cline, M. J.,** Monoclonal antibodies to HAL-A, B and IA-like antigens inhibit colony formation by human myeloid progenitor cells, *J. Immunol.*, 125, 2004, 1980.
42. **Quaranto, V., Walker, L. E., Pellegrino, M. A., and Ferrone, S.,** Purification of immunologically functional subsets of human Ia-like antigens on a monoclonal antibody (Q5/13) immunoadsorbent, *J. Immunol.*, 125, 1421, 1980.
43. **Beckman, I. G., Bradley, J., Brooks, D. A., Kupa, A., McNamara, P. J., Thomas, M., and Zola, H.,** Human lymphocyte markers defined by antibodies derived from somatic cell hybrids. II. A hybridoma secreting antibody against an antigen expressed by human B and null lymphocytes, *Clin. Exp. Immunol.*, 40, 1, 1980.
44. **Brooks, D. A., Beckman, I., Bradley, J., McNamara, P. J., Thomas, M. E., and Zola, H.,** Human lymphocyte markers defined by antibodies derived from somatic cell hybrids. I. A hybridoma secreting antibody against a marker specific for human B lymphocytes, *Clin. Exp. Immunol.*, 39, 477, 1980.
45. **Barnstable, G., Bodmer, W. F., Brown, G., Galfre, G., Milstein, C., Williams, A. F., and Ziegler, A.,** Production of monoclonal antibodies to group A erythrocytes, HLA and other human cell surface antigens—new tools for genetic analysis, *Cell*, 14, 7, 1978.

46. **Trucco, M. M., Stocker, J. W., and Ceppellini, R.,** Monoclonal antibodies against human lymphocyte antigens, *Nature (London),* 273, 666, 1978.
47. **Zola, H., Beckman, I. G., Bradley, J., Brooks, D. A., Kupa, A., McNamara, P. J., Smart, I. J., and Thomas, M. E.,** Human lymphocyte markers defined by antibodies derived from somatic cell hybrids. III. A marker defining a subpopulation of lymphocytes which cuts across the normal T-B-null classification, *Immunology,* 40, 143, 1980.
48. **Le Bien, T. W. and Kersey, J. H.,** A monoclonal antibody (TA-1) reactive with human T lymphocytes and monocytes, *J. Immunol.,* 125, 2208, 1980.
49. **Dalchau, R., Kirkley, J., and Fabre, J. W.,** Monoclonal antibody to a human leukocyte-specific membrane glycoprotein probably homologous to the leukocyte-common (L-C) antigen of the rat, *Eur. J. Immunol.,* 10, 737, 1980.
50. **Dalchau, R., Kirkley, J., and Fabre, J. W.,** Monoclonal antibody to a human brain-granulocyte-T lymphocyte antigen probably homologous to the W3/13 antigen of the rat, *Eur. J. Immunol.,* 10, 745, 1980.
51. **Levy, R., Dilley, J., Fox, R. I., and Warnke, R.,** A human thymus-leukemia antigen defined by hybridoma monoclonal antibodies, *Proc. Natl. Acad. Sci. U.S.A.,* 76, 6552, 1979.
52. **McMichael, A. J., Pilch, J. R., Galfre, G., Mason, D. Y., Fabre, J. W., and Milstein, C.,** A human thymocyte antigen defined by a hybrid myeloma monoclonal antibody, *Eur. J. Immunol.,* 9, 205, 1979.
53. **Ritz, J., Pesando, J. M., Notis-McConarty, J., Lazarus, H., and Schlossman, S. F.,** A monoclonal antibody to human acute lymphoblastic leukemia antigen, *Nature (London),* 283, 583, 1980.
54. **Ritz, J., Pesando, J. M., Notis-McConarty, J., and Schlossman, S. F.,** Modulation of human acute lymphoblastic leukemia antigen induced by monoclonal antibody *in vitro, J. Immunol.,* 125, 1506, 1980.
55. **Boumsell, L., Coppin, H., Pham, D., Raynol, B., Lemerle, J., Dausset, J., and Bernard, A.,** An antigen shared by a human T cell subset and B cell chronic lymphocytic leukemic cells, *J. Exp. Med.,* 152, 229. 1980.
56. **Royston, I., Majda, J. A., Baird, S. M., Meserve, B. L., and Griffiths, J. C.,** Human T cell antigens defined by monoclonal antibodies: the 65,000-Dalton antigen of T cells (T65) is also found on chronic lymphocytic leukemia cells bearing surface immunoglobulin, *J. Immunol.,* 125, 725, 1980.
57. **Wang, C. Y., Good, R. A., Ammirati, P., Dymbort, G., and Evans, R. L.,** Identification of a p69,71 complex expressed on human T cells sharing determinants with B-type chronic lymphatic leukemic cells, *J. Exp. Med.,* 151, 1539, 1980.
58. **Nadler, L. M., Stashenko, P., Hardy, R., and Schlossman, S. F.,** A monoclonal antibody defining a lymphoma associated antigen in man, *J. Immunol.,* 125, 570, 1980.
59. **Morimoto, C., Reinherz, E. L., Abe, T., Homma, M., and Schlossman, S. F.,** Characteristics of anti-T-cell antibodies in systemic lupus erythematosus: evidence for selective reactivity with normal suppressor cells defined by monoclonal antibodies, *Clin. Immunol. Immunopathol.,* 16, 474, 1980.
60. **Reinherz, E. L., Weiner, H. L., Hauser, S. L., Cohen, J. A., Distaso, J. A., and Schlossman, S. F.,** Loss of suppressor T cells in active multiple sclerosis. Analysis with monoclonal antibodies, *N. Engl. J. Med.,* 303, 125, 1980.
61. **Taetle, R. and Royston, I.,** Human T-cell antigens defined by monoclonal antibodies. Absence of T65 on committed myeloid and erythroid progenitors, *Blood,* 56, 943, 1980.
62. **Belitsky, P., Ghose, T., Aquino, J., Tai, J., and MacDonald, A. S.,** Radionuclide imagining in metastases from renal-cell carcinoma by ^{131}I-labelled antitumor antibody, *Radiology,* 126, 515, 1978.
63. **Ballou, B., Levine, G., Hakala, T. R., and Solter, D.,** Tumor location detected with radioactively labelled monoclonal antibody and external scintigraphy, *Science,* 206, 844, 1979.
64. **Bernstein, I. D., Tam, M. R., and Nowinski, R. C.,** Mouse leukemia: therapy with monoclonal antibodies against a thymus differentiation antigen, *Science,* 207, 68, 1980.

Chapter 11

MONOCLONAL ANTIBODIES TO THE MAJOR HISTOCOMPATABILITY ANTIGENS

Rosemary L. Betts and Ian F. C. McKenzie

TABLE OF CONTENTS

I. INTRODUCTION

In this review monoclonal antibodies reacting with histocompatibility antigens will be described and discussion will concentrate on those species against which the majority of antibodies have been produced (i.e., mouse, rat, man, and chicken). Thus monoclonal antibodies against antigens of wide distribution (e.g., H-2 K, D, L; HLA-A,-B,-C) will be described as well as those of restricted distribution (e.g., Ia, DR)—the criterion for inclusion in this review is that the gene coding for the determinant map within the major histocompatibility complex (MHC) of the species.

It is clear that monoclonal antibodies can be produced to the antigens of the MHC. This fact is evidenced by the extensive literature (to be reviewed herein) describing murine alloantibodies and xenoantibodies to the MHC of several species.[1–3] These appear to be produced with ease, but at this time it is premature to draw conclusions on their precise role in the analysis of the MHC and how informative they will be in comparison to conventionally produced alloantisera.

Monoclonal antisera certainly have many advantages (Table 1), such as the provision of unlimited volumes of high titered antibody of the same specificity, affinity and class, and freedom from contaminating antibodies either to other specificities, viruses, or autoantibodies. However, there are also a number of disadvantages, such as the noncytotoxicity of some antibodies, low affinity, and the problem of cross-reactivity (to be discussed below). These first two disadvantages can be overcome simply by discarding the line or fusing until the appropriate immunoglobulin class and antibody affinity emerge. Further disadvantages of monoclonal xenoantisera include the difficulty in producing the desired antibody (see below) and determining the relationship of the specificities detected to those defined by conventional alloantisera. In addition, monoclonal xenoantisera may be used in the future for in vivo diagnosis and treatment of disease in man and the longterm use of mouse protein in man may give rise to serum sickness. It is to be expected that these disadvantages will ultimately be overcome by producing only alloantisera, for example by employing human-human cell fusions. At present, the advantages of using monoclonal antisera, especially alloantisera (to mouse H-2 and Ia antigens) so far outweighs the disadvantages that production of antisera by the cell fusion method is now the method of choice and, if available, monoclonal antisera to H-2 and Ia antigens should be used in preference to conventional reagents. It will be

Table 1
ADVANTAGES AND DISADVANTAGES OF THE USE OF MONOCLONAL REAGENTS FOR THE ANALYSIS OF THE MHC

Advantages	Possible disadvantages
I. Alloantisera (e.g., mouse anti-H-2, Ia antibodies)	
Reaction with a single determinant	Noncytotoxicity
	Low affinity
No contamination with other antibodies	Cross-reactions
	pH and temperature dependence
Unlimited volumes	
High titer	
Same Ig class	
Same affinity	
II. Xenoantisera (e.g., mouse anti-HLA)	
Same as above	Same as above
	? all polymorphic determinants recognized
	Preponderance of monomorphic anti-HLA, β2-M antibodies
	? relationship to alloantibody
	Foreign protein (in vivo use)

noted that more information is provided on HLA/DR specificities than on H-2 and Ia and the reason for this is that the H-2 and Ia antibodies have largely confirmed existing data, whereas monoclonal HLA and DR antisera, are xenoantisera and provide a series of new reagents requiring greater characterization.

II. REACTIONS OF MONOCLONAL ALLOANTISERA AND XENOANTISERA

The use of monoclonal antisera for the analysis of cell membrane antigens has many advantages over the use of alloantisera or xenoantisera produced by the usual immunization procedures (Table 1). However, the differences between monoclonal antibodies and conventional antisera may lead to difficulties in interpretation and some of the potential problems and difficulties will be outlined here; it is also worth drawing attention to two monographs on the interpretation of serological data.[4,5]

A. Comparison of Monoclonal Alloantisera with Conventional Alloantisera

This comparison mainly refers to the H-2 and Ia alloantibodies since they are the most widely produced monoclonal alloantibodies. This first point to note is that monoclonal antibodies are directed to the same specificity (determinant) and consist of antibody molecules of identical isotype, affinity, and lability. By contrast, alloantisera are usually produced by pooling sera obtained from many mice and consist of a range of antibodies with varying specificity, isotype, and affinity. Furthermore, each immunized mouse may have a different array of antibodies each time it is bled, adding further to the list of variables.[6] In spite of all these variables, a workable system defining the H-2 and Ia antigens has emerged, although over the years there have been specificities defined which cannot easily be reproduced (e.g., H-2.22, Ia-6).

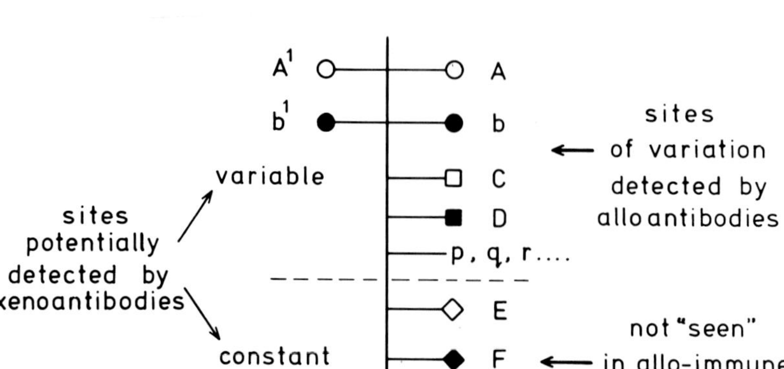

FIGURE 1. Conceptual diagram of MHC divided (for convenience only) into constant and variable regions. A, b, C, D = different alloantigenic determinants. E, F, G . . . determinants present in the "constant" region. A^1, b^1 = same molecules as A, b . . . but possibly seen differently in a xenogeneic immunization. (Note that the diagram is drawn thus only for discussion; there is no evidence for separate constant and variable regions as shown; they could well be the same sequences.)

Some attempts have been made to align the specificities detected by monoclonal antibodies with those detected by conventional antisera.[7–9] In other studies, a different nomenclature has been suggested for monoclonal antibodies.[9] The first approach of assigning the specificities detected by monoclonal antisera with existing numbers if they are found to be similar to conventional antisera is, in the long term likely to lead to further difficulties. For example, a molecule may bear a series of determinants, such as A, b, C, D . . . p, q, r in Figure 1. By conventional immunization, A, C, D are always detected, b is sometimes detected, and p, q, r are never detected because the antibody titers to these are too low and they escape detection. With monoclonal antibodies it is possible to obtain high titers to all these specificities (A, b, C, D . . . p, q, r) particularly if the antibody producing hybridomas are grown in vivo. For this reason monoclonal antibodies defining specificities previously undetected may emerge with titers in the order of 1: 5×10^6. In the future, when a sufficiently large panel of antisera is available, it is likely that H-2 and Ia specificities will be defined by only monoclonal antisera and these will become the standards, rather than conventional antisera. An advantage of this form of standardization is that large batches of identical antibodies can be assembled and distributed for world-wide use.

B. Comparison of Monoclonal Xenoantisera with Conventional Alloantisera

Several problems have emerged here and some disappointment expressed that mouse monoclonal antibodies have rarely recognized identical determinants to those found by alloimmunization. For example, there are few mouse anti-HLA monoclonal antibodies that recognize known polymorphic HLA specificities. There are several explanations for this—illustrated in Figure 1. For convenience, the molecule (e.g., HLA-A) has been divided into a constant and variable region, although at present there is no evidence to suggest that such a structure exists. "Monomorphic" antibodies can be produced which recognize the same determinants in all individuals (i.e., EFC in Figure 1). Whether these are distinct determinants on the "constant" portion of the molecule is not clear at present. These antibodies to monomorphic determinants could in fact recognize common features of the polymorphic determinants (A, b, C) which are not recognized in alloimmunizations. Two other variables may also occur. First, the mouse may recognize the same determinants as found in an alloimmunization or secondly, the mouse could "see" these same determinants in a different way so that determinant A could be seen as A^1 by the mouse. There are then, four possibilities for specificities to be detected by monoclonal xenoantibodies:

1. Monomorphic determinant—the common part of the MHC molecule and not recognized in alloimmunization (e.g., EFG of Figure 1).
2. Polymorphic determinant—identical to that recognized by conventional antisera (e.g., A of Figure 1).
3. Polymorphic determinant—similar to, but slightly different to that in (2) (e.g., A^1 of Figure 1).
4. A "new" determinant not usually detected by conventional antibody because the response is too weak (e.g., p, q, r of Figure 1).

The possibility also exists that the mouse in xenoimmunization may never recognize a determinant that is "seen" as different by two individuals in alloimmunization (i.e., there may be some HLA specificities that mice will never recognize). This is not unlikely, but it is premature to make this conclusion. Furthermore, mice may recognize limited polymorphisms and produce antibodies to the so-called "supertypic" determinants which are common to several specificities (e.g., the antibody, Genox 3.53[1] which reacts with the HLA-DR1, DR2, and DRw6 specificities). Thus, the use of monoclonal antisera has simplified the analysis of alloantigenic systems such as the mouse H-2 and Ia specificities. However, at present, these antibodies appear to complicate the analysis of other systems, such as HLA-DR, but with greater production, study, and improved technology (e.g., human-human fusions) all monoclonal antisera should be superior to conventional antisera.

III. NOMENCLATURE

At present there is no widely accepted nomenclature for separately identifying monoclonal antibodies and their relationship to the defined specificities. For the murine H-2 and Ia specificities, Klein and colleagues[9] have suggested that monoclonal antibodies be named in order of description (e.g., H-2m1, H-2m2; Ia-m1, Ia-m2). In this case H-2m1 is not related to the H-2.1 specificity defined by conventional alloantisera. In other systems, the "m" prefix has been used to demonstrate a monoclonal antibody of the same specificity as the conventional antiserum (e.g., Ly-m6.2[10]). Either nomenclature is suitable but to our mind, monoclonal alloantisera will eventually replace conventional antisera for the definition of unique specificities and therefore, will require an entirely new nomenclature. No nomenclature exists for monoclonal xenoantisera. However, the widespread use of terms such as "monomorphic", "polymorphic", and "supertypic" should be noted. In this context, monomorphic refers to a specificity present in all members of the species and should not be confused with "monospecific" (a term used operationally to define the restricted reactions of a conventional alloantisera; all monoclonal antibodies are monospecific, but like all antibodies, they may show variable degrees of cross-reactivity with other determinants). The term "polymorphic" refers to variable reaction in a population so that some members carry the specificity while others do not, and "supertypic" refers to the reaction of one antibody that appears to "include" several specificities.

IV. MONOCLONAL ANTIBODIES TO THE MURINE MHC: H-2K, D, L

A. General

The murine MHC is situated on chromosome 17 and consists of many loci, but for the purposes of this review, only loci whose products are detected serologically and to which monoclonal antibodies have been made will be discussed (i.e., the H-2K, D, L, and Ia loci). These loci code for cell membrane glycoproteins which are found on almost all tissues in the mouse. They consist of a heavy chain (45,000 mol wt) and a β2-microglobulin (β2M) light chain (12,000 mol wt). The heavy chain bears the allotypic specificities and β2M is considered to be "invariant" (although recently a polymorphism has been described[11–13]), the β2M locus being linked to H-3 on chromosome 2. The H-2K, D, L loci are similar in structure and function suggesting their common origin. The H-2L locus, the most recently described, is closely linked to H-2D and as yet cannot be separated by recombination although its products can be identified serologically and biochemically. The finding of close linkage of H-2L to H-2D has led to speculation of the presence of additional closely linked genes near H-2D and evidence is accumulating to support this (discussed further below). The specificities of these loci are conventionally classified as "private" or "public", the private occurring only in one haplotype and public in several haplotypes. In addition, antibodies can "cross-react" with the products of different loci (e.g., H-2.1, 28 can be coded for by the different alleles of the H-2K, D, or L loci).

A whole range of monoclonal antibodies to private and public specificities of these loci have been described and have originated from several sources,[7,8,14–25] (Table 2). In general, the reaction of these follow the conventional H-2 antisera. Antibodies to specificities of the b, d, k haplotype have been made, but since the majority of fusions have involved these haplotypes, this is not surprising. It is considered that all known H-2 antibodies could be produced as monoclonal reagents. In additional, several "new" specificities have been described (i.e., reactions not defined in the existing H-2 charts), but as noted above, antibodies to these specificities must have been present in sera produced by conventional immunization, but presumably were too weak to be detected.

B. Specific Antibodies

The antibodies described thus far are listed in Table 2.[7,8,14–25] The first of these described was the anti-H-2K^k antibody, 11-4.1 (probably anti-H-2.11 or a new specificity) described by Hertzenberg and colleagues[14–16] which has been extensively tested in many laboratories, especially as the cell line can be obtained at the Salk Institute and the antibody is available from a commercial source.

H-2^k antibodies—In addition to the 11-4.1 antibody, which appears to recognize a public specificity common to the k and q haplotypes (b, d, s are negative), monoclonal antibodies have also been described to the H-2^k "public" specificities: H-2.5, 11, 25 (all from several laboratories) and to the private specificity H-2K.23.[7,8,17–22] There is no monoclonal antibody as yet to H-2.32, the H-2D^k private specificity, but this antibody is diffcult to make as the appropriate Ir genes must be present in the recipient.[14] Several new anti-H-2^k public specificities have also been described from Sachs' laboratory (Table 2).

H-2^b antibodies—A number of anti-H-2^b monoclonal antibodies have been described to the H-2D^b private specificity H-2.2,[7,17,18,23] to the public specificities H-2.39, and also to a number of new specificities.[8,20–22] Recently, several anti-H-2K^b antibodies have been described but only one resembles the private H-2K.33 specificity, which is surprising in that anti-H-2K.33 antibody is usually easy to produce by conventional means.

Table 2
SUMMARY OF ANTI-H-2 MONOCLONAL ANTIBODIES DERIVED FROM VARIOUS SOURCES

H—2 haplotype	Specificity	Line	Donor	Recipient	Ref.
H—2^k	New	11—4.1	CKB	BALB/C	14—16
H—2^k	New (H—2m1)	H116—22.R7	CBA	BALB/C	7— 9
	H—2.11 (H—2m3)	H100—5.R3	CBA	BALB/C	7— 9
	H—2.25 (H—2m4)	H100—27.R9	CBA	BALB/C	7— 9
	H—2.5 (H—2m5)	H100—30.R3	CBA	BALB/C	7— 9
H—2^b	H—2.2 (H—2m2)	B22—249R1	C57BL/6	BALB.K	7— 9
H—2^f	H—2.5	P1—42	A.SW(SJL)	A.CA	19
H—2^k	H—2.23	P8—30	CBA	BALB/C	19
	H—2.11	P11—20	CBA	BALB/C	19
	New	P11—11	CBA	BALB/C	19
	New	P11—14	CBA	BALB/C	19
H—2^b	New	20—8—4s	C3H.SW	C3H	20—22
	New	23A—5—21s	C3H.SW	C3H	20—22
	New	28—8—6s	C3H.SW	C3H	20—22
	New	28—11—5s	C3H.SW	C3H	20—22
	H—2.39	28—13—3s	C3H.SW	C3H	20—22
	H—2.64	28—14—8s	C3H.SW	C3H	20—22
H—$2^{b/d}$	New	27—11—132	(C57BL/6 × DBA/2)F_1	C3H	20—22
H—$2L^d$	H—2.65	23—B—10—1s	BALB/C	BALB/C—dm^2	20—22
	H—2.65	30—5—7s	BALB/C	BALB/C—dm^2	20—22
H—2K	H—2.5	3—83P	C3H	BALB/C	20—22
	H—2.23	16—3—22s	C3H	C3H.SW	20—22
	New	12—2—2s	C3H	C3H.SW	20—22
		15—1—5p	C3H	C3H.SW	20—22
		15—3—1s	C3H	C3H.SW	20—22
		15—5—5s	C3H	C3H.SW	20—22
		16—1—2s	C3H	C3H.SW	20—22
		16—1—11s	C3H	C3H.SW	20—22
		16—3—1s	C3H	C3H.SW	20—22
H—2^b	H—2.2	194—2.2	B6.C—H—2^{bm12}	BALB/C	23
H—2^b		141—4.2	BALB.B	C58	23
		141—13.2	BALB.B	C58	23
		141—24.2	BALB.B	C58	23
		141—32.4	BALB.B	C58	23
H—2^d	H—2.31				25

A common finding of many of the anti-H-2^b antibodies has been their cross-reactivity with d and q haplotypes, either together or separately and some also cross-react with the H-$2L^d$ specificities.[8,20–24]

H-2^d antibodies—As the BALB/c myeloma lines used for fusion have the H-2^d antigens it was considered that "antiself" anti-H-2^d antibodies would not be produced, or would be absorbed onto the surface of the cells. However, several anti-H-2^d antibodies have been described, many of which react with public H-2 alloantigens;[7,8,14–25] obviously there is no barrier to the production of antibodies to these specificities.

H-2L antibodies—Monoclonal antibodies (anti-H-2.64 and 65) to the recently described H-2L locus have been described from several laboratories, and these resemble the specificities detected by conventional alloantisera.[8,20–23]

C. Description of Several New H-2 Antibodies

Several antibodies have been produced in our laboratory by fusing after the immunization C58 anti-BALB/c-H-2^b. In addition to several anti-Qa-2 antibodies[24] some of the anti-H-2 antibodies were of particular interest.

1. 141-42

This antibody reacted with H-2 haplotypes b and q but not with f, k, p, r, or s. Haplotype d gave a substantially weaker reaction than with b or q. Studies of appropriate recombinant strains mapped the reactions to the D^b, D^d, and D^q loci and the H-2L reaction of BALB/c could not be differentiated from that of the BALB/c-H-2^{dm2} mutant which lacks the H-2L^d locus. The antibody was similar to the 27-11-135 line which apparently recognizes a new H-2^b specificity (Table 2). The strong cross-reactivity of H-2^q and the weak cross-reactivity of H-2^d is of interest.

2. 141-13.2 and -24.2

These two monoclonal antibodies have similar reactions with strains bearing the b and q haplotypes and the reaction also maps to the D^b and D^q loci; again the reaction with H-2^d strains was weaker than that of the b and q haplotypes. However, although all strains bearing the D^d allele gave weaker reactions, there was a heirachy in reactivity: strains whose D^d allele originated from B10.A or A strain (e.g., B10.A, B10.A[5R]; B10.T[6R]; AQR; A.TL; A.TH) all had weaker reactions than BALB/c or B10.D2. The effect was not due to the adjacent Tla locus which can affect the expression of H-2D specificities[27] as there was no difference between Tla$^+$ and Tla$^-$ strains but may be due to the reaction of the antibody with the product of a different locus (possibly H-2M)[28] wherein B10.A lacks the appropriate specificity which is carried by BALB/c.

3. 141-32.4

This antibody reacts equally with haplotypes b, d, q but not with f, k, p, r, or s and also represents a new specificity.

Thus from the one fusion, three new specificities could be defined, possibly a new locus defined, the clear demonstration of variable patterns of cross-reactivity demonstrated, as well as the Qa-2 antibodies, a testament to the usefulness of the monoclonal antibody technique.

D. Some Observations Made with Monoclonal Anti-H-2 Antibodies

The use of monoclonal anti-H-2 antibodies has led to some interesting findings which have confirmed earlier controversial observations.

1. Cross-Reactions, Strong, and Weak Reactions

One of the features of monoclonal anti-H-2 antibodies has been the clear demonstration of cross-reactions between haplotypes, particularly those giving rise to strong and weak reactions. This was alluded to earlier but has been found with many H-2 monoclonal antibodies.[7,8,14–23] For example, the antibody 20-8-45 reacts with H-2 haplotypes b and d with a titer 1/512 - 1/1024 but with other haplotypes (e.g., s) the titer is 1/16. The weak reaction would be due to one of several reasons:

1. The specificities detected are not identical but related and the titer being a measure of the affinity of the antibody. If sufficient strains are examined, a hierachy of reactions may be observed from the strongest to the weakest thus representing a range of cross-reactions.

2. The determinant could be identical but due to other factors may be less accessible for binding; such factors could be the conformation of the H-2 molecule—this being different with different haplotypes.
3. Regulatory controls imposed at some stage in the glycoprotein synthetic pathway, as have been suggested to explain the differences in the detection of H-2D specificities in the presence or absence of Tla antigens.[27]

Cross-reactions of a variable strength have been noted with H-2 antisera for many years but have been difficult to analyze because of the complexity of the antisera, and monoclonal antibodies clearly have distinct advantages in examining these reactions.

2. The Concept of Specificity—Multideterminant vs. Single Determinant

Prior to the advent of monoclonal antibodies, H-2 specificities were allocated on the basis of a unique strain distribution pattern determined by direct testing and absorption. Monoclonal antibodies have now altered this approach. For example, the H-2.2 specificity, the private specificity of $H\text{-}2D^b$, was allocated this number on the basis of unique reactions of a panel of antisera. Four different monoclonal antibodies, emanating from two laboratories, were stated to react with H-2.2 on the basis of their reaction with the $H\text{-}2D^b$ of C57BL/6; however blocking studies with these antibodies have indicated that there are at least two separate sites on the same molecule reacting with the different monoclonal antibodies, both being detected by conventional antisera. It is clear that so-called monospecific antisera contain a family of antibodies each reacting to a unique determinant on the same molecule but which can be separately detected by monoclonal antibodies. In general, however, the studies with H-2 monoclonal antisera have confirmed the observations made with conventional antisera and have emphasized that H-2 serology has led to the correct interpretation of the structure of the H-2 complex.[18]

3. The Heterogeneity of H-2D and H-2K Loci

The use of monoclonal antibodies has thus far led to the description of several new loci due to the "splitting" of the H-2K, H-2D, and H-2L loci. The variable $H\text{-}2D^d$ reactions (which were referred to the above) may represent an example of the previously described H-2M locus.[28] A new locus, H-2R, which is closely linked to H-2D and H-2L loci has recently been defined by several monoclonal antibodies made when the $H\text{-}2L^d$ loss mutant, BALB/c-$H\text{-}2^{dm2}$ was immunized with BALB/c.[22] The resultant antisera could be resolved into two components by coprecipitation techniques wherein the same specificity could be detected on two different molecules—one coded for by H-2L and the other, by the new locus, H-2R.[29] The $H\text{-}2L^d$ molecule has the specificities H2.64 and 65 (identified by monoclonal antibodies 28-14-85 and 30-5-75, respectively) whereas the $H\text{-}2R^d$ molecule has only the H-2.64 specificity.

Two other studies suggest a heterogeneity of the $H\text{-}2K^k$ locus. First, when cells reacting with the monoclonal antibody 11-4.1 (described above) were removed from the spleen of $H\text{-}2^k$ mice, cells remained which reacted with a conventional anti-$H\text{-}2K^k$ antibody but not with the 11-4.1 antibody.[30] The studies were extended by coprecipitation analysis and the results indicated a different cellular and molecular distribution of determinants detected by the two antibodies, implying that the determinants were coded for by different $H\text{-}2K^k$ loci. In another study, two different monoclonal $H\text{-}2K^k$ antibodies were compared and by five separate criteria were considered to recognize distinct determinants on different molecules.[31] The determinants were considered to be separate on the basis of co-capping studies and by the fact that one antibody recognizes a carbohydrate determinant while the other recognizes a glycoprotein determinant.

4. The Relationship Between Serologically Detected Specificities and Target Determinants Detected by Alloreactive T Cells

Although alloreactive T cells and antibodies clearly react with H-2K, and D, and L locus antigens, it has not been clear whether they detect identical or closely related determinants on the same molecule or on different molecules. Blocking of T-cell mediated lysis by conventional antisera was taken as evidence that the determinants were identical, but such sera are complex and could conceivably contain antibodies to both sets of determinants. However, monoclonal anti-H-2 alloantisera can block lysis[32,33] indicating that the antigens detected serologically and those by T-cell lysis are either identical or closely related spatially so that they can be blocked by steric hinderance.

5. Reactions of Monoclonal Antisera with Wild Mice

The number of different H-2 alleles defined in inbred mice is very much a function of the number of strains examined and this depends, to some extent, on the production of congenic and recombinant strains wherein one gene product can be examined with the complex antisera available. Another approach for analysis is to use monoclonal antibodies to determine the extent of H-2 polymorphism. Using a panel of H-2 monoclonal antibodies, a series of wild mice were tested[19] and found to give different reactions when compared with those obtained with the laboratory inbred strains. These results suggest more extensive polymorphism of the murine MHC than formerly realized.

Thus, in the short time since their production, monoclonal anti-H-2 antibodies have been of great value from several different viewpoints. They have confirmed and extended the knowledge of H-2 determined by conventional antisera and have led to the possible description of three new loci. They have given a more precise understanding of the nature and complexity of H-2 determinants and their relationship to those detected in the cell assay. In addition, they have been of use in isolation and distribution of H-2 antigens,[34] analysis of the control of isotype expression and will clearly be of value in cloning the H-2 genes. However, no great alteration in our interpretation of the H-2 complex has resulted, but rather, the provision of a standard set of highly useful reagents which will, in time, replace the conventional alloantisera for the definition of the murine MHC.

V. MONOCLONAL ANTIBODIES TO MURINE Ia ALLOANTIGENS

A. General

The I region in the mouse has excited considerable interest because of its central role in immune responses. This region contains the Ir genes and genes coding for the serologically detected Ia alloantigenic specificities. In addition, it contains histocompatibility (H) genes and genes (Lad) coding for stimulating determinants in the mixed lymphocyte reaction, and other genes important for cell collaboration in the immune response.[4] The I region has been extensively reviewed in recent years[4,35,36] and only anti-Ia antibodies will be reviewed here. The I region consists of the subregions I-A, I-B, I-J, I-E, and I-C, and more recently, the I-N subregion has also been defined; the gene order within the I region being N, A, B, J, E, C. The I-A/I-E subregions code for specificities found on B cells whereas I-N, I-J, and I-C subregions code for specificities found on T cells. Little is known of the functional capabilities of the I-N and I-C antisera; the I-J antisera have been found to react with suppressor T cells in many different systems. Each subregion is complex and may contain several genes coding for different alloantigenic specificities, as has already been found for the I-A and I-J subregions, but as yet not for the other subregions and indeed no serologically defined

Table 3
SUMMARY OF ANTI-Ia MONOCLONAL ANTIBODIES DERIVED FROM VARIOUS SOURCES

Haplotypes and subregion	Specificity	Line	Donor	Recepient	Ref.
I—A^k	Ia—1.2	11—2.12	CKB	BALB/C	14—16
	Ia—1.2	11—5.2	CKB	BALB/C	14—16
I—A^k	Ia—1.17	10—2.16	C3H	CWB	14—16
	Ia—1.17	10—3.6	C3H	CWB	14—16
	Ia—1.17	11—3.25	CKB	BALB/C	14—16
I—A^k	Ia—1.17	N—22	C57.BR-cd	129	42
I—A^k	Ia—1.2(Ia.m1)	H118—49R2	CBA	BALB/C	7— 9
	Ia—1.2(Ia.m2)	B15—R4R5	AKR	BALB/C	7— 9
I—A^b	Ia—1.8(Ia.m3)	B17-263.R1	C57BL/6	AKR	7— 9
	Ia—1.9(Ia.m4)	B17-123.R2	C57BL/6	AKR	7— 9
I—A^k	Ia—1.15(Ia.m5)	17/227.R2	A.TL	A.TH	7— 9
	Ia—1.19(Ia.m6)	H116-32.R5	CBA	BALB/C	7— 9
I—E^k	Ia—5.7(Ia.m7)	13/18	A.TL	A.TH	7— 9
	Ia—5.7(Ia.m7)	13/14	A.TL	A.TH	7— 9
I^p	Ia.13	P47—42	B10.P	(A × B10)F$_1$	19
I—A^b	Ia.20	25-5-16s	C3H.SW	C3H	20—22
	Ia.20	25-9-3s	C3H.SW	C3H	20—22
	New	25-9-17s	C3H.SW	C3H	20—22
	Ia.8	28-16-8s	C3H.SW	C3H	20—22
	Ia.20	93-20	B6.PL-Thy-1^a	AKR	23
I—E/C^k	Ia.7	14-4-4s	C3H	C3H.SW	20—22
I—E^k	New	17-3-3s	C3H	C3H.SW	20—22
I—A^k	Ia.2	26-7-11s	A.TL	A.TH	20—22
	Ia.18	26-8-16s	A.TL	A.TH	20—22

specificity exists for the I-B subregion. Thus far, monoclonal antibodies have been defined for the specificities found on B cells and coded for by genes mapping to the I-A and I-E subregions;[8,14–29] there are also reports[37] of anti-I-J monoclonal antibodies (Table 3). No monoclonal antibodies have been described for the I-N and I-C subregions. In short, anti-Ia monoclonal antibodies appear to be readily produced and have all the properties ascribed to the conventional antisera. Their use has not greatly altered our understanding of the I region but to some extent, have clarified the controversy existing between the glycoprotein and glycolipid Ia antigens.

B. Specific Antibodies

The specific anti-Ia antibodies produced thus far are listed in Table 3 and have originated from the same laboratories producing monoclonal anti-II-2 alloantisera. The length of the list demonstrates that these antibodies are not difficult to make and one can confidently predict that all anti-Ia antibodies will shortly be made by the cell fusion method. A number of antibodies have been defined which recognize known Ia specificities, (e.g., Ia-2, 8, 9, 13, 15, 17, 18, 19, and 20 of the I-A subregion and Ia-7 of the I-E subregion). These antibodies appear to be precisely those defined by the conventional alloantisera. Antibodies to the private specificities I^k: Ia-2; I^b: Ia-20 have also been produced and a number of new specificities defined. The general properties of Ia monoclonal antisera are similar to those of H-2 antisera and have been discussed at length in the preceding section. For example a number of new specificities have been defined, but as stated, these antibodies must have been present in the conventional antisera, albeit not detected. In addition, cross-reactions have been noted, often to an extent not noted previously and due to the high titer of many of the monoclonal antibodies. It has also been found that pairs of antisera, given the same specificity designation by their identical reaction on a panel of inbred strains need not react with the identical determinant. For example, two monoclonal antibodies (25-5-16S and 25-9-3S) both appear to recognize the same specificity "Ia-20" by virtue of their identical strain distribution. However one reacts with rat cells, the other not, indicating a reaction with different determinants. Thus monoclonal antibodies select determinants on a molecular basic rather than on a statistical basis as is done with a strain distribution allocation. The monoclonal anti-Ia antibodies do not appear to be remarkable other than ease of production, standardization, etc. Thus the anti-Ia.2 and Ia.20 antibodies to private specificities react accordingly, as do the antibodies to the public specificities. Some of these appear to react with different biochemical determinants (see below) and the reaction of anti-B cell antibodies with T cells has also been clarified. One of the more important group of antisera to be produced will be the anti-I-J monoclonal antisera. There is little information available at present regarding these monoclonal antibodies[37] but their production is eagerly awaited. The I-J products are difficult to detect directly[15] and serological studies have to be done by tedious functional assays, which prevents a full analysis. In addition, there has been a suspicion that many of the functions attributed to I-J antisera are in fact due to contaminating antiviral antibodies, and the provision of monoclonal antisera should solve this controversy.

C. Reaction of Ia Monoclonal Antibodies with T Cells

It has been difficult to conclusively prove the presence of Ia antigens on T cells but monoclonal anti-Ia antibodies react with lymph node T cells. Using two fluorescent labels and the FACS with monoclonal antisera, it was clear that the same IA and IE subregion alloantigens are carried on both T and B cells.[17,18] In addition, Ia alloantigens could be readily detected on PHA-induced blast cells (T cells) with monoclonal antisera.[39]

D. Biochemical Analysis of Alloantigens Detected with Anti-Ia Antisera

The current convention states that Ia alloantigens are present on the protein portion of glycoprotein molecules which consist of two chains (α,β) which are nonconvalently linked and have molecular weight of 28,000 to 33,000.[4,35,36] It is not clear on which chain the allotypic specificities reside. More recently, considerable evidence has been presented which indicates that there are another class of antigens coded for by genes in the murine MHC and which code the specificities determined by carbohydrate.[40,41] The presence of this second class is controversial because of the difficulty in reproducing the findings in different laboratories and particularly as the difficult rosetting assay was used to define the second classes specificities. However, with the use of monoclonal antibodies, which can only recognize *one* determinant, the problem has been partially solved. Using five different criteria,[42] (Table 4) to separate protein from carbohydrate structures, anti–Ia antibodies could be shown to react with one type of determinant or the other (but not both). These criteria were

1. Sensitivity of the antigen to neuraminidase
2. Precipitation of protein—Ia antigens and their demonstration in SDS gels
3. Inhibition by protein extracts free of glycolipid
4. Inhibition by glycolipid extracts free of protein
5. Inhibition of their reactions by simple sugars

Table 4
ANALYSIS OF MONOCLONAL ANTIBODY TO DETECT Ia[p] (PROTEIN) ON Ia[c] (CARBOHYDRATE) ANTIGENS[a]

Specificity	Monoclonal antibody	Protein or SDS-PAGE	Inhibition by protein	Inhibition by glycolipid	N/dase[b] suscepti-ble	Sugar inhibition
Ia.2[b]	H118—49	+	+	—	—	—
Ia.2[c]	B15—124.R5	—	—	+	—	+
Ia.7[P]	13—4	+	+	—	—	—
Ia.7[P]	13—18	+	+	—	—	—
Ia.8[P]	B17—263.R6	±	+	—	—	—
Ia.9[c]	B17—123.R4	—	—	+	±	—
Ig.15[P]	17—227	+	+	—	—	—
Ia.17[c]	N—22	—	+	+	+	+
Ia.17[P]	11—3	+	+	—	—	—
Ia.19[P]	H116—32	+	+	—	—	—

[a] - Further details in Reference 42.
[b] - Neuraminidase.

A series of monoclonal antibodies were demonstrated to react with either one determinant or the other[42] (see Table 4). Thus, of the antibodies studied, two different monoclonal antibodies to Ia-2 were shown to react with different determinants: H.118-49 to react with protein whereas B15-124.R5 to react with carbohydrate. As well, two different Ia-17 antibodies, from two different sources were shown to react with either protein (11-3) or carbohydrate (N-22). It should be noted that these two pairs of antibodies apparently react with the same determinant as judged from a strain distribution involving inbred and recombinant strains, however, both clearly react with a different type of determinant. Of the other antibodies, two monoclonal Ia-7 antibodies were shown to react with a protein determinant, anti-Ia-8 with a protein and anti-Ia-9 with carbohydrate; Ia-15 and Ia-19 antisera with protein antigens. These determinants have been termed Ia[p] and Ia[c].[42] Thus, the monoclonal antibodies have contributed to resolving the controversy and at this time the data clearly points to the existence of two different types of determinants. However, what is not clear is the molecular interaction between these determinants or whether they are present on the same or different molecules, and whether one is the reflection of the conformation of the other or whether they represent two entirely different and unrelated systems which occur at the same time on the same cells. This latter possibility would appear to be unlikely and it may be that these are two entirely different structural systems which are linked in their function. Such a possibility could arise if the glycoprotein function is to act as a glycosyl transferase producing the specific structures detected with the anticarbohydrate monoclonal antibody.

Thus, as with all the other systems, the monoclonal antibodies have provided a major technical advance in the study of the murine MHC. There has been little conceptual alteration in the studies of the I region with the advent of the monoclonal antisera, however, certain obvious advantages have occurred, and these have been described.

VI. MONOCLONAL ANTIBODIES TO THE RAT MHC: RT1

A. General

The rat MHC (RT1) shares many features in common with the MHC of man and mouse being divided into three regions: A, B, and C.[43] The RT1.A locus codes for the classical transplantation antigens analagous to the mouse H-2K, D and human HLA-A, B antigens being glycoproteins (mol wt 45,000 daltons) and are expressed on the cell surface in association with β2-microglobulin.[44–46] The antigens coded for by the RT1.B locus are predominantly expressed on B lymphocytes, some thymocytes and kidney cells,[43] and are glycoproteins consisting of two chains of 33,000 and 28,000 daltons.[47] Serologically these behave like the DR and Ia antigens of man and mouse. Recent studies[47,48] suggest that there are at least two distinct B antigen species which are homologues of Ia antigens coded by the I-A and I-E subregions of the murine MHC. One of these rat Ia-like antigens may in fact be coded for by the C region.[49]

B. Description of Antibodies

Several groups are involved in the production of antirat RT1 monoclonal antibodies, usually by fusing with immunized rat spleen cells and a mouse myeloma line. It has been suggested that rat-mouse hybridomas have several advantages over mouse-mouse hybridomas; such as the stability of hybrids, their tendency not to interchange heavy and light chains with the myeloma proteins, the ease in which rat antibodies can be identified from mouse myeloma chains, and the relatively high yield of cytotoxic anti-MHC antibodies obtained.[3]

In addition to their conventional reactions, the antirat RT1 monoclonal antibodies show cross-reactions between rat, mouse, and human MHC determinants. For example, the MRC OX3 antibody binds to spleen cells from rat strains of RT1 haplotypes l and y, to mouse splenocytes of H-2 haplotypes b and s (this correlates with mouse Ia specificity 9), and to human B lymphoblastoid cell lines (LCL) bearing HLA-DR1, DR2, and DRw6 determinants.[50,51] Of note, is that MRC OX3 reacts with the same DR determinants defined by the anti-HLA-DR monoclonal antibody, Genox 3.53[1] but does not bind to normal B lymphocytes bearing the HLA-DR1, DR2, or DRw6 determinants. The MRC OX4 antibody binds to spleen cells from all rat strains tested and to mouse spleen cells of H-2 haplotypes k and s which correlates with mouse Ia specificities 17 or 18; it does not bind to any human B LCL or separated B lymphocytes. Previous studies [52,53] suggest that the determinants recognized by both MRC OX3 and MRC OX4 correspond to an antigen coded for by the mouse I-A subregion and therefore, implies that the HLA-DR1, DR2, and DRw6 antigens also share some homology with the murine I-A antigens. Results from work with the MRC OX4 antibody and a rat Ia alloantiserum give further evidence that there are at least two rat B antigen species which are the equivalents of the mouse I-A and I-E/C subregion products.[50] This is consistent with the biochemical data obtained for rat Ia antigens using conventional allo- and xenoantisera.[47,48]

A number of other antirat RT1 monoclonal antibodies have been described in the literature and these have also been shown to cross-react with the murine H-2 and human HLA complexes.[3,54] An interesting point which emerged from these studies was that some monoclonal antibodies defining polymorphic determinants of the rat A antigen reacted with a monomorphic determinant expressed by both mouse and man.

Howard et al.[55] have produced several anti-RT1A[a] monoclonal antibodies and using competitive inhibition binding studies describe two separate polymorphic sites, called the p and s sites, on the A antigen.[49] Furthermore, it was shown that the p and s sites segregated with different rat RT1 haplotyes indicating that not only are these two determinants topographically separate, but are also genetically independent. These same antibodies were also used to study cell lysis. It had previously been noted that the lytic behavior of some monoclonal antibodies did not completely agree with results obtained with direct binding assays.[55,56] This could, in part, be attributed to their monoclonality. However when two monoclonal antibodies, which alone were nonlytic, were mixed together they become cytotoxic for the target cell.[49] This synergistic lysis is dependent on each monoclonal antibody reating to a separate determinant expressed on the same antigenic molecule, such as the p and s sites in the RT1A^a haplotype. This observation may prove to be valuable to workers involved in the production of cytotoxic anti-HLA monoclonal reagents for routine tissue-typing. Since the occurrence of cytotoxic monoclonal antibodies to polymorphic HLA determinants seems fairly low (due to the antibody being noncomplement fixing or alternatively is potentially complement fixing but the determinant density on the cell surface is too low for effective lysis) the mixing of two anti-HLA antibodies in such a way to retain specificity may overcome this problem and would be an alternative to the antiglobulin method for inducing cytotoxicity.

In other studies the R3/13 monoclonal antibody, directed against rat RT1A^a antigens was used to enhance renal allograft survival with a full RT1^a difference.[57] Other workers[3,58] using different rat strain combinations and a different monoclonal antibody, D4/68, have also shown enhancement in some combinations. The demonstration that monoclonal antibodies can induce graft enhancement in the rat may be useful for similar studies in human allograft enhancement.

VII. MONOCLONAL ANTIBODIES TO THE HUMAN MHC: HLA AND β2-MICROGLOBULIN

A. General

The HLA complex is the most polymorphic system known in man and it is the maintenance of this polymorphism which suggests that its function is of importance to the survival of the species.[59–61] Briefly, the HLA-A, -B, and -C antigens are coded for by genes located on the short arm of human chromosome 6[62] and are analogous to the H-2K, D, and L loci of the mouse. These human histocompatibility antigens can be serologically defined using conventional human alloantisera. Biochemical studies have revealed that the HLA-A, -B, and -C antigens are glycoproteins which are noncovalently linked to β2M and have molecular weights of 44,000 and 12,000 daltons, respectively. It is the larger 44,000 dalton chain which bears the polymorphic determinants while the smaller β2M chain, which is coded for by a gene located on chromosome 15,[63] appears to be invariant. The HLA antigens are expressed on the surface of all normal cells with the possible exception of erythrocytes, trophoblast,[64] and spermatozoa.[65]

The implication of HLA antigens in transplantation and disease and their fundamental role in cell-cell recognition and immune function has encouraged intense studies which have frequently led to confusing results. However, monoclonal antibodies may be of help in solving some of these problems.

B. Monomorphic Anti-HLA Antibodies

Monoclonal antibodies to monomorphic determinants of the HLA antigenic complex occurs very often, and most laboratories doing xenogeneic mouse antihuman fusions would have produced several xenogeneic monoclonal antibodies to the "invariant" region of the HLA antigens (Table 5). The hybridoma line, W6/32[66] is the most fully characterized monomorphic HLA monoclonal antibody. The monoclonal antibody was produced after immunization of BALB/c mice with a human tonsil leukocyte membrane preparation and fusion with the myeloma line P3/X63-Ag8. The W6/32 antibody is of the IgG_{2a} subclass, is active in complement-dependent cytotoxicity and binds protein A. It has been screened on a large panel of human cell types including peripheral blood lymphocytes (PBL), T and B LCL, lines derived from malignant cells, and human spermatozoa. Notable exceptions of positive reactivity are Daudi, a B cell line which

Table 5
SUMMARY OF ANTI-HLA AND -β2M MONOCLONAL ANTIBODIES DERIVED FROM VARIOUS SOURCES

Cell line	Specificity	Ref.
W6/32	Monomorphic—HLA	69
PA2.5	Monomorphic—HLA	81
PA2.6	Monomorphic—HLA	81
S1.34	Monomorphic—HLA	2
169-IE4.3	Monomorphic—HLA	122
Q1/28	Monomorphic—HLA	74
PA2.1	HLA—A2	81
BB7.2	HLA—A2	1
FMC5	HLA—A2	84
118—1G1	HLA—A2	123
MA2.1	HLA—A2/B17	83
26A3	HLA—A3/All	124
F10.13/13	HLA—Aw19/B7/B8	85
BB7.1	HLA—B7	1
26C4	HLA—Bw6	125
241—6.7	HLA—unknown	126
BBM.1	β_2M	91
PA2.12	β_2M	81
BB7.3	β_2M	1
BB7.4	β_2M	1
S1.26	β_2M	2
22E641	β_2M	127
246E9E7	β_2M	127

lacks β2M and therefore cannot express HLA antigens at the cell surface,[67] a choriocarcinoma line, and spermatozoa. W6/32 has also been tested on a panel of mouse-human cell hybrids containing limited numbers of human chromosomes. Only hybrid cells containing chromosome 6 alone or chromosomes 6 and 15 bound W6/32.[68] Considerable effort has been taken to show that W6/32 reacts with a determinant common to all HLA-A, -B, and -C chains and that the noncovalent linkage of β2M to form the HLA/β2M complex is mandatory to the binding site of the W6/32 antibody.[69] Immunoabsorbent columns of W6/32 - Sepharose have been shown to bind individual solubilized preparations of HLA-A2, -B8, and -Cw2. Isolated ^{125}I-HLA-A2 chains bind very weakly to W6/32, while no binding of ^{125}I-β2M could be detected. When an excess of unlabeled β2M was added to the isolated ^{125}I-HLA-A2 chains, binding to W6/32 was considerably improved. This evidence, together with the fact that no monoclonal antibody against the HLA heavy chain alone has been described, suggests that β2M confers a significant conformational change to the HLA molecule and that the predominant immunogenic sites arise from this structural rearrangement. W6/32 has also been used to study the expression and relative density of HLA antigens on lymphoid and nonlymphoid cell populations. By quantitative absorption assays using homogenates of various tissues and cell preparations, it has been shown that in comparison to spleen, other tissues (kidney, liver, heart, brain, bone marrow, thymocytes, platelets, erythrocytes, reticulocytes, and chronic lymphatic leukemia (CLL) cells) have low densities of HLA.[70] Using an indirect radiobinding assay with W6/32, it was also demonstrated that human B-LCL express approximately nine times as much cell surface HLA as normal PBL.[69] In addition to these findings the absence of HLA-A, -B, and -C antigens from two choriocarcinoma cell lines has been verified using W6/32 in indirect binding studies and absorption assays.[64] Using W6/32 and surface-labeling techniques (immunofluorescence, immunoperoxidase, and autoradiography) the cellular distribution and differential expression of HLA antigens on thymic cell suspensions and tissue sections was studied.[71] HLA antigens were demonstrated to be present on the majority of thymic medullary cells while cortical thymocytes appeared to lack HLA antigens, which is analogous to the distribution of H-2 antigens in mouse thymus.[71]

Studies of evolutionary relationships involving the comparison of homologous proteins, such as HLA, from different species has also been aided by the use of monoclonal antibodies. The W6/32 antibody recognizes a determinant present on the cell surface of apes, Old World monkeys, and the owl monkey of karyotype VI.[72] Another monomorphic anti-HLA antibody, PA2.5 (Table 5), gave additional reactions with most New World monkeys and defined a polymorphism in the spider monkey. Such studies as these provide a simple way of defining different antigenic determinants of the HLA/β2M complex and further suggest that the amino acid sequence of HLA chains has been highly conserved since before the divergence of New and Old World monkeys. This is not so surprising since it has been found that the HLA-A, -B chains and the H-2 K, D chains share approximately 70% amino acid sequence homology.[73]

The number of antigenic determinants on HLA glycoproteins recognized in xenogeneic immunization schedules appears to be relatively small as monomorphic-HLA monoclonal antibodies seem to define the same specificity. Comparison by capping and inhibition studies with W6/32 and 169-1 E4.3 (Table 6) suggest that these two antibodies are detecting the same determinant on the HLA/β2M complex. Trucco et al.[2] comparing the reactivity of their monomorphic anti-HLA antibody, S1.34 with W6/32, have also arrived at this conclusion. S1.34 is a noncomplement fixing antibody of the IgG_1 class and was produced following fusion with the myeloma line, P3/NS1/1-Ag4-1 and spleen cells from DBA 2/J mice immunized against the LCL, WT 52. The monomorphic anti-HLA antibody, Q1/28 has been used to study the expression of HLA glycoproteins on human myeloid progenitor cells and during the cell cycle of human lymphoid cells. Using a colony-forming-unit (CFU-C) assay, it has been shown that HLA antigens are present on human myeloid progenitor cells.[74] Sarkar et al.[75] have synchronized cells of the human B cell line, WI-L2 by density dependent arrest in the G_1 phase and samples from the G_0, G_1, late S, and late G_2 phase were examined for expression of cell surface HLA antigens where it was found their density remained constant throughout the cell cycle.

At this point it is relevant to mention the monoclonal antibody, 5-4.8 produced in our laboratory.[76] This antibody is lymphocyte-specific, reacting with PBL from all donors, all CLL, and LCL including Daudi. Immunoprecipitation studies have shown that 5-4,8 reacts with a two chain complex with molecular weight 45,000 and 12,000 daltons which are similar to the molecular weights described for the HLA glycoproteins and β2M, respectively.[61] However, blocking, capping, and inhibition, studies using a monoclonal anti-β2M antibody and antimonomorphic HLA antibodies (results not shown) have indicated that the molecular complex defined by 5-4.8 is not associated with either β2M or HLA glycoproteins,

C. Polymorphic Anti-HLA Antibodies

The introduction of the hybridoma fusion technique was initially considered to be the solution for obtaining monoclonal antibodies specific to all the known HLA-A, -B, and -C specificities and thus alleviate the requirement for human alloantisera which are difficult to produce and characterize. However, the relative difficulty, so far encountered in producing good polymorphic-anti-HLA reagents was unpredicted. This is es-

Table 6
SUMMARY OF ANTIHUMAN MHC MONOCLONAL ANTIBODIES PRODUCED IN OUR LABORATORY[a]

Cell line	Specificity of antibody	Ig class	Complement binding	Protein A binding	Recipient mouse strain	Immunogen
246E9E7	Anti—β2M	N.T.[b]	+	+	CBA	T—ALL[c]
22E641	Anti—β2M	N.T.	+	+	CBA	T—ALL
169—1E4.3	Anti—HLA (monomorphic)	IgG_{2a}	±	+	C3H	PBL[d] + LCL[e]
246—B8	Anti—HLA (monomorphic)	N.T.	+	+	CBA	T—ALL
118—1G1	Anti—HLA—A2	N.T.	—	—	(BALB/C × 129)F_1	NHL[f](HLA—A2, A19, B5, B18)
241—6.7	Anti—HLA (polymorphic)	N.T.	—	—	BALB/C	PBL (HLA—A1, AW31; B7, BW44)
19—26.1	Anti—DR (polymorphic)	IgG_{2a}	+	+	CBA	Raji
169—1B5.1	Anti—Ia (monomorphic)	IgG_{2b}	+	+	C3H	PBL + LCL
203—B9	Anti—Ia (monomorphic)	N.T.	+	+	CBA	B—CLL[g]

[a] All fusions with P3/NS1/1-Ag4-1 myeloma.
[b] N.T. = not tested.
[c] T-ALL = T-cell acute lymphatic leukemia.
[d] PBL= peripheral blood lymphocytes
[e] LCL = lymphoblastoid cell lines.
[f] NHL = non-Hodgkins lymphoma.
[g] B-CLL = B-cell chronic lymphatic leukemia.

pecially surprising since several workers[77–80] have shown that it is possible to produce xenoantisera specific to some HLA determinants previously defined by conventional alloantisera.

Of the few polymorphic-HLA monoclonal antibodies described, anti-HLA-A2 has occurred several times. The PA2.1 antibody[81] (Table 5) was produced following fusion with the mouse myeloma line, P3/NSI/1-Ag4-1 and spleen cells from BALB/c mice immunized with purified papain-solublized HLA-A2 antigen prepared from the cell line JY. This antibody is of the IgG_1 class, is noncomplement fixing, and does not bind protein A. PA2.1 is specific for all cells typed as HLA-A2 and a HLA-A28 variant determinant which has only been found on the IDF cell line.[1,81] Of interest is the cytotoxic BB7.2 antibody which although produced in a different fusion to PA2.1 displays exactly the same reactivity patterns including binding to the IDF cell line.[1] McMichael et al.[82] have used PA2.1 and their MA2.1 monoclonal antibody,[83] which reacts with a determinant common to HLA-A2 and B17 antigens, to show that the HLA molecules are the restriction elements for influenza virus-specific cytotoxic T cells. By coating influenza virus-infected target cells with the monoclonal anti-HLA antibodies, lysis by sensitized cytotoxic T cell could be specifically blocked.

In our laboratory, a monoclonal antibody, 118-1 G1 (Table 6) has been produced which appears to be specific for HLA-A2. Of the 33 different donor cells tested, 17 (all of which have been typed as HLA-A2) were positive with 118-1 G1 and 16, which were HLA-A2 negative, did not react. The FMC5 antibody[84] and several antibodies described by Parham and Bodmer[81] define supertypic determinants found on HLA-A2 and several other HLA specificities.

The BB7.1 antibody[1] was produced following fusion with the mouse myeloma line, P3/NSI/1-Ag4-1 and BALB/c mouse spleen cells immunized with papain—purified HLA-A2, B7. It is of the IgG_1 class and therefore does not bind protein A or complement. Of interest is that this antibody appears to be specific for HLA-B7 and does not bind to cells of the common serological cross-reactive specificity, HLA-B40. Westphal et al.[125] (personal communication) have produced a cytotoxic monoclonal antibody, 2BC4 which is reactive against HLA-Bw6, a supertypic determinant linked to several HLA-B specificities. This antibody should prove to be valuable in understanding the mechanisms defining the HLA-Bw4/Bw6 specificities.

Monoclonal antibodies which show cross-reactions between HLA specificities are of considerable interest and may be potentially useful in accurately delineating the complexities of the HLA system. In particular, are the MA2.1 (mentioned above), 26A3, and F10.13/13 (Table 5) antibodies. The 26A3 antibody shows specific reactivity for HLA-A3 and A11. It was raised against PBL from an acute myeloid leukemia patient (HLA-A2, A3; B5; Cwl) in BALB/c mice and fusion was with the P3/X63-653 myeloma line. The antibody is of the IgG2a subclass, is cytotoxic and binds protein A. The F10.13/13 antibody[85] was produced following fusion with P3/NSI/1-Ag4-1 myeloma and spleen cells from BALB/c mice immunized with T cells (HLA-A2, Aw24; B8, B13; C-). It is of the IgG3 class and active in complement-dependent cytotoxicity. By the "lysostrip" technique, F10.13/13 reacts with HLA-Aw19, B7, and B8 and more weakly with B40, Bw41, and Cw3. The reactivity of this antibody is complex and different reactions indicate variable degrees of cross reactivity with different determinants, but the maximal affinity of the antibody is for the determinant common to HLA-Aw19, B7, and B8. The fact that monoclonal antibodies are being produced which recognize cross reacting determinants associated with both HLA-A and -B loci is of interest and suggests similarities between the mouse and human MHC systems.

The production of monoclonal antibodies which detect previously undefined HLA specificities is likely such as shown by the monoclonal antibody, 241-6.7 which reacts with a small population of normal individuals (Table 6). Capping studies with monomorphic anti-HLA antibodies (W6/32 and 169-1 E4.3) have shown 241-6.7 recognizes a determinant associated with the HLA antigens. A family study of the immunizing donor suggests that it is linked to the paternal HLA-haplotype, HLA-Aw31, Bw44 and HLA-typed cells from over 30 unrelated individuals, some of which were HLA-Aw31 or Bw44 positive were all unreactive with 241-6.7.

Murine monoclonal antibodies specific to the polymorphic determinants of HLA are yet to be proven suitable typing reagents as so few are available for this, and it will be several years before a complete panel of monoclonal typing sera will be available. In the meantime, monoclonal anti-HLA antibodies (both monomorphic and polymorphic) are proving to be valuable tools for the biochemical analysis of HLA chains[86] and their synthesis[87] and the data which has accumulated from studies using monoclonal anti-HLA antibodies suggests that they will be of further use in defining the HLA system.

D. Anti-β2-Microglobulin Antibodies

The generally accepted criterion for identification of a monoclonal antibody to β2M as opposed to a determinant of the HLA/β2M complex is that it must be inhibited by purified, free β2M. On this basis, several monoclonal anti-β2M antibodies have been described (Table 5). Early work suggested that human β2M is highly immunogenic in xenogeneic immunization schedules.[2] However, it is the experience of our laboratory that the HLA/β2M complex has an equal or greater potentiality to be immunogenic than the β2M chain alone.

The antibody S1.26, was produced following immunization of DBA 2/J mice with the LCL, WT 52 and fusing the spleen cells with the P3/NSI/1-Ag4-1 myeloma line.[88,89] It is of the IgG2a subclass and binds both complement and protein A and has been used for the quantitative analysis of HLA antigens on the surface of lymphoid cells.[90] By contrast to previously published data,[91] it was found that some β2M molecules on B cells are not bound to the HLA heavy chains, but it was generally agreed that there is a greater excess of free β2M on the surface of human T cell lines than on B cells. An immunoabsorbent column with the S1.26 monoclonal antibody coupled to Sepharose beads was used to study the temperature dependent elution of β2M as a potential method for the isolation of pure HLA molecules.[92] The work suggests that antigen elution by increasing the temperature enables improved recovery of antigenic activity than is usually obtained when conventional acid or base elution procedures are employed.

The BBM.1 anti-β2M antibody was produced by immunizing mice with MOLT 4 cells and fusing with the myeloma line, P3/X63-Ag8.[91] The IgG2b antibody binds protein A and complement. Studies with this antibody[91] have shown that the determinant recognized is not as highly conserved as that recognized by the W6/32 monomorphic HLA antibody. In contrast to W6/32, BBM.1 reacted only weakly with gibbon, orangutan and rhesus fibroblasts, and baboon lymphocytes, suggesting that β2M is under considerable evolutionary selection.

The BBM.1 antibody has also been used to immunoprecipitate low levels of β2M from extracts of a human choriocarcinoma cell line.[64] Previous studies[93] using the same antibody but different techniques had failed to detect the presence of either β2M or HLA antigens on the surface of the same cell line. The results suggested that mechanisms operate to control and prevent the production and expression of HLA antigens on the surface of the normal trophoblast and other HLA-negative tissues.

In our laboratory, two anti-β2M antibodies, 22E6 41 and 246 E9E7 have been produced (Table 6).

Table 7
SUMMARY OF ANTI-HLA-DR MONOCLONAL ANTIBODIES DERIVED FROM VARIOUS SOURCES

Cell line	Specificity	Ref.
DA2	Monomorphic—DR	96
S1.5	Monomorphic—DR	2
S1.19	Monomorphic—DR	2
E17/3	Monomorphic—DR	2
E18/3	Monomorphic—DR	2
Q5/13	Monomorphic—DR	100
Q2/70	Monomorphic—DR	99
2.06	Monomorphic—DR	105
L227	Monomorphic—DR	102
L203	Monomorphic—DR	102
FMC4	Monomorphic—DR	84
7.2	Monomorphic—DR	114
169-1B5.1	Monomorphic—DR	128
OKI1	Monomorphic—DR	115
FMC2	HLA—DR4 (split)	112
Genox 3.53	HLA—DR1, 2, W6	1
Genox 3.32	All DR except DR7	1
Q2/80	All DR except DR5	98
Q5/6	All DR except DR7	101
E15/4	HLA—DR3, 5, w6	2
17.15	HLA—DR4, 5	113
19—26.1	HLA—DR (unknown)	129

It is of interest to consider whether a polymorphism, such as has been detected for murine β2M,[11-13] will also be found for the human analogue. With the use of several monoclonal antihuman β2M reagents, this could prove to be the case.

VIII. MONOCLONAL ANTIBODIES TO THE HUMAN MHC: HLA-DR

A. General

The HLA-DR locus of the human MHC codes for serologically defined determinants which are considered to be the analogues of the murine Ia antigens. They have a restricted tissue distribution, being found on B lymphocytes, monocytes, and various nonlymphoid tissues, but are not detected on T lymphocytes, erythocytes, or platelets.[94] Biochemical analysis has shown that the membrane-associated HLA-DR antigens are comprised of two noncovalently linked glycoprotein chains, molecular weight 28,000 and 33,000 (gp 28.33).[95]

A number of laboratories have produced monoclonal antibodies to HLA-DR determinants (Table 7) and it is already evident that the HLA-DR locus is far more complex than is presently suggested by typing with conventional human alloantisera. The relative abundance in which monoclonal anti-HLA-DR antibodies have been produced suggest that, at least for the mouse, human HLA-DR antigens are good immunogens.

B. Monomorphic Anti-HLA-DR Antibodies

Several monomorphic anti-HLA-DR monoclonal antibodies have been described (Table 7). One of these is the noncytotoxic DA2 antibody,[96] which has been used to determine the amount of HLA-DR antigens on a variety of human tissues.[70] The studies indicated that like spleen, the kidney has a relatively high density of these antigens while all other tissues studied (e.g., heart, liver, brain) have very low levels.

Competition experiments with several other monomorphic HLA-DR antibodies[2] suggested that there are at least three distinct groups of monomorphic anti-HLA-DR antibodies:

1. Those which compete with each other and therefore detect an identical or spatially close determinant on the same HLA-DR polypeptide
2. Those which are noncompetitive and are directed against determinants far apart on the same HLA-DR polypeptide such that no steric hindrance occurs
3. Those which are noncompetitive and are directed against determinants on separate HLA-DR polypeptide chains

These separate polypeptide chains may refer to the recognized gp28.33 chains or to polypeptides coded for by an undefined HLA-linked locus such as that suggested elsewhere.[97]

These studies have been extended using four different monomorphic anti-HLA-DR antibodies, Q2/70, Q2/80, Q5/6, and Q5/13[98] (Table 7). Comparison of their reactivity with a polyclonal rabbit anti-HLA-DR serum and quantitative binding assays have shown that all four monoclonal antibodies detect subsets of Ia-like antigens. Q5/13 has the widest reactivity, recognizing 75% of Ia-like antigens, Q5/6 has an intermediate reactivity while Q2/70 and Q2/80 detect only 30% of Ia-like antigens. Inhibition studies suggest that the determinants detected by Q2/70, Q2/80, and Q5/13 are spatially close to each other but distinct from that recognized by Q5/6. Q2/70[99] and Q5/13[100] are reactive with all HLA-DR allospecificities but the determinant recognized by Q5/6[101] is not detected on HLA-DR7 and similarly, Q2/80[98] does not react with the HLA-DR5 specificity. Based on these results at least five different Ia-like antigens can be described and with other studies with monoclonal antibodies,[102] suggest that more than one locus codes for the Ia-like antigens of man. Immunodepletion and immunoprecipitation studies using the L203 and L227 antibodies (Table 7) have also revealed that both antibodies recognize the gp.28.33 moiety, but L227 also defines a specificity on a 25,000 molecular weight chain.[102] This third Ia chain is thought to represent a second population of human Ia-like molecules and confirms earlier work.[97] The cytotoxic monoclonal antibody, 169-1 B5.1 (Table 6) produced in our laboratory shows similar reactivity to the L227 antibody in that it precipitates three chains of molecular weights 33,000, 28,000, and 25,000 daltons. Several other monomorphic anti-Ia antibodies have also been produced recently and their reactivity in competitive binding assays with 169-1 B5.1 will make an interesting study.

In other studies the noncytotoxic S1.5 monoclonal antibody (Table 7) has been used[103] in a rosetting technique to separate and enrich for HLA-DR-antigen-bearing cells. Although this method has not been adopted for routine T and B cell separation it serves to illustrate the potential usefulness of monoclonal antibodies in immunological procedures. In several studies a monomorphic anti-HLA-Dr antibody, 2.06 was used to analyze the HLA-D region-associated antigens by two-dimensional polyacrylamide gel electrophoresis (2D-PAGE) where HLA-D related electrophoretic polymorphism in the basic and smaller gp28 chain was found and it was suggested that the patterns corresponded to allele-specific markers of different HLA-D genotypes.[104,105] These results are in agreement with those obtained using rabbit anti-HLA-DR sera with 2D-PAGE and also with amino acid sequencing and peptide mapping data.[106–108] Other workers, however, consider the heavier gp33 chain to carry the polymorphic specificities.[109–111] More work is required before an answer to this problem can be found, but monomorphic-HLA-DR antibodies will play a major role in the structural analysis of the HLA-DR antigens.

C. Polymorphic Anti-HLA-DR Antibodies

Contrasting with the high frequency of monomorphic anti-HLA-DR antibodies produced, few monoclonal antibodies to polymorphic-HLA-DR specificities have been described (Table 7). The only monoclonal antibody to a single, already defined HLA-DR specificity described in the literature to date is the FMC2 antibody[112] which is thought to detect a split of the HLA-DR4 specificity. Although, the data regarding this antibody is limited.

All the other polymorphic anti-HLA-DR monoclonal antibodies described thus far detect at least two HLA-DR specificities or "supertypic" determinants (Table 7). It is of interest that the monoclonal antibodies, Genox 3.53,[1] E15/4,[2] and 17.15[113] react with determinants of previously established cross-reactive groups of HLA-DR specificities.[94] The noncytotoxic, Genox 3.53 antibody detects a determinant common to the HLA-DR1, DR2, and DRw6 specificities; E15/4 is cytotoxic and reacts with cells bearing the specificities, HLA-DR3, DR5, or DRw6, and the cytotoxic 17.15 antibody recognizes a supertypic determinant found on HLA-DR4, DR5, and some DR7 and DRw9 positive cells. This suggests that cross-reactivity is not an artifact of complex alloantisera but a real phenomenon.

Several polymorphic anti-Ia monoclonal antibodies have been produced in our laboratory which do not appear to fit any previously defined HLA-DR specificities. Further analysis of the reaction patterns of these antibodies in population, family, and disease studies is in progress. Of particular interest is the cytotoxic monoclonal antibody, 19-26.1 (Table 6) which was produced following fusion of spleen cells from CBA mice immunized with Raji LCL. The accumulated data from studies with this antibody are in accordance with it detecting a HLA-DR determinant. However, the fact that no definite HLA-DR specificity can be assigned to 19-26.1 suggests that the determinant recognized may be coded for by an undefined Ia-locus. Coprecipitation analysis with 19-26.1 and HLA-DR alloantisera failed to conclusively verify whether the determinant defined by 19-26.1 is located on the HLA-DR molecule or on a separate "new" Ia-like moiety. Although results from our work and others[97,98,102] suggest the existence of a second Ia-like locus, its positive identification is difficult.

Retrospective analysis of previously discarded "multispecific" HLA-DR alloantisera may in fact indicate reaction patterns similar to those defined by the anti-HLA-DR monoclonal antibodies which recognize supertypic determinants. However, the redefinition of the HLA-DR specificities by xenogeneic monoclonal antibodies seems to be inevitable and the likely outcome is a series of HLA-DR specificities resembling those already defined for the murine Ia antigens.

IX. MONOCLONAL ANTIBODIES TO THE MHC OF OTHER SPECIES

A. Chicken

The MHC of the chicken, the B system, displays significant similarities to the mammalian MHC in that it is composed of two classes of antigens:[116] (1) the 44,000 molecular weight heavy chain of the B antigen and a 12,000 molecular weight molecule which presumably represents the β2M analogue and (2) the 26,000 molecular weight chain, which is thought to represent the Ia analogue, is called the B-L antigen. Amino acid sequence data has also shown that the B antigens share a high degree of homology with mammalian histocompatibility antigens and suggest that the B system is the evolutionary homologue of the mouse H-2, human HLA, and guinea pig GPLA systems.[117] A more detailed discussion of the chicken MHC can be found elsewhere.[118,119]

One extensive study has led to the production of several mouse antichicken MHC monoclonal antibodies,[120] a number of which detect polymorphic-antigenic specificities. A strong, preferential response to produce antichicken MHC antibodies was noted when mice were immunized with chicken erythrocytes. This observation is in accordance with the finding that normal mouse serum contains strong "natural" antibodies against chicken MHC antigens suggesting a pre-existing immunity. These studies were extended[121] and showed that the apparent specificity of the monoclonal antibody can be altered by changing the conditions of reaction such as pH and temperature. These findings are of particular significance when considering the use of monoclonal antibodies as typing reagents for highly polymorphic systems, such as the MHC, where only one or a few amino acids may differ between an antigenic specificity and the occurrence of cross-reactions is considerably high. It should be stressed that these seemingly anomalous reactions need not be regarded as a disadvantage since it is possible to alter the assay conditions enough to reduce the cross-reactions below the level of detection but still retain the ability to detect the desired specificity. Consequently, it is suggested that the conditions of assay be specified for each monoclonal antibody and considerable care taken when changing assay systems. The fact that altered apparent specificity with pH changes was observed for all five monoclonal anti-B antigen antibodies studies suggests that this may be a common feature of antichicken MHC monoclonal antibodies and may also hold true for monoclonal antibodies against MHC determinants of other species.

B. Other Species

Murine monoclonal antibodies have also been produced to the horse and bovine MHC (W. Davis, personal communication[130]) and also to the lizard MHC (J. Wetherall, personal communication[131]). Few details are available concerning these antibodies at this time.

With the advent of monoclonal antibodies, it seems likely that the MHC of many species previously "unexplored" will be studied in considerable detail. This will not only result in a more informed knowledge of individual species' MHC, but will also give a broader concept of the significance and functional role of MHC in relation to all species.

X. CONCLUSIONS

Monoclonal antibodies to the MHC of several different species have been described, each produced by immunizing mice and fusing their spleen cells with a HAT sensitive mouse myeloma. Several conclusions can be made: (1) monoclonal alloantibodies produced against murine antigens recognize systems that were previously described: H-2 and Ia antigens. Several new loci and new specificities have been described, emphasizing the power of this new technique for antibody production, (2) monoclonal xenoantibodies have also been produced to be MHC of other species and include anti-HLA-A, -B, and anti-β2M antibodies. These have the advantage of large volumes of active and monoclonal material. However the reagents are xenogeneic antibodies and this imposes certain restrictions on the specificity of the antibodies produced, and it appears that the mouse is not easily able to recognize all of the alloantigenic specificities defined. Nonetheless the mouse can recognize human cell surface polymorphisms and it remains to be seen whether monoclonal antibodies to these determinants are of the same biological significance as the alloantibodies to MHC antigens, particularly in transplantation and in studies of disease in man.

ACKNOWLEDGMENTS

The original work quoted was supported by funds obtained from the National Health and Medical Research Council of Australia, Australian Tobacco Research Foundation and the Anti-Cancer Council of Victoria. We acknowledge the work in our laboratory of Mark Hogarth, Hilary Vaughan, Peter Thurlow, Chris Thompson, Margaret Henning, Gillian Edwards, and Sue Douglas.

REFERENCES

1. **Brodsky, F. M., Parham, P., Barnstable, C. J., Crumpton, M. J., and Bodmer, W. F.,** Monoclonal antibodies for analysis of the HLA system, *Immunol. Rev.,* 47, 3, 1979.
2. **Trucco, M. M., Garotta, G., Stocker, J. W., and Ceppellini, R.,** Murine monoclonal antibodies against HLA structures, *Immunol. Rev.,* 47, 219, 1979.
3. **McKearn, T. J., Fitch, F. W., Smilek, D. E., Sarmiento, M., and Stuart, F. P.,** Properties of rat anti-MHC antibodies produced by cloned rat-mouse hybridomas, *Immunol. Rev.,* 47, 91, 1979.
4. **Klein, J.,** *Biology of the Mouse Histocompatibility—2 Complex,* Springer-Verlag, New York, 1975, 81.
5. **Snell, B. D., Dausset, J., and Nathenson, S. G.,** *Histocompatability,* Academic Press, New York, 1976, 401.
6. **Iványi, P. and De Greeve, P.,** Individual mice of one inbred strain produce anti-H-2 antibodies of different specificities, in *Origins of Inbred Mice,* Morse, H. C., Ed., Academic Press, New York, 1978, 633.
7. **Lemke, H., Hämmerling, G. J., and Hämmerling, U.,** Fine specificity analysis with monoclonal antibodies of antigens controlled by the major histocompatibility complex and by the Qa/TL region in mice, *Immunol. Rev.,* 47, 175, 1979.
8. **Ozato, K., Mayer, N., and Sachs, D. H.,** Hybridoma cell lines secreting monoclonal antibodies to mouse H-2 and Ia antigens, *J. Immunol.,* 124, 533, 1980.
9. **Klein, J., Götze, D., Hämmerling, G. J., and Lemke, H.,** Nomenclature of H-2 and Ia antigens defined by monoclonal antibodies, *Immunogenetics,* 9, 503, 1979.
10. **Kimura, S., Tada, N., Nakayama, E., and Hämmerling, U.,** Studies of the mouse Ly-6 alloantigen system. I. Serological characterization of mouse Ly-6 alloantigen by monoclonal antibodies, *Immunogenetics,* 11, 373, 1980.
11. **Michaelson, J., Rothenberg, E., and Boyse, E. A.,** Genetic polymorphism of murine β2-microglobulin detected biochemically, *Immunogenetics,* 11, 93, 1980.
12. **Goding, J. W. and Walker, I. D.,** Allelic forms of β2-microglobulin in the mouse, *Proc. Natl. Acad. Sci. U.S.A.,* 77, 7395, 1980.
13. **Goding, J. W.,** Evidence for linkage of murine β2-microglobulin to H-3 and Ly-4, *J. Immunol.,* 126, 1644, 1981.
14. **Oi, V. T., Jones, P. P., Goding, J. W., Hertzenberg, L. A., and Hertzenberg, L. A.,** Properties of monoclonal antibodies to mouse Ig allotypes, H-2, and Ia antigens, *Curr. Top. Microbiol. Immunol.,* 81, 115, 1978.
15. **Ledbetter, J. A. and Hertzenberg, L. A.,** Xenogeneic monoclonal antibodies to mouse lymphoid differentiation antigens, *Immunol. Rev.,* 47, 63, 1979.
16. **Goding, J. W., Oi, V. T., Jones, P. P., Hertzenberg, L. A., and Hertzenberg, L. A.,** Monoclonal antibodies to alloantigens and to immunoglobulin allotypes, in *Cell of Immunoglobulin Synthesis,* Academic Press, New York, 1979, 309.
17. **Hämmerling, G. J., Hämmerling, U., and Lemke, H.,** Isolation of twelve monoclonal antibodies against Ia and H-2 antigens. Serological characterization and reactivity with B and T lymphocytes, *Immunogenetics,* 8, 433, 1979.
18. **Klein, J., Huang, H. J. S., Lemke, H., Hämmerling, G. J., and Hämmerling, U.,** Serological analysis of H-2 and Ia molecules with monoclonal antibodies, *Immunogenetics,* 8, 419, 1979.

19. **Vollmers, H. I., Eulitz, M., and Götze, D.,** Reactivity of hybridoma antibodies specific for H-2 antigens with cells of inbred and wild mice, *Immunogenetics,* 8, 447, 1979.
20. **Ozato, K., Hansen, T. H., and Sachs, D.,** Monoclonal antibodies to the H-2L^d antigen, the products of the third polymorphic locus of the mouse MHC., *J. Immunol.,* 125, 2473, 1980.
21. **Ozato, K. and Sachs, D. H.,** Monoclonal antibodies to mouse MHC antigens. III. Hybridoma antibodies reacting to antigens of the H-2^b haplotype reveal genetic control of isotype expression, *J. Immunol.,* 126, 317, 1981.
22. **Ozato, K., Epstein, S. L., Henkart, P., Hansen, T. H., and Sachs, D. H.,** Studies on monoclonal antibodies to mouse MHC products, *Transplant. Proc.,* XIII, 958, 1981.
23. **Hogarth, P. M., Sutton, V., Crewther, P., and McKenzie, I. F. C.,** Analysis of the murine MHC with monoclonal antibodies, *Transplantation,* in press.
24. **Hogarth, P. M., Crewther, P., Edwards, G., and McKenzie, I. F. C.,** The Qa-2 system: description with monoclonal antibodies, *Eur. J. Immunol.,* in press.
25. **Kimura, S., Tada, N., Nakayama, E., Liu, Y., Taylor, B. A., and Hämmerling, U.,** A new mouse cell surface antigen (La-3) controlled by a gene linked to Mls locus, and defined by monoclonal antibodies, *Immunogenetics,* in press.
26. **Shinohara, N., Ricks, J., Hansen, T. H., and Sachs, D. H.,** Genetic control of immune response to the H-2D^k private specificity, H-2.32, *J. Immunol.,* 119, 1732, 1977.
27. **Boyse, E. A., Stockert, E., and Old, L. J.,** Isoantigens of the H-2 and Tla loci of the mouse. Interactions affecting their representation on thymocytes, *J. Exp. Med.,* 128, 85, 1968.
28. **Iványi, D. and Démant, P.,** Complex genetic effect of the B10.D2 (M504) (H-2^{dm1}) mutation, *Immunogenetics,* 8, 539, 1979.
29. **Hansen, T. H., Ozato, K., Melino, M. R., Coligan, J. E., Kindt, T. J., Jandinski, J. T., and Sachs, D. H.,** A gene cluster in the H-2D region: evidence in two haplotypes for at least three D region encoded molecules, D,L,R, *J. Immunol.,* in press.
30. **Eskinazi, D. P., Molinaro, G. A., Reisfeld, R. A., and Ferrone, S.,** Cellular and molecular heterogeneity of H-2K^k antigens detected with a monoclonal antibody, *J. Immunogenet.,* 8, 101, 1981.
31. **O'Neill, H. C. and Parish, C. R.,** Monoclonal antibody detection of two classes of H-2K^k molecules, *Mol. Immunol.,* 18, 713, 1981.
32. **Lindahl, K. F. and Lemke, H.,** Inhibition of killer—target cell interaction by monoclonal anti-H-2 antibodies, *Eur. J. Immunol.,* 9, 526, 1979.
33. **Epstein, S. L., Ozato, K., and Sachs, D. H.,** Blocking of allogeneic cell—mediated lympholysis by monoclonal antibodies to H-2 antigens, *J. Immunol.,* 125, 129, 1980.
34. **Hermann, S. H. and Mescher, M. F.,** Purification of the H-2K^k molecule of the murine major histocompatibility complex, *J. Biol. Chem.,* 254, 8713, 1979.
35. **Moller, G., Ed.,** *Transplant. Rev.,* 30, 1, 1976.
36. **Schwartz, B. D. and Cullen, S. E.,** Chemical characteristics of Ia antigens, *Semin. Immunopathol.,* 1, 85, 1978.
37. **Murphy, D. B.,** The I-J subregion of the murine H-2 gene complex, *Semin. Immunopathol.,* 1, 111, 1978.
38. **Parish, C. R. and McKenzie, I. F. C.,** Direct visualization of T lymphocytes bearing Ia antigens controlled by the I-J subregion, *J. Exp. Med.,* 146, 332, 1977.
39. **Michaelides, M. M. and McKenzie, I. F. C.,** Detection of Ia alloantigens on PHA-T blast cells, *Transplantion,* 31, 330, 1981.
40. **Higgins, T. J., Parish, C. R., and McKenzie, I. F. C.,** Comparison of antigens recognized by xenogeneic and allogeneic anti-Ia antibodies. Evidence for two classes of Ia antigens, *Immunogenetics,* 6, 343, 1978.
41. **Higgins, T. J., Parish, C. R., and McKenzie, I. F. C.,** Carbohydrate-defined antigens controlled by the I region, in *Current Trends in Histocompatibility,* Reisfeld, R. A. and Ferrone, S., Eds., Plenum Press, New York, in press.
42. **Higgins, T. J., Parish, C. R., Hogarth, P. M., McKenzie, I. F. C., and Hämmerling, G. J.,** Demonstration of carbohydrate- and protein-determinant Ia antigens by monoclonal antibodies, *Immunogenetics,* 11, 467, 1980.
43. **Günther, E. and Stark, O.,** The major histocompatibility system of the rat, *Transplant. Proc.,* 11, 1550, 1979.
44. **Blankenhorn, E. P., Cecka, J. M., Götze, D., and Hood, L.,** Partial N-terminal amino acid sequence of rat transplantation antigens, *Nature (London),* 274, 90, 1978.
45. **Nilsson, S. F. and Wigzell, H.,** Isolation and partial characterization of rat lymphoid cell surface histocompatibility antigens and immunoglobulins, *Scand. J. Immunol.,* 7, 307, 1978.
46. **Haustein, D. and Günther, E.,** Biochemical analysis of gene products of major histocompatibility recombinant haplotypes in the rat, *Eur. J. Immunol.,* 10, 615, 1980.

47. **Cecka, J. M., Blankenhorn, E. P., Götze, D., and Hood, L.,** Microsequence analysis of Ia antigens from three strains of rats, *Eur. J. Immunol.*, 10, 140, 1980.
48. **Blankenhorn, E. P., Cecka, J. M., Frelinger, J., Götze, D., and Hood, L.,** Structure of Ia antigens from the rat. Mouse alloantisera demonstrate at least two distinct molecular species, *Eur. J. Immunol.*, 10, 145, 1980.
48. **Howard, J. C., Butcher, G. W., Galfrè, G., Milstein, C., and Milstein, C. P.,** Monoclonal antibodies as tools to analyze the serological and genetic complexities of major transplantation antigens, *Immunol. Rev.*, 47, 139, 1979.
50. **McMaster, W. R. and Williams, A. F.,** Monoclonal antibodies to Ia antigens from rat thymus: cross reactions with mouse and human and use in purification of rat Ia glycoproteins, *Immunol. Rev.*, 47, 117, 1979.
51. **McMaster, W. R., Winearls, B. C., and Parham. P.,** A monoclonal mouse anti-rat Ia antibody which cross reacts with a human HLA-DRw determinant, *Tissue Antigens,* 14, 453, 1979.
52. **Cook, R. G., Vitetta, E. S., Uhr, J. W., and Capra, J. D.,** Structural studies on the murine Ia alloantigens. V. Evidence that the structural gene for the I-E/C beta polypeptide is encoded within the I-A subregion, *J. Exp. Med.*, 149, 981, 1979.
53. **Allison, J. P., Walker, L. E., Russel, W. A., Pellegrino, M. A., Ferrone, S., Reisfeld, R. A., Frelinger, J. A., and Silver, J.,** Murine Ia and human DR antigens: homology of amino-terminal sequences, *Proc. Natl. Acad. Sci. U.S.A.*, 75, 3953, 1978.
54. **Smilek, D. E., Boyd, H. C., Wilson, D. B., Zmijewski, C. M., Fitch, F. W., and McKearn, T. J.,** Monoclonal rat anti-major histocompatibility complex antibodies display specificity for rat, mouse and human target cells, *J. Exp. Med.*, 151, 1139, 1980.
55. **Howard, J. C., Butcher, G. W., Galfrè, G., and Milstein, C.,** Monoclonal anti-rat MHC (H-1) alloantibodies, *Curr. Top. Microbiol. Immunol.*, 81, 54, 1978.
56. **Galfrè, G., Howe, S. C., Milstein, C., Butcher, G. W., and Howard, J. C.,** Antibodies to major histocompatibility antigens produced by hybrid cell lines, *Nature (London),* 266, 550, 1977.
57. **Gallico, G. G., Butcher, G. W., and Howard, J. C.,** The role of subregions of the rat major histocompatibility complex in rejection and passive enhancement of renal allografts, *J. Exp. Med.*, 149, 244, 1979.
58. **Stuart, F. P., McKearn, T. J., and Fitch, F. W.,** Enhancement of rat renal allografts with monoclonal antibody, *Surgery,* 86, 30, 1979.
59. **Amos, D. B. and Kostyu, D. D.,** HLA-A central immunological agency of man, *Adv. Human Genet.*, 10, 137, 1980.
60. **Krangel, M. S., Orr, H. T., and Strominger, J. L.,** Structural function, and biosynthesis of the major human histocompatibility antigens. (HLA-A and HLA-B), *Scand, J. Immunol.*, 11, 561, 1980.
61. **Barnstable, C. J., Jones, E. A., and Crumpton, M. J.** Isolation, structural and genetics of HLA-A, -B, -C and -DRw (Ia) antigens, *Brit. Med. Bull.*, 34, 241, 1978.
62. **Francke, U. and Pellegrino, M. A.,** Assignment of the major histocompatibility complex to a region of the short arm of human chromosome 6, *Proc. Natl. Acad. Sci. U.S.A.*, 74, 1147, 1977.
63. **Goodfellow, P. N., Jones, E. A., Van Heyningen, V., Solomon, E., Bobrow, M., Miggiano, V. C., and Bodmer, W. F.,** The β2-microglobulin gene is on chromosome 15 and not in the HLA region, *Nature (London),* 254, 267, 1975.
64. **Trowsdale, J., Travers, P., Bodmer, W. F., and Patillo, R. A.,** Expression of HLA-A, -B, and -C and β2-microglobulin antigens in human choriocarcinoma cell lines, *J. Exp. Med.*, 152, 11s, 1980.
65. **Law, H. Y. and Bodmer, W. F.,** Use of microimmunobilisation and microagglutination assays for attempted detection of HLA antigens and β2-microglobulin on human sperm, *Tissue Antigens,* 12, 249, 1978.
66. **Barnstable, C. J., Bodmer, W. F., Brain, G., Galfrè, G., Milstein, C., Williams, A. F., and Ziegler, A.,** Production of monoclonal antibodies to group A erythrocytes, HLA and other human cell surface antigens—new tools for genetic analysis, *Cell,* 14, 9, 1978.
67. **Arce-Gomez, B., Jones, E. A., Barnstable, C. J., Solomon, E., and Bodmer, W. F.,** The genetic control of HLA-A and B antigens in somatic cell hybrids: requirements for β2-microglobulin, *Tissue Antigens,* 11, 96, 1978.
68. **Solomon, E. and Jones, E. A.,** Monoclonal antibodies as tools for human genetic analysis, in *Monoclonal Antibodies Hybridomas: a new dimension in biological analyses,* Kennett, R. H., McKearn, T. J., and Bechtol, K. B., Eds., Plenum Press, New York, 1980, chap. 6.
69. **Parham, P., Barnstable, C. J., and Bodmer, W. F.,** Use of monoclonal antibody (W6/32) in structural studies of HLA-A, B, C antigens, *J. Immunol.*, 123, 342, 1979.
70. **Williams, K. A., Hart, D. N. J., Fabre, J. W., and Morris, P. J.,** Distribution and quantitation of the HLA-A, B, C and DR (Ia) antigens on human kidney and other tissues, *Transplantation,* 29, 274, 1980.

71. **Brown, G., Biberfeld, P., Christensson, B., and Mason, D. Y.,** The distribution of HLA on human lymphoid bone marrow and peripheral blood cells, *Eur. J. Immunol.*, 9, 272, 1979.
72. **Parham, P., Sehgal. P. K., and Brodsky, F. M.,** Anti-HLA-A, B, C monoclonal antibodies with no alloantigenic specificity in humans define polymorphisms in other primate species, *Nature (London),* 279, 639, 1979.
73. **Orr, H. T., Lopez de Castro, J. A., Parham, P., Ploegh, H. L., and Strominger, J. L.,** Comparison of amino acid sequences of two human histocompatibility antigens, HLA-A2 and HLA-B7. Location of putative alloantigenic sites, *Proc. Natl. Acad. Sci. U.S.A.*, 76, 4395, 1979.
74. **Fitchen, J. H., Ferrone, S., Quaranta, V., Molinaro, G. A., and Cline, M. J.,** Monoclonal antibodies to HLA-A, B and DR antigens inhibit colony formation by human myeloid progenitor cells, submitted.
75. **Sarkar, S., Glassy, M. C., Ferrone, S., and Jones, O. W.,** Cell cycle and the differential expression of HLA-A, B and HLA-DR antigens on human B lymphoid cells, *Proc. Natl. Acad. Sci. U.S.A.*, 77, 7297, 1981.
76. **Vaughan, H. A., Thompson, C. H., Henning, M. M., Hogarth, P. M., Betts, R. L., and McKenzie, I. F. C.,** A human lymphocyte glycoprotein antigen defined by a monoclonal antibody, *Eur. J. Immunol.*, in press.
77. **Einstein, A. B., Jr., Mann, D. L., Gordon, H. G., Trapani, R. J., and Fahey, J. L.,** Heterologous antisera against specific HL-A antigens, *Transplantation,* 12, 299, 1971.
78. **Robb, R. J., Humphreys, R. E., Strominger, J. L., Fuller, T. C., and Mann, D. L.,** Rabbit anti-HL-A2 sera, *Transplantation,* 19, 445, 1975.
79. **Allison, J. P., Belvedere, M., Reisfeld, R. A., Pellegrino, M. A., and Ferrone, S.,** Serologic and immunochemical characterization of HLA-A9 xenoantisera, *J. Immunol.*, 121, 579, 1978.
80. **Schäfer, K., Albert, E. D., Rodt, H., and Thierfelder, S.,** Serological analysis of xenogeneic anti-lymphoblastoid cell-line sera with sepcificity against HLA-B12, *Immunogenetics,* 10, 595, 1980.
81. **Parham, P. and Bodmer, W. F.,** Monoclonal antibody to a human histocompatibility alloantigen, HLA-A2, *Nature (London),* 276, 397, 1978.
82. **McMichael, A. J., Parham, P., Brodsky, F. M., and Pilch, J. R.,** Influenza virus-specific cytotoxic T-lymphocytes recognize HLA molecules. Blocking by monoclonal anti-HLA antibodies, *J. Exp. Med.*, 152, 195s, 1980.
83. **McMichael, A. J., Parham, P., Rust, N., and Brodsky, F. M.,** A monoclonal antibody that recognizes an antigenic determinant shared by HLA A2 and B17, *Human Immunol.*, 1, 121, 1980.
84. **Zola, H.,** Monoclonal antibodies against human cell membrane antigens: a review, *Pathology,* 12, 539, 1980.
85. **Richiardi, P., Amoroso, A., Crepaldi, T., Ceppellini, R., and Trucco, M.,** A xenogeneic monoclonal antibody recognizing specificities controlled by HLA-A and B alleles, *Immunogenetics,* 12, 615, 1981.
86. **Parham, P.,** Purification of immunologically active HLA-A and -B antigens by a series of monoclonal antibody columns, *J. Biol. Chem.*, 254, 8709, 1979.
87. **Ploegh, H. L., Cannon, L. E., and Strominger, J. L.,** Cell-free translation of the mRNAs for the heavy and light chains of HLA-A and HLA-B antigens, *Proc. Natl. Acad. Sci. U.S.A.*, 76, 2273, 1979.
88. **Trucco, M. M., Stocker, J. W., and Ceppellini, R.,** Monoclonal antibodies against human lymphocyte antigens, *Nature (London),* 266, 666, 1978.
89. **Trucco, M. M., Stocker, J. W., and Ceppellini, R.,** Monoclonal antibodies to human lymphocyte membrane antigens, *Curr. Top. Microbiol. Immunol.*, 81, 66, 1978.
90. **Trucco, M., De Petris, S., Garotta, G., and Ceppellini, R.,** Quantitative analysis of cell surface HLA structures by means of monoclonal antibodies, *Human Immunol.*, 1, 233, 1980.
91. **Brodsky, F. M., Bodmer, W. F., and Parham, P.,** Characterization of a monoclonal anti-β2-microglobulin antibody and its use in the genetic and biochemical analysis of major histocompatibility antigens, *Eur. J. Immunol.*, 9, 536, 1979.
92. **Garotta, G. and Trucco, M.,** HLA antigens temperature dependent elution from specific monoclonal antibody columns, in *Protides of the Biological Fluids,* Peeters, H., Ed., Pergamon Press, 1980.
93. **Jones, E. A. and Bodmer, W. F.,** Lack of expression of HLA antigens on choriocarcinoma cell lines, *Tissue Antigens,* 16, 195, 1980.
94. **Bodmer, J. G.,** Ia antigens. Definition of the HLA-DRw specificities, *Br. Med. Bull.*, 34, 233, 1978.
95. **Snary, D., Barnstable, C. J., Bodmer, W. F., Goodfellow, P. M., and Crumpton, M. J.,** Cellular distribution, purification and molecular nature of human Ia antigens, *Scand, J. Immunol.*, 6, 439, 1977.
96. **Brodsky, F. M., Parham, P., and Bodmer, W. F.,** Monoclonal antibodies to HLA-DRw determinants, *Tissue Antigens,* 16, 30, 1980.

97. **Tosi, R., Tanigaki, N., Centis, D., Ferrara, G. B., and Pressman, D.,** Immunological dissection of human Ia molecules, *J. Exp. Med.,* 148, 1592, 1978.
98. **Quaranta, V., Pellegrino, M. A., and Ferrone, S.,** Serological and immunochemical characterization of the specificity of four monoclonal antibodies to distinct antigenic determinants expressed on sulpqullation of human Ia-like antigens, *J. Immunol.,* 126, 548, 1981.
99. **Quaranta, V., Indiveri, F., Glassy, M. C., Ng, A., Russo, C., Molinaro, G. A., Pellegrino, M. A., and Ferrone, S.,** Serological functional, and immunological characterization of a monoclonal antibody (McAb Q2/70) to human Ia-like antigens, *Human Immunol.,* 1, 211, 1980.
100. **Quaranta, V., Walker, L. E., Pellegrino, M. A., and Ferrone, S.,** Purification of immunologically functional subsets of human Ia-like antigens on a monoclonal antibody (Q5/13) immunoadsorbent, *J. Immunol.,* 125, 1421, 1980.
101. **Quaranta, V., Tanigaki, N., and Ferrone, S.,** Distribution of antigenic determinants recognized by three monoclonal antibodies (Q2/70, Q5/6 and Q5/13) on human Ia-like alloantigens and on their subunits, *Immunogenetics,* 12, 175, 1981.
102. **Lampson, L. A. and Levy, R.,** Two populations of Ia-like molecules on a human B cell line, *J. Immunol.,* 125, 293, 1980.
103. **Stocker, J. W., Garotta, G., Hausmann, B., Trucco, M., and Ceppellini, R.,** Separation of human cells bearing HLA-DR antigens using a monoclonal antibody rosetting method, *Tissue Antigens,* 13, 212, 1979.
104. **Charron, D. J. and McDevitt, H. O.,** Analysis of HLA-D region associated molecules with monoclonal antibody, *Proc. Nat. Acad. Sci. U.S.A.,* 76, 6567, 1979.
105. **Charron, D. J. and McDevitt, H. O.,** Characterization of HLA-D-region antigens by two-dimensional gel electrophoresis. Molecular genotyping, *J. Exp. Med.,* 152, 18s, 1980.
106. **Shackelford, D. A. and Strominger, J. L.,** Demonstration of structural polymorphism among HLA-DR light chains by two-dimensional gel electrophoresis, *J. Exp. Med.,* 151, 144, 1980.
107. **Silver, J., Walker, L. E., Reisfeld, R. A., Pellegrino, M. A., and Ferrone, S.,** Structural studies of murine I-E and human DR antigens, *Mol. Immunol.,* 16, 37, 1979.
108. **Silver, J. and Ferrone, S.,** Structural polymorphism of human DR antigens, *Nature (London),* 279, 436, 1979.
109. **Klareskog, K., Rask, L., Fohlman, J., and Peterson, P. A.,** Heavy HLA-DR (Ia) antigen chain is controlled by the MHC region, *Nature (London),* 275, 762, 1978.
110. **Barnstable, C. J., Jones, E. A., Bodmer, W. F., Bodmer, J. G., Arce-Gomez, B., Snary, D., and Crumpton, M. J.,** Genetics and serology of HLA-linked human Ia antigens, *Cold Spring Harbor Symp. Quant. Biol.* 41, 443, 1977.
111. **Snary, D., Barnstable, C., Bodmer, W. F., Goodfellow, P., and Crumpton, M. J.,** Human Ia antigens—purification and molecular structure, *Cold Spring Harbor Symp. Quant. Biol.,* 41, 379, 1977.
112. **Zola, H., Bradley, J., Macardle, P., McEvoy, R., and Thomas, M.,** A hybridoma antibody which reacts with human cells carrying the DRw4 tissue type. Evidence for heterogeneity of DRw4, *Transplantation,* 29, 72, 1980.
113. **Hansen, J. A., Martin, P. J., Kamoun, M., Nisperos, B. N., and Thomas, E. D.,** A supertypic HLA-DR specificity (DRW4 + 5) defined by murine monoclonal antibody, *Human Immunol.,* 2, 103, 1981.
114. **Hansen, J. A., Martin, P. J., and Nowinski, R. C.,** Monoclonal antibodies identifying a novel T-cell antigen and Ia antigens of human lymphocytes, *Immunogenetics,* 10, 247, 1980.
115. **Reinherz, E. L., Kung, P. C., Pesando, J. M., Ritz, J., Goldstein, G., and Scholssman, S. F.,** Ia determinants on human T-cell subsets defined by monoclonal antibody. Activation stimuli required for expression, *J. Exp. Med.,* 150, 1472, 1979.
116. **Ziegler, A. and Pink, J.,** Chemical properties of two antigens controlled by the major histocompatibility complex of the chicken, *J. Biol. Chem.,* 251, 5391, 1976.
117. **Vitetta, E. S., Uhr, J. W., Klein, J., Pazderka, F., Moticka, E. J., Ruth, R. F., and Capra, J. D.,** Homology of (murine) H-2 and (human) HLA with a chicken histocompatibility antigen, *Nature (London),* 270, 535, 1977.
118. **Pazderka, F., Longenecker, B. M., Law, G. R. J., and Ruth, R. F.,** The major histocompatibility complex of the chicken, *Immunogenetics,* 2, 101, 1975.
119. **Pink, J. R. L., Droege, W., Hála, K., Miggiano, V. C., and Ziegler, A.,** A three-locus model for the chicken major histocompatibility complex, *Immunogenetics,* 5, 203, 1977.
120. **Longenecker, B. M., Mossman, T. R., and Shiozawa, C.,** A strong, preferential response of mice to polymorphic antigenic determinants of the chicken MHC, analyzed with mouse hybridoma (monoclonal) antibodies, *Immunogenetics,* 9, 137, 1979.

121. **Mossman, T. R., Gallatin, M., and Longenecker, B. M.,** Alteration of apparent specificity of monoclonal (hybridoma) antibodies recognizing polymorphic histocompatibility and blood group determinants, *J. Immunol.*, 125, 1152, 1980.
122. **Betts, R. L. and McKenzie, I. F. C.,** unpublished data, 1981.
123. **Vaughan, H. A., Thurlow, P. J., Betts, R. L., and McKenzie, I. F. C.,** unpublished data, 1981.
124. **Billing, R. and Terasaki, P.,** personal communication, 1981.
125. **Westphal, E.,** personal communication, 1981.
126. **Betts, R. L., Vaughan, H. A., and McKenzie, I. F. C.,** unpublished data, 1981.
127. **Betts, R. L., Thurlow, P. J., Vaughan, H. A., and McKenzie, I. F. C.,** unpublished data, 1981.
128. **Betts, R. L., Vaughan, H. A., and McKenzie, I. F. C.,** unpublished data, 1981.
129. **Thompson, C. H., Vaughan, H. A., Potter, T. A., and McKenzie, I. F. C.,** The definition of a HLA-DR specificity by a monoclonal antiserum, in preparation.
130. **Davis, W.,** personal communication.
131. **Wetherall, J.,** personal communication.

INDEX

A

B

C

D

E

F

G

H

I

J

K

L

M

N

O

P

R

S

T

U

V

X

Z

S/NVQ Level 2

Health & Social Care

Yvonne Nolan

www.heinemann.co.uk
✓ Free online support
✓ Useful weblinks
✓ 24 hour online ordering

01865 888058

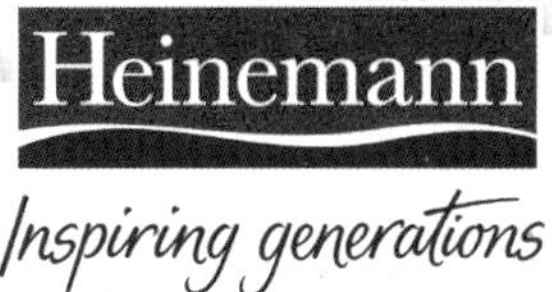

Heinemann Educational Publishers
Halley Court, Jordan Hill, Oxford OX2 8EJ
Part of Harcourt Education

Heinemann is the registered trademark of
Harcourt Education Limited

First published 2005

10 09 08 07 06
10 9 8 7 6 5

British Library Cataloguing in Publication Data is available
from the British Library on request.

10-digit ISBN: 0 435450 69 7
13-digit ISBN: 978 0 435450 69 4

Edited by Jan Doorly
Designed by Wooden Ark
Typeset by Ken Vail Graphic Design
Illustrated by Graham-Cameron Illustration (Steph Dix)

Cover design by Wooden Ark
Printed in China by Everbest Printing Co. Ltd
Cover photo: © Getty Images

Acknowledgements
Every effort has been made to contact copyright holders of material reproduced in this book. Any omissions will be rectified in subsequent printings if notice is given to the publishers.

Tel: 01865 888058 www.heinemann.co.uk